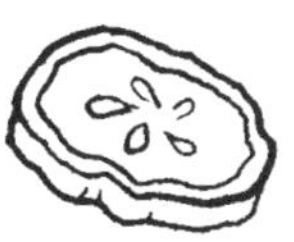

PICKLE PACKET II

STORIES, ACTIVITIES, & LESSONS FOR GRADES K-4

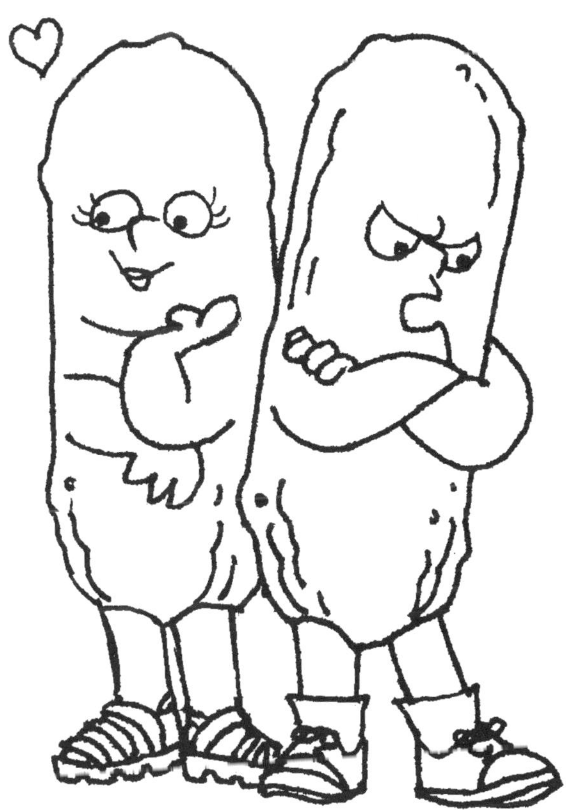

WRITTEN BY

PATRICIA KIENZLE

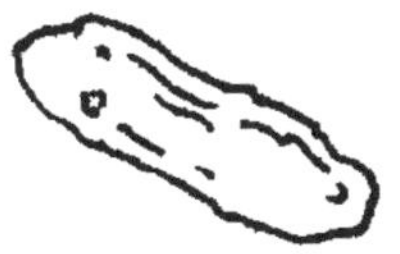

ILLUSTRATED BY

HARRY NORCROSS

ABOUT THE AUTHOR

Patricia Taylor Kienzle has a bachelor's degree in education and a master's degree in counseling. After teaching for 10 years at Farmington Elementary School in Fayetteville, Arkansas, she became an elementary counselor. She is the recipient of the Christa McAuliffe Fellowship for Arkansas. Pat is married and the mother of two sons.

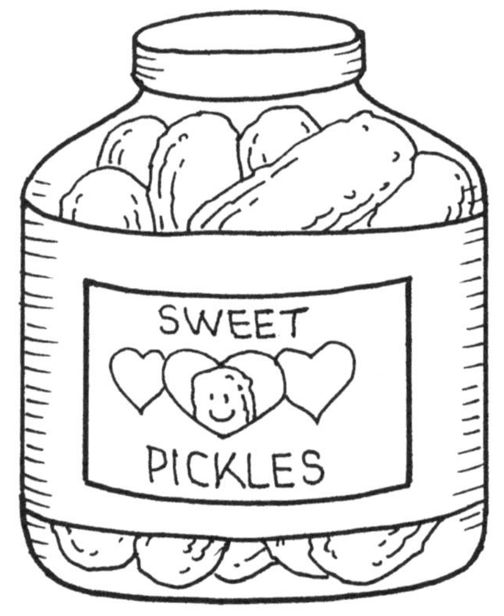

mar*co products, inc.
1443 Old York Road
Warminster, PA 18974
1-800-448-2197

ISBN: 1-57543-124-6

DEDICATION

This book is dedicated to elementary school counselors who share both the smiles and tears of our children.

I would also like to recognize my husband, David. This book was completed the month of our 30th wedding anniversary. David, thank you for putting up with *pickle* stuff all over the house, sharing my time with my projects, and being called the *Pickle Lady's* husband.

A MESSAGE FROM THE AUTHOR

Welcome to a new *Pickle Packet.* The purpose of this book is to enhance the *Life Is Like A Pickle* theme already in place and expand it to encompass new topics. Every topic in this book is based on an actual situation, but the book covers only a fraction of the situations that counselors encounter. Most of the pages in the first book still work, and it was hard for me not to include them here. Since writing that book, though, I've had 15 more years' experience as an elementary counselor and I've gained a deeper appreciation of how numerous and varied those encounters are.

In Washington, D.C. to attend the Christa McAuliffe Fellowship Conference, I was treated very well by the hotel staff. But as I stepped off the elevator one afternoon, I noticed that the lobby was being roped off and all the elevators were being held for a major league football team. It was so evident that those men were paid many times what we educators earn, and also get top billing in public. Some of them are great people and do wonderful things. But you do wonderful things all the time for the children of our country.

It is you, the elementary school counselor, who makes life a little sweeter in schools across the country.

HOW TO USE
PICKLE PACKET II

Each activity listed in the *Introduction* is identified by two codes. One code identifies the appropriate use for the activity. The other code identifies the appropriate grade levels. While reading the codes, remember that the grade levels can overlap, just as ability levels vary from school to school, and that some activities are most appropriate at certain times of the year.

The following codes are used for the activities:

I	Individual Use
SG	Small-Group Use
C	Classroom Use
PH	Parent Handout

Classroom materials can also be used with small groups or with individuals. An activity marked **SG** or **I** is designed to provide personal attention to an individual or a small number of students.

The following codes are used to indicate appropriate grade levels:

K 1 2 3 4

Although the activities will be designated for use between kindergarten and grade 4, many have been used with grades 5 and 6 as a review for students who have used the themes in earlier years.

Sample lesson plans on various topics are provided on pages 267-293. These guidelines may be adapted to your own personal situation.

To assist in lesson planning, the book also incudes a topical index on pages 294-296. This section will quickly guide you to materials relevant to specific topics.

INTRODUCTION

CHAPTER 1: Basics For *Life Is Like A Pickle* 37-46

Introducing *Life Is Like A Pickle* 38

C K-3

This activity requires a jar of sweet pickles, sour pickles, and sweet gherkins. Before meeting with the students, fill in the blank spaces on the activity sheet (page 38) by writing your name and where you can be found. Then reproduce the activity sheet for each student.

Show the students the jar of sweet pickles and the jar of sour pickles. Tell them which is which. Discuss feelings that are sweet and those that are sour, explaining that it's normal to have *sour pickle* feelings sometimes. Distribute the activity sheet and read it with the students. When you have finished reading, ask the students whether the feelings listed on their activity sheet are *sweet* or *sour*. You may want to have them explain their answers and give examples of what they mean. Review what you have written on the bottom of the activity sheet and remind the students that *a counselor is always a friend.* Display the jar of sweet gherkins. Tell the students their little fingers are sweet gherkins and wave. Tell them this is the way to say "hello" when they see you.

The Pickle Pledge 39

C K-3

Reproduce *The Pickle Pledge* for each student. Teach the students the words to the pledge, then recite it with the students. When you have finished the session, tell the students they may take the activity sheet home.

Actions For The Pickle Pledge 40

C K-2

For variety, teach young students to perform actions as they recite *The Pickle Pledge*. This is a fun activity that can be used for a parent presentation.

Pickle Routine 41-42

C K-3

This routine is used with *pickle* toys. If toys are not available, the routine may be used to accompany the actions to the pledge.

Discussion Guide **43**

▶ **C K-4**

Reproduce the activity sheet for yourself and each student. Keep it handy until you are familiar with the basic lesson. When you are ready to begin the lesson, distribute the activity sheet and a pencil to each student. Then review each point and have the students write answers to the questions. When everyone has completed the activity, tell the students to keep their guide where they can refer to it easily. Conclude the activity by telling the students that counselors, like other people, get angry sometimes. Explain that when you get angry, you have to ask yourself the same questions children ask themselves: If I get mad, will I hurt anyone? Will I destroy things? Will I use words that will get me in trouble with anyone? Will I stay mad for a long time? You may want to share this sheet to help other adults at school understand the guidance theme.

The Role Of The School Counselor **44**

▶ **PH K-4**

This handout may be used at the beginning of the year, at a Parent Night, or during School Counselor Week. Write your name and telephone number in the spaces provided. Then reproduce as many sheets as you need.

Parent Letter **45**

▶ **PH K-2**

Parents are sometimes confused when they hear their children talk about *pickles*. To clarify what you are doing and what parents may be hearing, reproduce this letter and send it home with students when you are teaching the pickle theme.

Pickle Stick Puppet Patterns **46**

▶ **I SG C K-4**

Sweet and sour puppets may be made from these patterns.

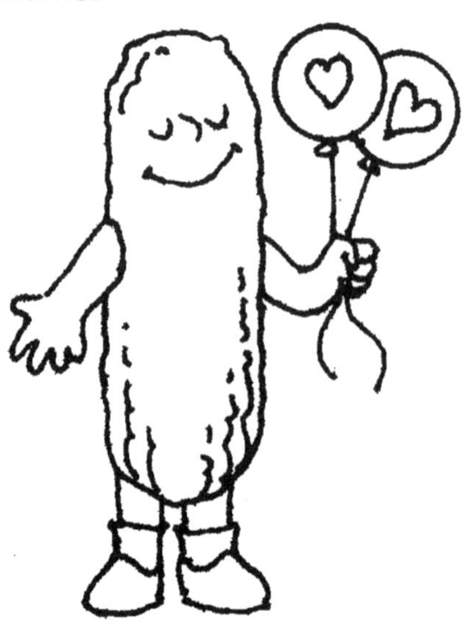

C 2-4

This activity sheet introduces pickles. Reproduce it for each student. Distribute the activity sheet and a pencil to each student and review it with the group. When everyone has completed the activity sheet, have the students circle all the different kinds of pickles they have tried. Tell them to place an "X" next to the name of their favorite.

C K-1

Reproduce the activity sheet for each student. Distribute the activity sheet and a pencil to each student. Explain that six feeling words are hidden in the *word search*. Each of the words is spelled across, from left to right. Tell the students to find and circle each of the six words. For the youngest students, you may want to underline the first letter of each word in the word search. When everyone has completed the activity sheet, discuss the meaning of each feeling word.

C 1-2

Reproduce the activity sheet for each student. Distribute the activity sheet and a pencil to each student. Explain that there are two pickle *word searches* on this page. One is for *sweet pickle words* and the other is for *sour pickle words*. Each of the words is spelled across, from left to right. Tell the students to find and circle the words. When everyone has completed the activity sheet, discuss the meaning of each feeling word. (*Note:* For students who have recently started first grade, you may want to cut the activity sheet apart and make this two activities.)

SG C 2-4

This *word search* encourages students to expand their *feeling words* vocabulary. Reproduce the activity sheet for each student. Distribute the activity sheet and a pencil to each student. Tell the students to look across, down, and diagonally for the hidden words and circle them. When everyone has completed the activity sheet, discuss the meaning of each feeling word. (*Note:* This activity may also be used as a cooperative activity.)

Pickle Puzzles 52

▶ **C K-1**

Reproduce the puzzles on green paper. If you use white paper, have the students lightly color over the words with a green crayon. Distribute the activity sheet, an envelope, and scissors to each student. Read each unfinished sentence on the puzzles and allow the children to volunteer ways that each might end. Have the students cut the puzzles apart and put them back together. Direct the students to put the puzzle pieces in an envelope, take the envelope home, and ask someone at home to finish the sentences with them. (*Note:* If there's not enough time for cutting during the guidance lesson, that activity may be done in the classroom before the guidance lesson or later at home. If you are only presenting the activity and not reproducing the puzzles for student use, make two puzzles out of posterboard to introduce the sentences. Kindergarten students may be able to work on only one puzzle at a time.)

Sonny's Birthday (Picture Story) 53

▶ **C K-2**

Reproduce the story and distribute a copy to each student. Review the words represented by the pictures at the top of the page. Tell the students:

> "We are going to work together while we read a story showing how our feelings change. I will read the words and stop whenever I come to a picture. You should be looking at your paper while I'm reading. When I stop, look at the picture and say the word that the picture represents. When we have finished reading the story, I will have some questions for you."

Read the story. Then ask the following questions:

- Does it have to be a bad day because the sun isn't shining? *(No.)*
- Why was Sonny upset when he saw the lightning? *(He thought he might not get to ride his new bike.)*
- What are some good manners Sonny might have used when he opened his presents? *(He might have opened one present at a time and thanked the person who gave it to him before opening another present.)*
- What surprised Sonny at the end of the story? *(The lightning was gone, and there was a rainbow in the sky.)*
- Can you think of a time you were surprised? *(Accept any appropriate answers.)*

For kindergarten students, read the story again in the same manner. First-graders may be ready to read it with you.

Kate's Cat (Picture Story) 54

C K-2

Reproduce the story and distribute a copy to each student. Review the words represented by the pictures at the top of the page. Tell the students:

> "We are going to work together while we read a story showing how our feelings change. I will read the words and stop whenever I come to a picture. You should be looking at your paper while I'm reading. When I stop, look at the picture and say the word that the picture represents. When we have finished reading the story, I will have some questions for you."

Read the story. Then ask the following questions:

- What made Mom upset with the cat? *(The cat dug up her flowers.)*
- Did she stay upset a long time? *(No.)*
- When Mom got upset with the cat, did she hurt anyone or destroy anything? *(No.)*
- What was the funny thing the cat did? *(The cat chased a dog.)*
- How did Kate feel when they couldn't find the cat? *(Accept any appropriate answers.)*
- Do you think Kate had a hard time going to sleep? *(Accept any appropriate answers.)*
- Was Kate happy when she woke up? *(No.)*
- Who found the cat? *(Kate and the dog.)*
- Who was happy then? *(Kate, the dog, and the cat.)*
- In the story, even though the cat and dog are different, they care about each other. Can people who are different care about each other? *(Yes.)*

For kindergarten students, read the story again in the same manner. First-graders may be ready to read it with you.

Sweet Pickles 55

C 1-3

Reproduce the activity sheet for each student. Distribute the activity sheet and a pencil to each student. Explain that this is a jar of sweet pickles and it should include only pickles that have something sweet to say. Direct the students to check the jar and mark an "X" on the pickles that do not belong. For the youngest students, it may be necessary to read the statements on the pickles aloud. Older students can do this activity independently and may be encouraged to draw other pickles outside the jar and write *sweet pickle sentences* on them. After everyone has completed the activity sheet, ask the students to think of sweet pickle situations they have experienced. Call on volunteers to share their experiences with the class. An added feature could be a *Sweet Pickle Bulletin Board* on which students could write personal sweet pickle situations on a cutout of a pickle.

Sour Pickles 56

▶ **C 1-3**

Follow the instructions for *Sweet Pickles* (page 9), eliminating the bulletin board suggestion.

What Are Bread And Butter Pickles? 57

▶ **C 2-4**

Reproduce the activity sheet for each student. Show the students a jar of bread and butter pickles. Explain that the pickles in this jar are neither very sweet nor very sour. Distribute the activity sheet and a pencil to each student. Then read the first three paragraphs on the activity sheet with the group. Tell the children that many things in life are neither good nor bad by themselves—they are in the middle. We can complain about those situations or make the best of them. For example, suppose it's a very snowy day and the roads are icy. We could complain that we could not get out of the house or we could just make the best of it and find something to do inside. Read the directions on the activity sheet. Have the students underline the sentences. When everyone has completed the activity sheet, review each answer, not comparing answers, but having the students explain the reasons for their choices.

Bread And Butter Choices 58

▶ **C 1-4**

Reproduce the activity sheet for each student. Distribute the activity sheet and a pencil to each student. Read the information at the top of the page with the group, then have the students complete the activity sheet. When everyone has completed the activity sheet, have the students share their answers.

Bread And Butter Poem 59

▶ **C 1-3**

The purpose of this activity is to create an opportunity to discuss situations that are neither good nor bad. Reproduce the activity sheet for each student. Distribute the activity sheet and crayons to each student. Read the poem with the group, then ask the students to describe times when things did not go their way. After each situation is described, discuss what could have been done to make the day worse and what could have been done to make the day better. Conclude the lesson by developing the concept that when things aren't as you want them to be, you can choose to have either a sweet pickle day or a sour pickle day. Then allow the students to color the border on their activity sheet. Encourage them to take their sheets home and display them in a place where they can be reminded of the lesson.

Secret Code Sheets 1-3 60-62

C PH 1-3

Reproduce the activity sheet(s) to be used with the children. Distribute the activity sheet(s) and a pencil to each student. Introduce the lesson by making some familiar hand signs (waving, pointing, thumbs up, etc.) and having the students identify their meaning. Then ask if anyone knows what it means if we say a person is *deaf.* Once the students realize that people who are deaf are people who cannot hear, expand the concept by saying that because they are unable to hear, people who are deaf talk with their hands as we did in the beginning of the lesson. Tell the students people who are deaf have a hand sign for each letter of the alphabet. Have the students look at the top of the activity sheet to see the different hand signs used to identify letters. Ask them to find the first letter of their first name and then form the letter with their hands. Then have all the students show their hand signs at the same time. Tell the students that the hand signs at the top of the page are like a secret code, and that they are to write the letter that matches the hand sign above each picture. When they are finished, they will have the answer to the secret code. Allow the students to complete the activity sheet(s). Then discuss each saying.

Secret Code #1—Have a sweet pickle day. Look for the good things.
Secret Code #2—Life is like a pickle. Sweet. Sour.
Secret Code #3—Everybody feels sad at times. It is okay to ask for help.

Pickle Pop-Up 63

C K-3

This is a listening and physical activity that lends itself to a discussion of feelings. Read the directions, then choose one or more stories to have the students practice listening and following directions. When you have completed the activity, you may wish to let the students make up one or more stories of their own, using the sweet pickle and sour pickle theme.

Sweet And Sour Feelings 64

I K-4

This activity is designed to help you learn more about an individual student. Reproduce the activity sheet. Tell the student you will read the beginning of a sentence and he/she is to finish it. You, not the student, should do the writing. Begin with the two introductory incomplete sentences to acquaint the student with the process. Then read all the sentences. Use the space at the bottom of the page for more notes, especially about the composition of the student's family. Analyzing the student's answers can provide a better perspective of the student's self-esteem as well as insight into some of the problems the student is coping with. Although intended for individual use, this activity could be used with small groups and classes if the students are able to write their own answers.

How Do You Feel About School? 65

C K-4

Reproduce the activity sheet for each student. Tell the students that the expressions on our faces can often reveal how we feel about something. Draw several circles on the chalkboard. Tell the students that the circles represent faces. Then ask how a face would look if a person were happy, sad, angry, excited, frustrated, etc. As each feeling is named, have a volunteer come to the board and draw the appropriate expression on one of the faces. Distribute the activity sheet and a pencil to each student. Tell the students to look at each pickle and at the word written beneath it. Then tell them to draw a mouth on each pickle that shows how they feel about the word(s) written below the drawing. When everyone has completed the activity, review each word by having two or three students explain the reason for their drawing. The blanks at the bottom of the activity sheet can be filled in with words not covered in the activity sheet.

Just Thinking 66

I K-4

Reproduce the activity sheet and give it to the student. Explain that you will be reading some incomplete sentences and that the student should complete the statements with the first thing that comes to mind. Read the first sentence and write the student's reply on the blank line. Do the same for each of the other sentences. Continue until finished. Throughout the activity, carefully watch the student's expressions. This will give you further insight into the student and his/her concerns.

Pickle Path Game 67-69

SG 1-4

Reproduce a gameboard and the game cards, on cardstock if possible, for yourself and for each student. Cut the game cards apart and laminate both the gameboard and the cards. When you have completed the activity, allow each student to take his/her new game home. Use one game for the activity. Shuffle the game cards and place them in a pile, face down. Distribute a piece of wrapped candy to each player and have the players place the candy at "Start." Decide who will go first, then move around the gameboard counterclockwise. Have the first player draw a card, follow its directions, and then place it at the bottom of the pile. The gameboard has one *Bread and Butter Pickle* space. When a player draws a card that sends him/her to the *Bread and Butter Pickle* space, the player must tell whether the situation described on the card would make his/her day better or worse. The player should then describe a response to the situation that would have made his/her day worse. Play continues with the next player. As each player reaches "Finish," he/she may eat the candy. Give each player a game to take home.

Service project: Students can make *Pickle Path Games* to give to hospitals, waiting rooms, abused women's shelters, needy families, etc.

Pickle Memory Game 70-71

I SG K-3

Reproduce two copies of the activity sheets for each game, using cardstock, if possible. Cut the cards apart and laminate them for durability. Shuffle the cards and lay them unstacked, face down, on a table or desk. Decide who will play first. The first player draws two cards. If the cards are a match, the player describes a time he/she had that particular feeling. Then the cards are placed in the player's pile. The player then continues to take turns until the two cards drawn are not a match. If the cards drawn are not a match, the player shows the cards to the other players and replaces them, face down, in the same space. The game continues until all the cards have been matched. The winner is the player with the most cards. If possible, make a set of cards for each student to take home.

Service project: Students can make *Pickle Memory Games* to give to hospitals, waiting rooms, daycare centers, after-school programs, needy families, etc.

Sherry's Walk (Simple Maze) 72

C K-1

Reproduce an activity sheet for each student. Tell the class a short story about Sherry and how she has lost her library book. Ask the students to describe how they think Sherry feels. Distribute the activity sheet and a pencil to each student. Explain that Sherry now has found her book and must return it to the library. It is the students' task to find a path (without crossing any lines) from the playground to the library. When everyone has completed the activity sheet, have the students share their finished work. Then ask the questions at the bottom of the activity sheet.

"In A Pickle" Pictures 73

C K-2

Reproduce an activity sheet for each student. Tell the students that being "in a pickle" means that you are in trouble or have a problem. Distribute the activity sheet and a pencil to each student. Look at each set of pictures with the students. Discuss which picture would put a person "in a pickle" and have the students circle that picture. If available, read *Arthur In A Pickle* by Marc Brown (ISBN 0-679-888469-6).

"In A Pickle" Situations 74

C 1-4

Reproduce an activity sheet for each student. Distribute the activity sheet and a pencil to each student. Read the directions with the students. Then have the students complete the activity sheet and, when finished, share their answers.

"In A Pickle" Sentence Puzzles 75

▶ **C PH 1-4**

Reproduce an activity sheet for each student. Distribute the activity sheet, scratch paper (optional), and a pencil to each student. Read the directions with the students and explain that these sentences have hidden meanings. Divide the students into groups and have them work together to decide what each sentence should be. You may provide scratch paper for each group to write down its answer. When everyone has completed the activity sheet, discuss each sentence and its meaning. An alternate way to use this activity sheet would be to reproduce it and send it home with the students to complete with their family members.

"In A Pickle" And Other Silly Sayings 76

▶ **C PH 2-4**

Reproduce an activity sheet for each student to use at school or at home. If you are presenting the activity at school, distribute the activity sheet and a pencil to each student. Explain that this is a *matching* activity. Tell the students they are to read the silly saying on the left and find its true meaning from the sentences in the second column. Then they are to write the letter that explains the true meaning of the sentence on the blank next to the silly saying. When everyone has completed the activity sheet, have the students share their answers. The answers are: 1-E, 2-D, 3-A, 4-H, 5-G, 6-B, 7-C, 8-L, 9-I, 10-J, 11-K, 12-F.

How To Get Out Of A Pickle 77

▶ **C 2-4**

Reproduce an activity sheet for each student. Distribute the activity sheet and a pencil to each student. After discussing or reviewing the meaning of *in a pickle*, introduce the four steps to decision making as the way to get *out of a pickle*. Tell the students to read the four steps at the bottom of the activity page, then number them in the order that would help a person get *out of a pickle.* When everyone has completed the activity sheet, review the answers. Then present some *in a pickle* situations for the students to practice the four steps of decision making. The answers are: 2, 3, 1, 4.

"In A Pickle" Bookmarks 78

▶ **C 2-4**

Copy or glue a copy of the sheet onto cardstock. Cut the bookmarks apart and give them to the students after they have completed *How To Get Out Of A Pickle* (page 77).

CHAPTER 3: Pickle Mountain School Stories 79-152

This chapter is a collection of stories to be used in grades K-4 as classroom lessons, small-group counseling sessions, or individual counseling contacts. The stories should be read aloud to students in grades K-1 and reproduced for students in grades 2-4 to read. Each story includes follow-up questions to be discussed, and some stories include other activities. If you are reproducing the questions for students, cover the answers before making copies. The children may draw pictures to illustrate each of the stories.

Individual students in grades 3-4 may read a story to K-1 students as peer helpers. If you choose to do this, select a topic that will benefit one or both students. Have the older student lead a discussion based on the questions that follow the story or have the students draw pictures relating to the story.

Following the title of each story is a list of correlating topics. If there is an activity sheet directly related to the story, it will also be listed. Other related activities can be found in Chapter 4.

Character Education At Pickle Mountain School 93-97

▶ **I SG C K-4**

Correlating Topics: Problem solving, creativity

Additional Activities: Chapter 3, reproducible poster, *Three Care Rules* (page 97); Chapter 4, *Caring With Pennies* (page 168), *We Care About Each Other Phrases* (page 188), *We Care About Each Other Pictures* (page 189), *We Care About Ourselves Phrases* (page 190), *We Care About Ourselves Pictures* (page 191), *We Care About The Earth Phrases* (page 192), *We Care About The Earth Pictures* (page 193); Chapter 5, *Jobs At School* (page 206), *Occupations At School* (page 207); Chapter 6, *Sentences On Safety* (page 221)

Grateful Gary's Gifts 98-102

▶ **I SG C K-4**

Correlating Topics: Appreciation, courtesy, adaptability, divorce, nature study

Additional Activities: Chapter 3, *Grandpa & Grandma's Birdhouse* (page 102); Chapter 4, *Sweet Pickle Tips For Opening Gifts* (page 164)

Packed Pickle Goes To The Hospital 103-107

▶ **I SG C K-4**

Correlating Topics: Compassion, cooperation, hospital careers

Additional Activities: Chapter 3, *Packed Pickle Activities* (page 107); Chapter 5, *All Jobs Are Important* (page 196), *Jobs At A Hospital* (page 202), *Occupations At A Hospital* (page 203)

The Pickle Sweep 108-113

▶ **I SG C K-4**

Correlating Topics: Compassion, adaptability, cooperation, responsibility, drug education

Additional Activities: Chapter 3, *The Pickle Sweep Song* (page 113); Chapter 4, *Pickle Sweep Activity* (page 165), *Keep Or Sweep Out* (page 166), *Sweep Out* (page 167)

Big And Bigger Field Trips 114-117

▶ **I SG C K-4**

Correlating Topics: Responsibility, cooperation, airline and airport careers

Additional Activities: Chapter 3, *The Airport* (page 117); Chapter 5, *All Jobs Are Important* (page 196), *Jobs At An Airport* (page 204), *Occupations At An Airport* (page 205)

Lunch For Susan's Grandmother 118-121

▸ **I SG C K-4**

Correlating Topics: Compassion, appreciation, citizenship, respect, community service

Additional Activities: Chapter 3, *Meals On Wheels* (page 121); Chapter 4, *Caring With Pennies* (page 168)

Packed Like Pickles 122-126

▸ **I SG C K-4**

Correlating Topics: Compassion, cultural differences, adaptability, community service

Additional Activities: Chapter 4, *Packed Like Pickles* (page 169); Chapter 5, *Jobs At School* (page 206), *Occupations At School* (page 207)

The "Unempty" House 127-131

▸ **I SG C K-4**

Correlating Topics: Disabilities, adaptability, diversity

Secret Code Activities: Chapter 2, *Secret Code #1* (page 60), *Secret Code #2* (page 61), *Secret Code #3* (page 62); Chapter 4, *Secret Code-Manners* (page 163), *Manual Alphabet* (page 170), *Saying Words Three Ways* (page 171), *Secret Code-Laughing* (page 176), *Secret Code-Tattling* (page 182)

Language Activity: Chapter 4, *Manual Alphabet* (page 170), *Saying Words Three Ways* (page 171)

Career Activities: Chapter 5, *Jobs At School* (page 206), *Occupations At School* (page 207), *Jobs For Building Houses* (page 208), *Occupations For Building Houses* (page 209)

There are five stories in the following "WHEN" section. Instructions for using "WHEN" brand pickles are in Chapter 4, page 172.

Penny Pauses (When To Ask For Things) 132-135

▸ **I SG C K-4**

Correlating Topics: Careers at school, contemplation, problem solving, respect

Additional Activities: Chapter 4, *"When" Should You Ask? Pickles* (page 173), *"When" Should You Ask? Pictures* (page 174); Chapter 5, *Jobs At School* (page 206), *Occupations At School* (page 207)

I SG K-4

Reproduce an activity sheet for each student. Distribute the activity sheet and a pencil to each student. Read the text at the top of the page with the students. Then have the students circle the house that is most like theirs, write their family composition in the large empty house, and use the other empty house on Candied Dill Lane if they have a parent living in another house. Watch the students' expressions, which may be as valuable as their verbal responses. This is an activity sheet you might choose to keep for your personal information. (*Note:* This activity may be used to promote a discussion on family differences: divorce, death, imprisoned parent, adoption, etc.)

C K-2

This activity can be used to help the youngest students walk in an orderly fashion from place to place in the school. Reproduce an activity sheet for each student. Distribute the activity sheet and crayons to each student. Review each action and the reason for it with the students. Then practice walking in lines with the students. After the students have finished practicing walking in a line, tell them to color the activity sheet. If any of the signs on the activity sheet do not fit your school, change them.

C 1-3

This page is a lesson to be taught by adult leaders. It tells of the importance of holding the door for the person behind you, not slamming it, or letting it close on the next person.

C 1-3

This activity should be presented after *No Sour Pickles At The Door* (page 162). Reproduce an activity sheet for each student. Distribute the activity sheet and a pencil to each student. Have the students use the manual alphabet at the top of the page to decode the message at the bottom of the page. The answer is *Hold the door for the person behind you. Smile.*

SG C K-2

This activity can be used alone or with the story *Grateful Gary's Gifts* (pages 98-102). Review the lesson with the teacher before presenting it to the class. Reproduce an activity sheet for each student, but do not distribute it until the lesson is over. Have imaginary gifts (or real ones, if you want to wrap that many gifts) and pretend to open each, using bad manners. For example, with the package that says, *Look at the card first!* open the package, ignoring the card. After each package is opened, ask the students what you did wrong. Distribute the activity sheet and review each of the polite ways to behave when opening a gift. Then give the teacher a gift to open. It can be something for the class (game, activity papers, snacks, etc.) or something for the teacher. It can even be something that already belongs to the teacher that the children didn't know about. The teacher will then model the polite way to receive a gift.

Pickle Sweep Activities (Drug Education) 165-167

SG K-4

These activities may be used with *The Pickle Sweep* story (pages 108-113). The theme of these activities is making healthy choices by sweeping out things that we don't want. They are appropriate for Red Ribbon Week. Begin by following the directions for the lesson (page 165). Then reproduce and distribute copies of *Keep Or Sweep Out* (page 166) for grades 3 and 4 or *Sweep Out* (page 167) for grades K-2 and a pencil to each student. Review the directions for the activity sheet and have the students complete it. Review the students' answers when everyone has completed the activity sheet.

Additional Activity: Chapter 6, *Sentences On Safety* (page 221)

Caring With Pennies (Compassion Or Thankfulness) 168

C K-4

This is an instruction page for adults. It may be used with the story *Lunch For Susan's Grandmother* (pages 118-121).

Packed Like Pickles (Caring) 169

C K-4

This is an instruction page for adults. It may be used with the story *Packed Like Pickles* (pages 122-126).

Manual Alphabet (Communication) 170

C K-4

Reproduce the activity sheet for each student. Explain that this alphabet is the means by which deaf people communicate. This activity sheet can be used with the story *The "Unempty" House* (pages 127-131).

Saying Words Three Ways (Communication) 171

▶ **C K-4**

Reproduce the activity sheet for each student. Explain that there are different ways to communicate. Sometimes we communicate in our own language or in a foreign language. Sometimes we use signing, the language of the deaf. Review the words on the activity sheet in English. Then use the *Manual Alphabet* (page 170) to demonstrate the different hand signs used for letters. Review the signing actions for the words on the activity sheet. Then review the foreign-language words.

"When" Brand Pickles 172

▶ **SG C K-4**

This is a leader instruction page for a series of lessons relating to the *When* stories (pages 132-152). Review the instructions and follow the directions for copying the *When* labels for jars.

"When" Should You Ask? Pickles 173

▶ **C K-4**

If possible, reproduce the activity sheet on green paper. Cut the questions out in the shape of pickles. Place the questions in the pickle jar labeled "When should you ask people to give you things?" To review the lesson, reproduce this activity sheet for the students and have them read the statements on the pickles and answer the questions individually or in small groups. This activity can be used with the story *Penny Pauses* (pages 132-135).

"When" Should You Ask? Pictures 174

▶ **C K-1**

If possible, reproduce the activity sheet on green paper. If you are using a jar, cut out the pictures in a pickle shape and place them in the pickle jar labeled "When should you ask people to give you things?" As the students draw pictures from the jar, have them tell if it would be all right to ask someone to give you the item pictured to keep. You may also reproduce this activity sheet for students to complete individually or in small groups. This activity can be used with the story *Penny Pauses* (pages 132-135).

"When" Should You Laugh? Pickles 175

▶ **C K-4**

Reproduce the activity sheet on green paper. Cut the questions out in the shape of pickles. Place the questions in the pickle jar labeled "When Should You Laugh?" To review the lesson, reproduce this activity sheet for the students and have them read the statements on the pickles and answer the questions individually or in small groups. This activity can be used with the story *Laughing Leaves* (pages 136-138).

Secret Code (Laughing) **176**

▶ **C 2-4**

Reproduce an activity sheet for each student. Distribute the activity sheet and a pencil to each student. If this is the first secret code sheet you have used, explain sign language. Tell the students to use the key at the top of the page to decode the message below. The answer is: Before you laugh at a person, see if he is laughing too.

"When" Should You Tell? Pickles **177-178**

▶ **C K-4**

Reproduce the activity sheets on green paper. Cut the questions out in the shape of pickles. Place the questions in the pickle jar labeled "When should you tell on another student?" To review the lesson, reproduce this activity sheet for the students and have them read the statements on the pickles and answer the questions individually or in small groups. This activity can be used with the story *Thursday, The Third Day Of Third Grade* (pages 143-147).

Playground Reporting **179**

▶ **C K-2**

Reproduce an activity sheet for each student. Read the story *Thursday, The Third Day Of Third Grade* (pages 143-147) or discuss the differences between *tattling* and *reporting*. Distribute the activity sheet and a pencil to each student. Read the directions with the students and have them complete the activity sheet. When everyone has completed the activity sheet, review the answers together.

Tattling/Reporting Guidelines **180**

▶ **C PH K-4**

Reproduce an activity sheet for each student. Review the text. Then tell the students to take the activity sheet home and go over it with their parents. The purpose of taking it home is to help parents understand that children are supposed to report some things.

Stoplight For Tattles And Reports **181**

▶ **C K-2**

Reproduce an activity sheet for each student. Distribute the activity sheet and crayons to each student. Have the students color their stoplight. Explain to the students the meaning of the three colors—red, yellow, and green. Have the students put their fingers on the appropriate color as you read the rhyme from the activity sheet. Once they understand the concept, have them practice, using examples from the previous activity sheets or ones you have made up.

Secret Code (Tattling) 182

▶ **C 2-4**

Reproduce an activity sheet for each student. Distribute the activity sheet and a pencil to each student. If this is the first secret code sheet you have used, explain sign language. Tell the students to use the key at the top of the page to decode the message below. The answer is: Adults do not like it when you tattle. Adults do like reports.

"When" Should You Tell A Secret? Pickles 183-184

▶ **I C K-4**

Reproduce the activity sheets on green paper. Cut the questions out in the shape of pickles. Place the questions in the pickle jar labeled "When should you tell a secret?" To review the lesson, reproduce this activity sheet for the students and have them read the statements on the pickles and answer the questions individually or in small groups. This activity can be used with the story *Snow Days Secrets* (pages 139-142). (*Note:* If this activity is used in a classroom, caution the students not to tell you sour pickle secrets in class, but to talk with you later.)

So Many Choices 185

▶ **C 2-4**

Reproduce an activity sheet for each student for use in a discussion about which choices are important. Read the activity sheet with the students and answer the questions orally. This activity sheet can be used with the story *Choices In The City* (pages 148-152). (*Note:* This activity may be used to help students deal with perfectionism.)

"When" Is A Choice Important? Pickles 186-187

▶ **I SG C K-4**

Reproduce the activity sheets on green paper. Cut the questions out in the shape of pickles. Place the questions in the pickle jar labeled "When is a choice important?" To review the lesson, reproduce this activity sheet for the students and have them read the statements on the pickles and answer the questions individually or in small groups. This activity can be used with the story *Choices In The City* (pages 148-152). (*Note:* This activity may be used to help students deal with perfectionism.)

"We Care About" Lessons 188-193

▶ **C K-4**

The activities on pages 188-193 accompany the story *Character Education At Pickle Mountain School* (pages 93-97). The pages should be reproduced and distributed to the students after they have heard the story and sung the song. There are two activity sheets for each concept—We Care About Each Other, We Care About Ourselves, We Care About The Earth. The picture activity sheets are for use with students in grades K-2. The other activity sheets are for use with students in grades 2-4.

CHAPTER 5: Career Education 195-209

This chapter provides materials you can use to incorporate career education into your other lesson topics.

All Jobs Are Important 196

C 2-4

This activity focuses on the interrelationship of jobs and the idea that each job has value. Reproduce an activity sheet for each student. Distribute the activity sheet and a pencil to each student. Have the students complete the activity sheet. When everyone has completed the activity sheet, discuss each job circled and explain its importance.

Occupations List 197-199

C 2-4

This is a list of brief job descriptions that accompany the lessons in this section. It may be used in two ways.

1. Reproduce the *Occupations List* and distribute a copy to each student. Tell the students they may use the activity sheets for reference during the game. Divide the class into teams. Read a job description aloud. The first student who stands up and is able to correctly name the job associated with the description earns a point for his/her team. Play continues until one team reaches a predetermined number of points or until the allotted time has elapsed.

2. Divide the class into teams, but do not give the students copies of the list. For this game, students are to depend on what they know and must identify the jobs without any references. Play the game as described above.

(*Note:* At the end of the list, there is a *Supplementary Occupations List*. The jobs on this list are not referred to in this section, but the list may be used when you feel it is appropriate for your class.)

Jobs At A Pickle Factory 200

C K-1

Reproduce an activity sheet for each student. Distribute the activity sheet and a pencil or crayon to each student. Tell the students to look at the pictures and circle those pictures of workers who might work at a large pickle factory every day. Emphasize that being there every day means that these workers don't just come to the factory once in a while. This activity sheet may be used with the stories *How Pickle Mountain Got Its Name* (pages 80-83) or *Snow Days Secrets* (pages 139-142).

Occupations At A Pickle Factory 201

▸ **C 2-4**

Reproduce an activity sheet for each student. Distribute the activity sheet and a pencil to each student. Tell the students to circle the names of those workers who might work at a large pickle factory every work day. Emphasize that being there every day means that these workers don't just come to the factory once in a while. If the students were given the *Occupations List* for the previous activity (game #1, page 25), allow them to use it as a reference. (*Note:* You may extend this lesson by having the students relate the occupations at the pickle factory to other factory occupations.)

Jobs At A Hospital 202

▸ **C K-1**

Reproduce an activity sheet for each student. Distribute the activity sheet and a pencil or crayon to each student. Tell the students to look at the pictures and circle the pictures of workers who might work at a hospital every work day. Emphasize that being there every day means that these workers don't just come to the hospital once in a while. This activity sheet may be used with the stories *Packed Pickle Goes To The Hospital* (pages 103-107) or *Choices In The City* (pages 148-152).

Occupations At A Hospital 203

▸ **C 2-4**

Reproduce an activity sheet for each student. Distribute the activity sheet and a pencil to each student. Tell the students to circle the names of those workers who might work at a hospital every work day. Emphasize that being there every day means that these workers don't just come to the hospital once in a while. If the students were given the *Occupations List* for the previous activity (game #1, page 25), allow them to use it as a reference. (*Note:* You may extend this lesson by having the students relate the occupations at the hospital to other health-career occupations.)

Jobs At An Airport 204

▸ **C K-1**

Reproduce the activity sheet for each student. Distribute the activity sheet and a pencil or crayon to each student. Tell the students to look at the pictures and circle the pictures of workers who might work at an airport every work day. Emphasize that being there every day means that these workers don't just come to the airport once in a while. This activity sheet may be used with the story *Big And Bigger Field Trips* (page 114).

Occupations At An Airport 205

▸ **C 2-4**

Reproduce an activity sheet for each student. Distribute the activity sheet and a pencil to each student. Tell the students to circle the names of those workers who might work at a large airport every work day. Emphasize that being there every day means that these workers don't just come to the airport once in a while. If the students were given the *Occupations List* for the previous activity (game #1, page 25), allow them to use it as a reference. (*Note:* You may extend this lesson by having the students relate the occupations at the airport to other transportation occupations.)

C K-1

Reproduce an activity sheet for each student. Distribute the activity sheet and a pencil or crayon to each student. Tell the students to look at the pictures and circle the pictures of workers who might work at a school every work day. Emphasize that being there every day means that these workers don't just come to the school once in a while. This activity sheet may be used with the stories *Tired Of Stinky Pickle* (pages 84-87), *Fight For A Frog* (pages 88-92), *Character Education At Pickle Mountain School* (pages 93-97), *Packed Like Pickles* (pages 122-126), *Penny Pauses* (pages 132-135), *Laughing Leaves* (pages 136-138), and/or *Snow Days Secrets* (pages 139-142).

C 2-4

Reproduce an activity sheet for each student. Distribute the activity sheet and a pencil to each student. Tell the students to circle the names of those workers who might work at a school every work day. Emphasize that being there every day means that these workers don't just come to the school once in a while. If the students were given the *Occupations List* for the previous activity (game #1, page 25), allow them to use it as a reference.

C K-1

Reproduce an activity sheet for each student. Distribute the activity sheet and a pencil or crayon to each student. Tell the students to look at the pictures and circle the pictures of workers who might build or repair houses. This activity sheet may be used with the story *The "Unempty" House* (pages 127-131).

C 2-4

Reproduce an activity sheet for each student. Distribute the activity sheet and a pencil to each student. Tell the students to circle the names of those workers who might work at building or repairing houses. If the students were given the *Occupations List* for the previous activity (game #1, page 25), allow them to use it as a reference. (*Note:* You may extend this lesson by having the students relate the occupations for building houses to other construction occupations.)

CHAPTER 6:
Integrating Math And Literacy 211-228

Academic subjects are already a part of guidance lessons, even though the relationship isn't always acknowledged. This chapter will help you strengthen the connection of all subjects. When you write lesson plans, you may want to specify a math or literacy point you want to make.

Punctuation Pickles 212-216

C K-4

Reproduce and laminate (if you wish) pages 213-216 to make a set of wall posters for the counselor's area (when available) and for teachers who request them. Refer to the wall set when reading or writing during a guidance lesson. Reproduce the activity sheet (page 212) for the students. Review the information on each pickle. Tell the students to keep their activity sheets for reference during a writing lesson.

Finding Punctuation Marks 217

C K-2

This is a lesson on following instructions as well as recognizing punctuation marks. Reproduce the activity sheet for kindergarten students near the end of the year and work with them on the activity sheet. Reproduce the activity sheet for instructional purposes for first-grade students and for review for second-grade students. Distribute the activity sheet and crayons or markers to each student. When everyone has completed the activity sheet, review the answers. Make the activity available for teachers who wish to include it in their classroom presentation on punctuation.

Sentences About Pickles 218

C 1-2

Reproduce an activity sheet for each student. Have the *Punctuation Pickle* posters or student activity sheet available for student reference. Distribute the activity sheet and a pencil to each student. Review the directions with the students and have them complete the activity sheet. When everyone has completed the activity sheet, review the answers. Teachers can also present this activity.

Sentences About Anger 219

C 1-4

Reproduce an activity sheet for each student. Have the *Punctuation Pickle* posters or student activity sheet available for student reference. Distribute the activity sheet and a pencil to each student. Review the directions with the students and have them complete the activity sheet. You may need to do the activity with first-grade students. This activity sheet may be used with the *Using "Pickle Cat"* lesson (page 156). When everyone has completed the activity sheet, review the answers. Teachers can also present this activity.

Sentences On Tattling/Reporting 220

C 1-4

Reproduce an activity sheet for each student. Have the *Punctuation Pickle* posters or student activity sheet available for student reference. Distribute the activity sheet and a pencil to each student. Review the directions with the students, then have them complete the activity sheet. You may need to do the activity with first-grade students. This activity sheet may be used with the story *Thursday, The Third Day Of Third Grade* (pages 143-147) or the tattle/report activities (Chapter 4, pages 177-184). When everyone has completed the activity sheet, review the answers. Teachers can also present this activity.

Sentences On Safety 221

C 1-4

Reproduce an activity sheet for each student. Have the *Punctuation Pickle* posters or student activity sheet available for student reference. Distribute the activity sheet and a pencil to each student. Review the directions with the students, then have them complete the activity sheet. You may need to do the activity with first-grade students. This activity sheet may be used with the *Pickle Sweep* lesson (page 165), *We Care About Ourselves Phrases* (page 190), or *We Care About Ourselves Pictures* (page 191). When everyone has completed the activity sheet, review the answers. Teachers can also present this activity.

Ten Pickles Jars (Song) 222

C K-1

Sing this song, to the tune of *100 Bottles Of Soda (Pop) On the Wall,* with the students during guidance time. If you can, make 10 plastic pickle jars for the children to pass to one another during the song. Make copies of the song for those teachers who request them.

Pickle Math 223

C K-1

This activity correlates with math. Reproduce an activity sheet for each student to work on during a guidance lesson. Distribute the activity sheet and a pencil to each student and tell the students to complete it. When everyone has completed the activity sheet, review the answers. Make copies for those teachers who wish to use the activity in their classroom.

Sweet And Sour Pickle Problems **224**

▶ **C K-1**

This activity correlates with math. Reproduce an activity sheet for each student to work on during a guidance lesson. Distribute the activity sheet and a pencil to each student and tell the students to complete it. When everyone has completed the activity sheet, review the answers. Make copies for those teachers who wish to use the activity in their classroom.

Mrs. Smith's Pickles **225**

▶ **C 1-2**

This activity correlates with math. Reproduce an activity sheet for each student to work on during a guidance lesson. Distribute the activity sheet and a pencil to each student and tell the students to complete it. When everyone has completed the activity sheet, review the answers. Make copies for those teachers who wish to use the activity in their classroom.

Pickles For Lunch **226**

▶ **C 2-3**

This activity correlates with math. Reproduce an activity sheet for each student to work on during a guidance lesson. Distribute the activity sheet and a pencil to each student and tell the students to complete it. When everyone has completed the activity sheet, review the answers. Make copies for those teachers who wish to use the activity in their classroom.

Pickle Collection **227**

▶ **C 3-4**

This activity correlates with math. Reproduce an activity sheet for each student to work on during a guidance lesson. Distribute the activity sheet and a pencil to each student and tell the students to complete it. When everyone has completed the activity sheet, review the answers. Make copies for those teachers who wish to use the activity in their classroom.

Mr. Brown's Pickle Project **228**

▶ **C 4+**

This activity correlates with math. Reproduce an activity sheet for each student to work on during a guidance lesson. Distribute the activity sheet and a pencil to each student and tell the students to complete it. When everyone has completed the activity sheet, review the answers. Make copies for those teachers who wish to use the activity in their classroom.

CHAPTER 7: Vocabulary Activities.................................. 229-249

Discovery List Of Words For Sweet, Sour, And In-Between Feelings 230-236

C 2-4

Reproduce each page for each student. The pages can be used many times to help students expand their vocabulary for expressing feelings. Reproduce a couple of sets for teachers to keep in the classroom. This list is not comprehensive, but it includes some words for every letter of the alphabet.

Discovery List Of Words For Sweet And Sour Feelings.................. 237-241

C K-2

This starter list for grades K-2 includes at least one word for each letter of the alphabet. For kindergarten, use this list to introduce words to go with letters of the alphabet. Make a copy for the teacher, but not for the students. For students who have recently started first grade, use the list as an instructional tool. When the students begin independent writing, make copies for them as well as for the teacher.

Your Name... 242

C PH 1-4

Reproduce an activity sheet for each student. Distribute the activity sheet and a pencil to each student. Write your name on the chalkboard to demonstrate the activity. Reinforce the activity by reviewing the example on the activity sheet. Tell the students to use their vocabulary lists (pages 230-236 or 237-241) for reference. When everyone has completed the activity sheet, have the students share their answers. This is an activity the students may do at home with their parents.

Vocabulary Search 243

C PH 3-4

Reproduce an activity sheet for each student. Distribute the activity sheet and a pencil to each student. Review the directions and have the students complete the *word search.* Tell the students to use their vocabulary lists (pages 230-236) for reference. This is an activity the students may do at home with their parents.

Synonyms And Antonyms 244

▶ **C 3-4**

Reproduce an activity sheet for each student. Distribute the activity sheet and a pencil to each student. Review the directions and have the students complete the activity sheet. Tell the students to use their vocabulary lists (pages 230-236) for reference. When everyone has completed the activity sheet, have the students share their answers.

How Many Words Can You Write? 245

▶ **C 2-4**

Reproduce an activity sheet for each student. Distribute the activity sheet and a pencil to each student. Tell the students to use their vocabulary lists (pages 230-236) to help them complete the activity sheet. When everyone has completed the activity sheet, have the students share their answers. Discuss the different feelings that can arise in any one situation.

Find The Word 246

▶ **C 1-2**

Reproduce an activity sheet for each student. Distribute the activity sheet and a pencil to each student. Tell the students to use their vocabulary lists (pages 237-241) to help them complete the activity sheet. When everyone has completed the activity sheet, have the students share their answers.

Sweet And Sour Words 247

▶ **C 1-2**

Reproduce an activity sheet for each student. Distribute the activity sheet, a pencil, and crayons to each student. Tell the students to use their vocabulary lists (pages 237-241) to help them complete the activity sheet. When everyone has completed the activity sheet, have the students share their answers.

Sweet And Sour Feelings Crossword **248**

C 1-2

Reproduce an activity sheet for each student. Distribute the activity sheet and a pencil to each student. Tell the students to use their vocabulary lists (pages 237-241) to help them complete the crossword. When everyone has completed the crossword, have the students share their answers. The answers are:

Across:	Down:
3. Thankful	1. Grumpy
6. Lonely	2. Curious
7. Safe	4. Angry
	5. Kind

Feelings Crossword **249**

C 2-4

Reproduce an activity sheet for each student. Distribute the activity sheet and a pencil to each student. Tell the students to use their vocabulary lists (pages 230-236) to help them complete the crossword. When everyone has completed the crossword, have the students share their answers. The answers are:

Across:	Down:
1. Overwhelmed	2. Exhausted
4. Discouraged	3. Adaptable
7. Tolerant	5. Ecstatic
8. Victorious	6. Bewildered
9. Industrious	

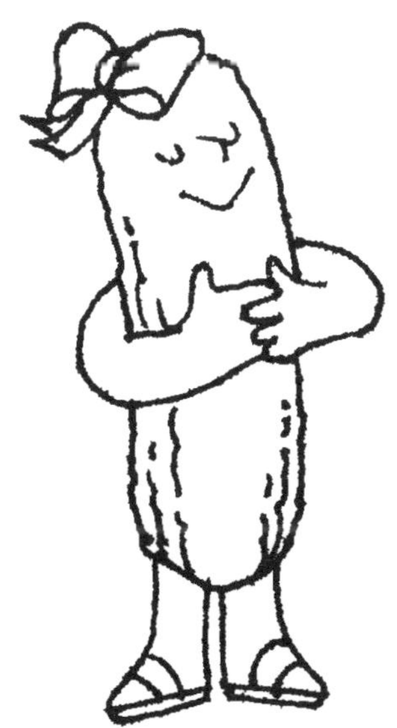

CHAPTER 8: Parent Involvement 251-265

The activities and information in this chapter are for parent education or for parent involvement with their children.

PH 1-4

This is an activity for parents to enjoy with their children. Make a copy for each student to take home and complete with a parent's help. When the completed activity sheet is returned, review the answers to the questions and make a class list of all the kinds of pickles mentioned.

PH 1-4

This is an activity for parents to enjoy with their children. Make a copy for each student to take home and complete with a parent's help. When the completed activity sheet is returned, review the answers to the questions and make a class list of all the kinds of pickles mentioned.

PH 2-4

This is an activity for parents to enjoy with their children. Make a copy for each student to take home and complete with a parent's help. Possible answers are: pie, pies, pick, picks, pike, pile, pikes, peck, pecks, sick, lick, licks, is, like, likes, lip, lips, sip, speck, lei, lisp, slip, spice.

PH K-4

Make a copy for each child to take home and make with a parent's help.

PH 2-4

This is a reproducible handout for children to take home to their parents as a follow-up to *Pickle Cat* (page 157) or other anger-management lessons. An explanation of what was learned in class is followed by the *Appropriate Ways To Handle Anger* word find. Make a copy for each student.

To help you more effectively use the ideas in *Pickle Packet II,* we have included 13 sample lesson plans. These lesson plans will help you realize how much can be accomplished during one 30-minute period. The included topics are: *Introducing the Pickle Theme, Bullying, Conflict Resolution, Anger Management, Tattling/Reporting, Drug/Alcohol Education, Feelings, Manners, Character Education,* and *Career Education.*

To help you more effectively use the ideas in *Pickle Packet II,* we have included 11 sample lesson plans. These lesson plans will help you realize how much can be accomplished during one 30-minute period. The included topics are: *Anger Management, Bullying, Conflict Resolution, Tolerance, Attitude, Character Education, Feelings,* and *Career Education.*

This section includes an index of topics found in *Pickle Packet II.*

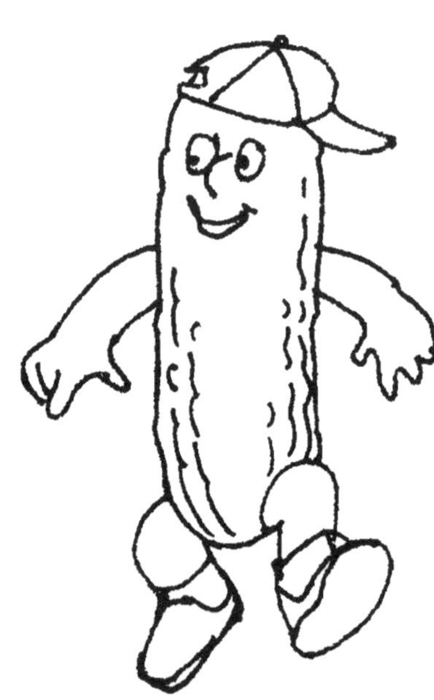

CHAPTER 1

BASICS FOR LIFE IS LIKE A PICKLE

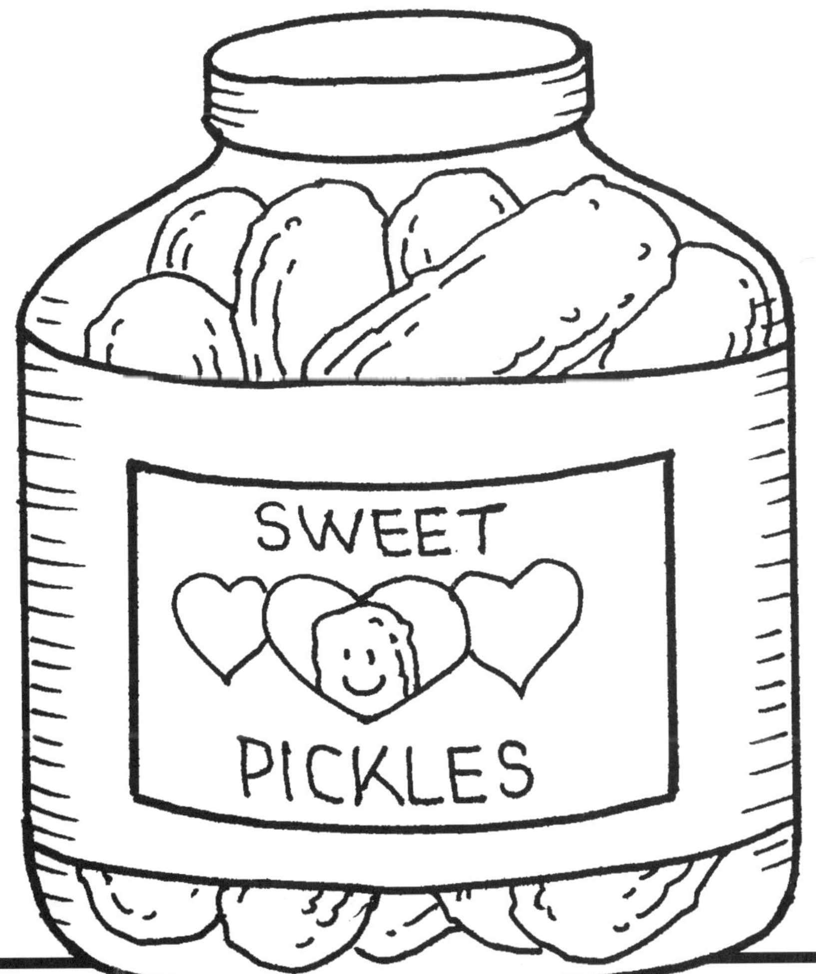

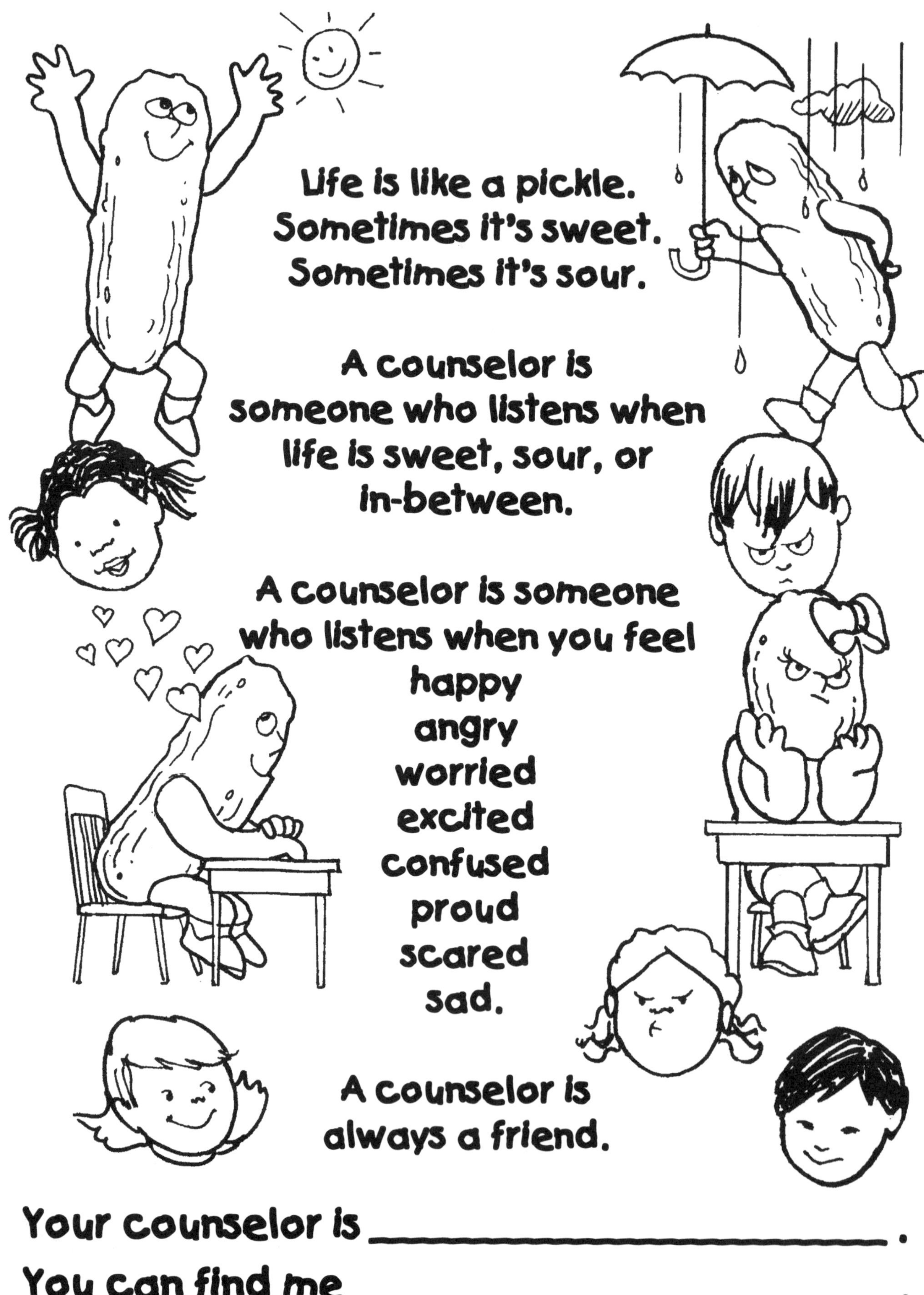

Life is like a pickle.
Sometimes it's sweet.
Sometimes it's sour.

A counselor is
someone who listens when
life is sweet, sour, or
in-between.

A counselor is someone
who listens when you feel
happy
angry
worried
excited
confused
proud
scared
sad.

A counselor is
always a friend.

Your counselor is ________________________.

You can find me ________________________.

THE PICKLE PLEDGE

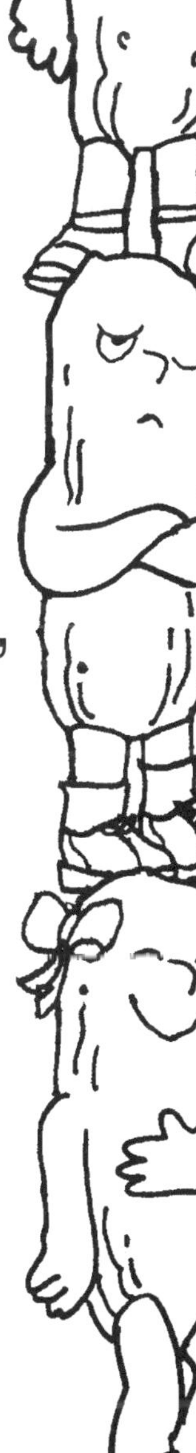

CHORUS

There are sweet pickles, sour pickles,
And some are in-between.
Life is like a pickle.
That doesn't mean it's green.
That doesn't mean it's green!

VERSE 1

Life is like a sour pickle
When I'm feeling sad.
And sometimes when I feel scared,
Confused, worried, or mad.

(REPEAT CHORUS)

VERSE 2

Life is like a sweet pickle
When days are filled with joy.
For I have lots of good feelings,
Like every girl and boy.

(REPEAT CHORUS)

ACTIONS FOR
THE PICKLE PLEDGE

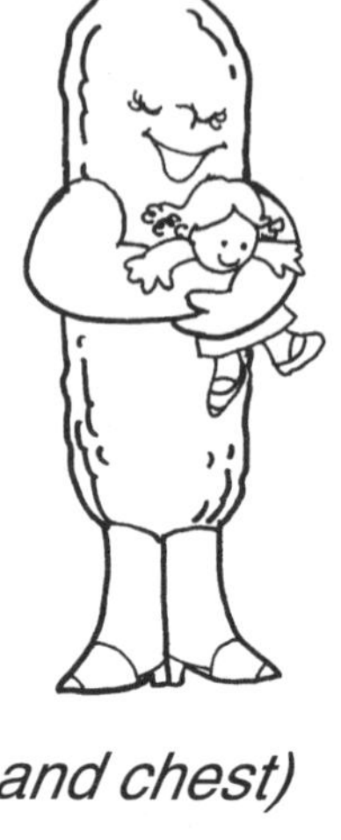

CHORUS

There are sweet pickles, *(hands in front of body, chest high)*

sour pickles, *(hands in front of body, at waist)*

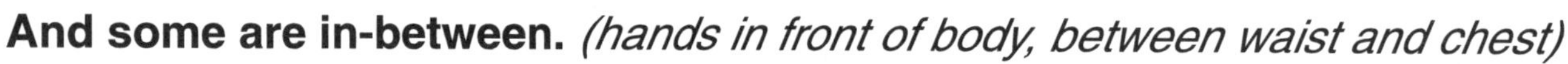

And some are in-between. *(hands in front of body, between waist and chest)*

Life is like a pickle. *(slightly move one hand up, the other down, repeat)*

That doesn't mean it's green. *(shake head "no")*

That doesn't mean it's green! *(shake head "no")*

VERSE 1

Life is like a sour pickle *(draw a frown with finger)*

When I'm feeling sad. *(frown)*

And sometimes when I feel scared, *(put hands up by head, make scared look)*

Confused, worried, or mad. *(put hands on hips as if mad)*

(REPEAT CHORUS)

VERSE 2

Life is like a sweet pickle *(draw a smile with finger)*

When days are filled with joy. *(wave hands in air as if celebrating)*

For I have lots of good feelings, *(point to self)*

Like every girl and boy. *(point to a girl and a boy)*

(REPEAT CHORUS)

PICKLE ROUTINE

Primary-age children like routine. I want to share with you the way I start almost all of my lessons. If I am doing a special project that does not begin this way, the students usually remind me that I have forgotten to do something.

During 17 years as the Pickle Lady, I have collected and given *pickle* names to a variety of toys. Most of them are stuffed animals. I have enough toys to let each child hold one while we say *The Pickle Pledge* (page 39) and review the pickle theme: "Life is like a pickle. Sometimes it's sweet. Sometimes it's sour." When using toys, these are two rules I learned the hard way:

1. Take the toy that is handed to you. You may say, "No, thank you," but you do not get another toy.
2. Keep the toys away from your head. (Yes, I have to teach about head lice, too. Therefore: *If it's something we share, it doesn't go in your hair.)*

My toys include:

- Pickle Monkey—stuffed monkey or puppet with a plastic pickle in its mouth instead of a banana
- Pickle in the Hat—stuffed pickle with a hat made by a parent
- Polka-Dot Pickle—large stuffed frog or puppet with black spots
- Pickle Puppet—purchased from Mar*co Products or made from pattern on page 46
- Pickle Wand—plastic pickle on the end of a dowel rod
- Pickle Pig—stuffed green mechanical pig with batteries removed so it can't be turned on during the lesson
- Cold Pickle—stuffed penguin or puppet with green scarf
- Slow Pickle—stuffed turtle or puppet
- Pickle Elephant—elephant puppet with a pickle eraser sewn to its trunk
- Pickle Pup—green stuffed puppy
- Lots of Teddy Bears named Sweet Gherkin, Sweet Pickle, Pickle Bear (wears a small pickle shirt), Pickle Bear's Friend, Sparkly Pickle, Tall Pickle

As you can tell, you can add a touch of green to many things you already have and give them *pickle* names. If time is short, I do not distribute toys for the children to hold while we say *The Pickle Pledge* (page 39) or during the discussion that follows. Instead, we perform *Actions For The Pickle Pledge* (page 40).

After reciting the pledge with the students, ask the following questions:

1. "Is it okay to be sad sometimes?" *(Yes. No one in the world is happy all the time.)* When you are really, really sad, will you stay sad forever? *(No.)* When you are really, really sad, whom can you talk with? *(This is the most elementary kind of suicide-prevention lesson, even though we never use that term.)*
2. "Is it okay to be scared sometimes?" *(Yes. Even grown-ups sometimes get scared. Being scared can sometimes keep you safe. I hope you are too scared to run across the road in front of a big truck or play on a swing set during a lightning storm. When you are scared, talk with an adult who cares about you.)*

3. "Is it okay to be mad sometimes?" *(Yes. Everybody gets angry sometimes. In fact, there are times you* should *be angry. When you are angry, you have to be careful what you do. You can show your anger, but you can't hurt anyone, destroy things, or use words that will get you in trouble with the principal, your teacher, or your parents. You don't want to stay mad for a long time.)*

At this point, I explain that counselors can get mad sometimes, too. I tell the students that when I get mad, I ask myself the following questions. They help me control my anger.

"Will I hurt anyone?"
"Will I destroy anything?"
"Will I use words that will get me in trouble with anyone?"
"Will I let you know I am mad?"
"Will I stay mad for a long time?"

If time allows, recite *The Pickle Pledge* again. Then collect the toys and end the lesson. Or continue with whatever activity you have planned.

VALUE OF USING THE PICKLE ROUTINE IN MOST K-2 LESSONS

First of all, children like and learn from predictability.

The *Pickle Routine* provides the opportunity to relate to any very sad event the children may have heard about. For example, it can be used to help children see there are various levels of sadness. Say:

"If I read a newspaper story about the death of a boy I didn't know, who had lived in a faraway state, I would be a little sad. *(Hold your two index fingers about an inch apart.)* I would think about his family, his teacher, and his friends. If I read about the death of a girl I didn't know, who had lived in the city where I lived, I would be more sad. *(Hold your fingers about six inches apart.)* And, if I read that a child who attended our school had died, I would be even sadder. *(Hold your hands about two feet apart.)* If that child was a member of my own family, I would be saddest of all. *(Hold your arms as far apart as possible.)* People who were very close to that child will be very, very sad for a very long time. Will they be sad all day, every day from now on?" *(No. The discussion about not being sad forever lays the foundation for suicide prevention, although the topic is not directly approached in these early years.)*

You can relate the question, "Is it okay to be scared sometimes?" to scary secrets or to being offered drugs. Emphasize that being scared can help keep you safe. Point out that adults are also scared sometimes.

When asking, "Is it okay to be mad sometimes?" you can get into a deeper lesson on anger or simply remind the students that counselors can get mad, too. Then review these points: It's okay to get mad, but you have to be careful what you do. You can't hurt anyone, destroy things, or use words that will get you in trouble with the principal, your teacher, or your parents.

DISCUSSION GUIDE

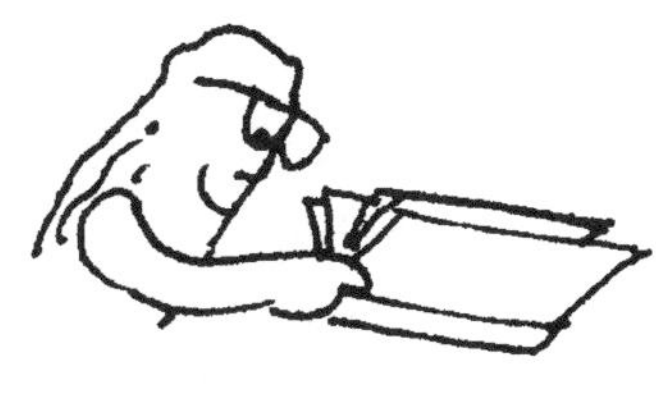

Are people supposed to be happy all the time? Why? Why not?

____

____

When you are sad, with whom can you talk?

____

When you are really, really sad, will you stay sad forever? Why? Why not?

____

____

Is it okay to be scared sometimes? Why? Why not?

____

____

When can being scared help keep you safe?

____

____

I hope you are too scared to:

- stay in a swimming pool during a thunderstorm
- get into a car with a stranger
- cross a street with traffic coming
- take a pill your mother or father did not give you

Is it okay to be mad sometimes? Why? Why not?

____

____

It is okay to be mad, but you can't:

- hurt anyone
- destroy things
- use words that will get you in trouble

Life is like a pickle. Sometimes it's sweet. Sometimes it's sour.

A school counselor cares for students when life is sweet or sour or in-between.

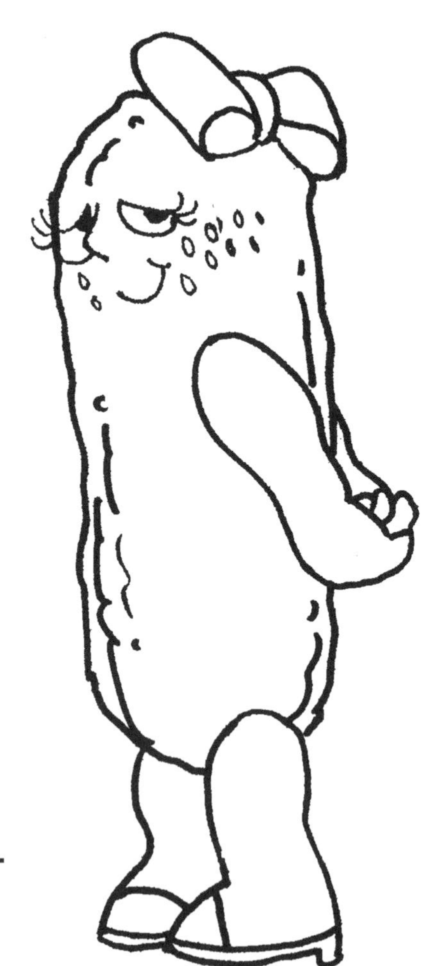

School counselors:

- help meet students' special needs
- promote a positive school atmosphere
- present classroom guidance lessons
- provide programs for parents
- counsel individual students
- meet with small groups of students
- consult with teachers
- confer with parents
- help in a crisis.

School counselors care about the emotional, social, and educational development of students.

Your school counselor is ______________________________.

Your school counselor's telephone number is ____________________

Dear Parents,

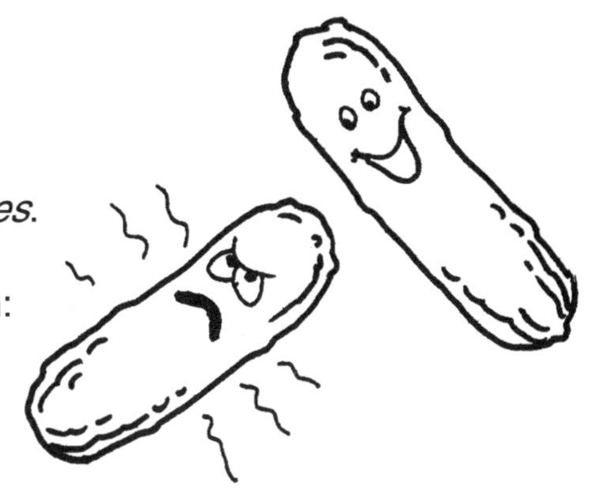

You may be surprised to hear children talking about *pickles*.
No, we are not eating lots of pickles at school.
Pickles are used in our guidance program when we teach:

Life is like a pickle.
Sometimes it's sweet.
Sometimes it's sour.

Students are learning that life is not supposed to be happy all the time and that it is okay to be sad. However, they are also learning that even when they are very, very sad, they will not stay sad forever. They are encouraged to express their sadness to an adult who loves them.

The children are learning that everyone is scared at times. Being scared can sometimes help keep children safe. We hope a child is too scared to run out into traffic or get into a car with a stranger. Students are taught to tell an adult they trust when they are very scared. Caring adults can reassure children without making them feel guilty for being scared.

Anger is another feeling we experience at times. There are some very good reasons for being angry. Students learn that it is okay to be angry and show anger, but that they must be careful what they do when they are angry. They cannot hurt people, destroy things, or use words that will get them in trouble.

During our lessons, students learn *The Pickle Pledge*. It's one you may have heard your children say.

> *(CHORUS)* There are sweet pickles, sour pickles, and some are in-between. Life is like a pickle. That doesn't mean it's green. That doesn't mean it's green!
>
> Life is like a sour pickle when I'm feeling sad. And sometimes when I feel scared, confused, worried, or mad.
> *(REPEAT CHORUS)*
>
> Life is like a sweet pickle when days are filled with joy. For I have lots of good feelings, like every girl and boy.
> *(REPEAT CHORUS)*

Don't be surprised if you hear some nicknames that include the word *pickle*. It's quite okay because it helps reinforce the lessons.

Caring about your children when life is sweet, sour, or in-between, ____________________,
(SIGNATURE)
your elementary counselor.

____
(PRINT NAME)

____
(TELEPHONE #)

PICKLE STICK PUPPET PATTERNS

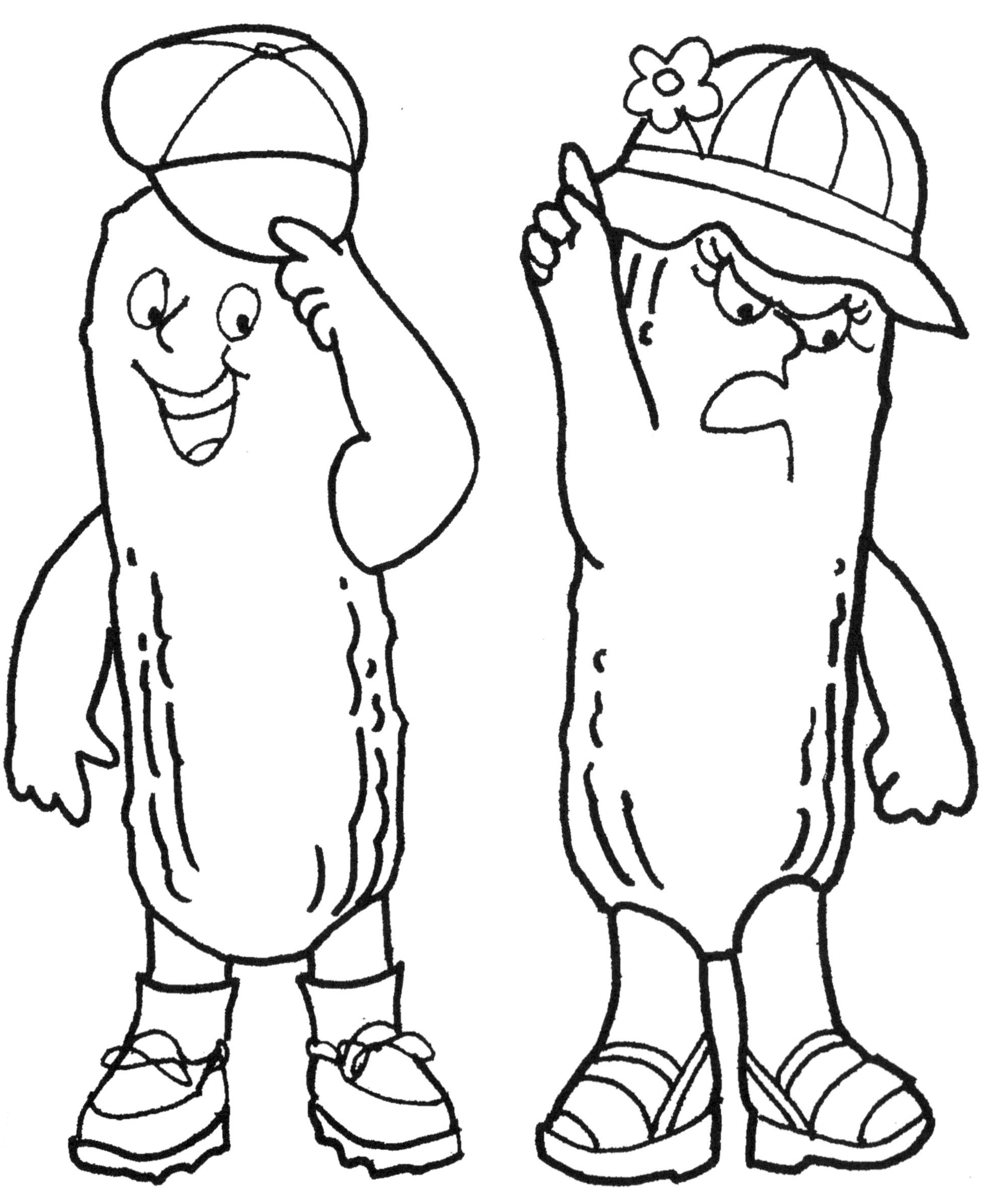

CHAPTER 2

JUST PICKLES

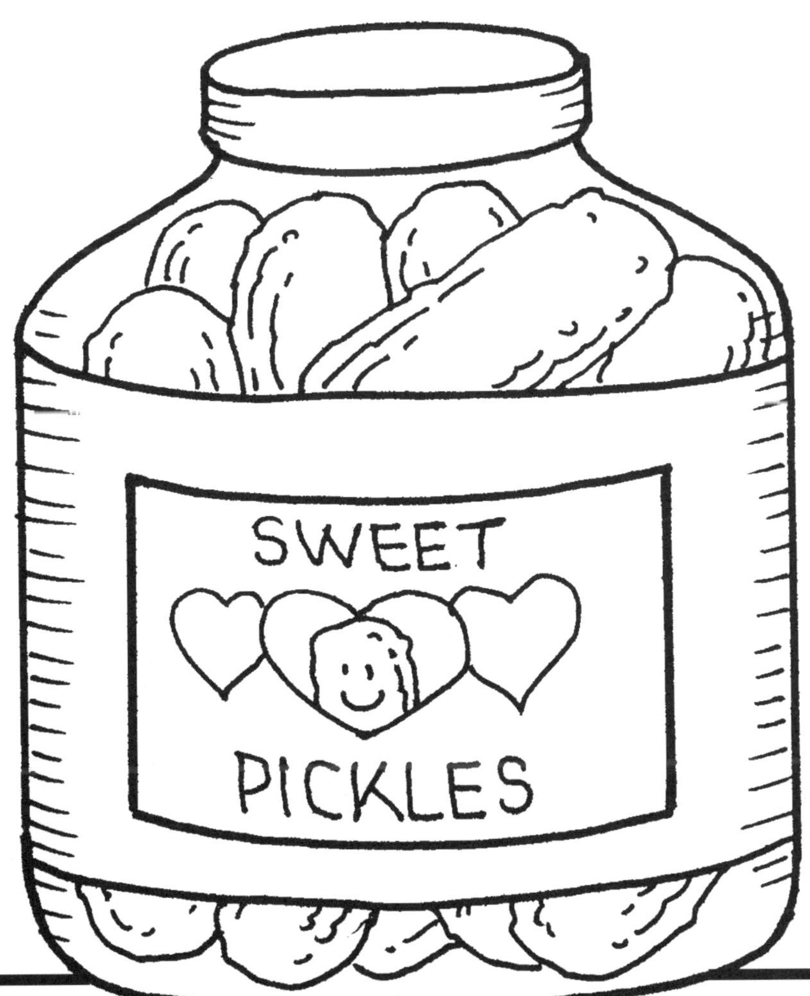

Name ______________________________

WHAT IS PICKLE?

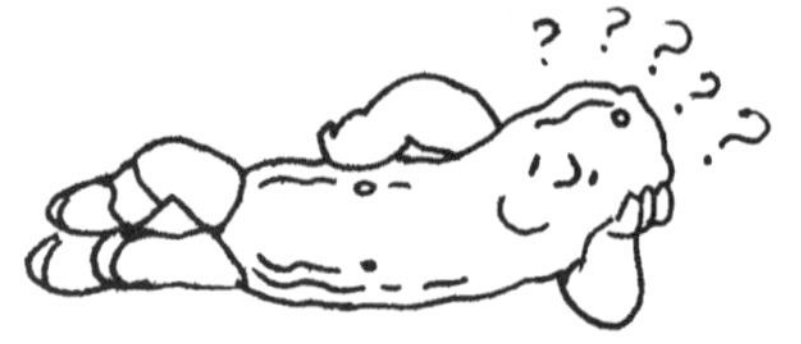

Pickle is a liquid, such as saltwater or vinegar, that is used to preserve meat or vegetables. Cucumbers preserved in such a liquid are called *pickles*. Other ingredients are added to give pickles different flavors.

Pickle is a word that can also mean *difficulty*. Maybe that is because having a problem can make a person feel trapped, like a cucumber sealed in the pickle solution.

Here are some foods found in cookbooks under the word *pickle:*

dill pickles	mustard pickles	bread and butter pickles
cantaloupe pickles	pickled okra	hot dill pickles
sweet pickle sticks	garlic dill pickles	pickled eggs
pickled vegetables	watermelon pickles	spiced pickled peaches
pickled jalapenos	pickled crab apples	

Here are some pickles found in a grocery store:

sweet gherkins	sweet and tangy	Polish dill
Kosher dill	garlic dill	zesty bread and butter
sweet pickle mix	sweet tiny midgets	hot and spicy garden mix

Besides coming in different flavors, pickles are shaped in many different ways. There are:

relish	whole	chips
chunks	sandwich slices	spears

Go back over this page and circle the kinds of pickles you have tried. Put an ✘ by your favorite.

Are there some people in your class who do not like pickles? ______________________

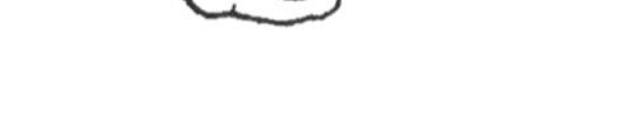

Did you know …

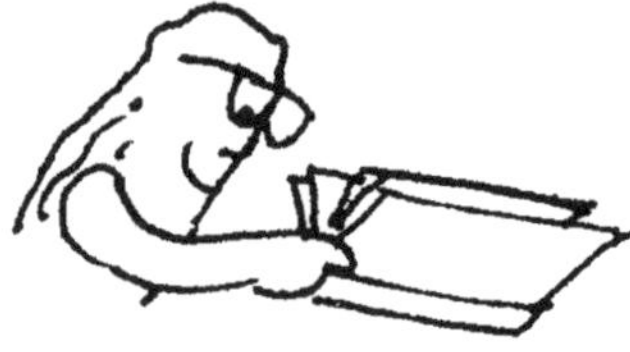

Our country's namesake, Amerigo Vespucci, was actually a pickle peddler. He supplied ships with pickled vegetables to prevent sailors from getting the sickness known as *scurvy*. Today we know that scurvy comes from a lack of Vitamin C, which is found in fruits and vegetables.

Name ______________________________

LITTLE PICKLE WORD SEARCH

The following words are hidden in the pickle below. Find and circle them. Hint: The words are hidden across.

HAPPY SAD SCARED LOVED MAD EXCITED

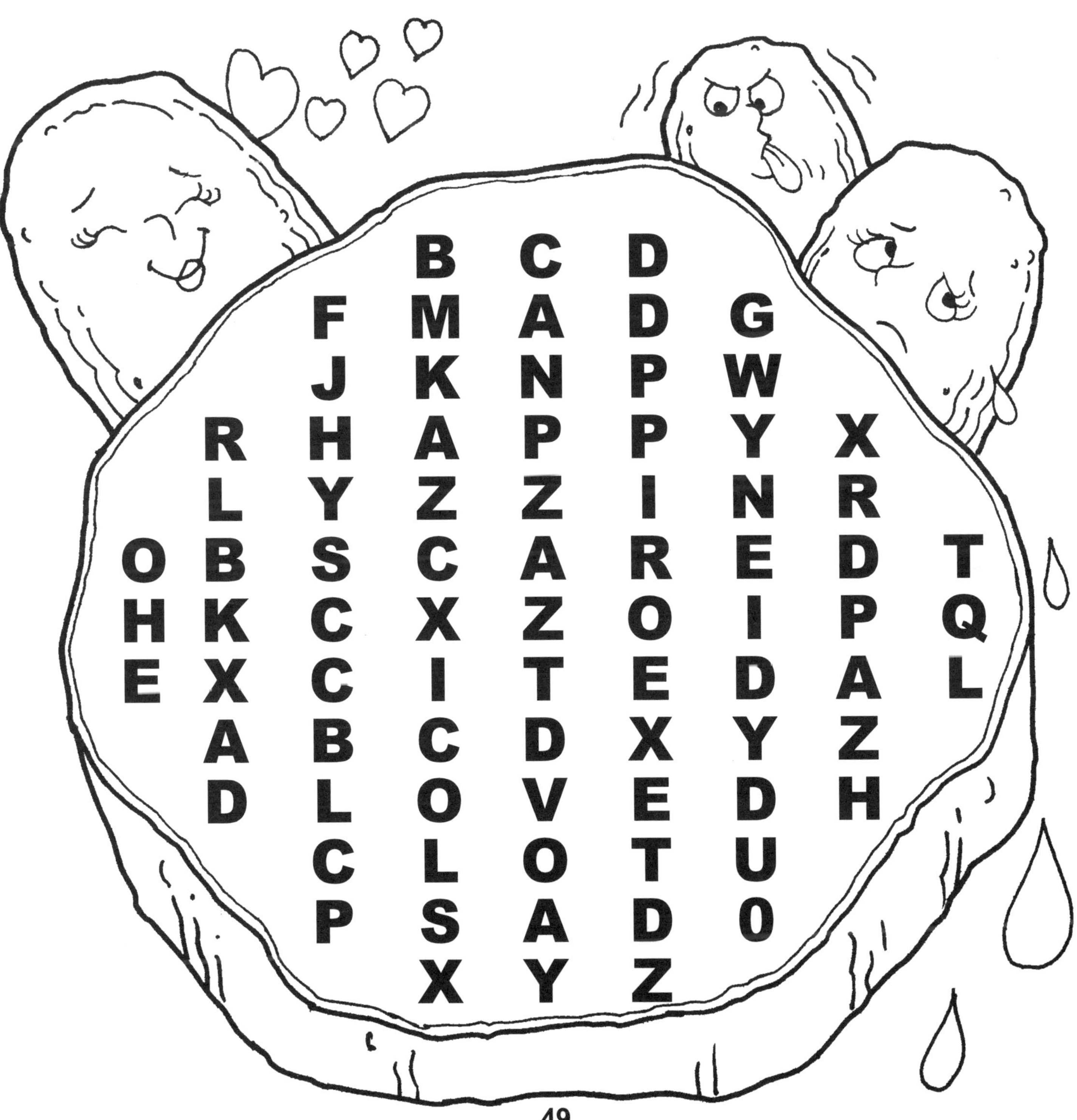

Name ______________________________

SWEET PICKLE, SOUR PICKLE
WORD SEARCHES

Below are two word searches. One contains *sweet pickle words* and the other contains *sour pickle words.* Find and circle the hidden words. Each word is spelled across, from left to right.

Can you find the *sweet pickle words?*

HAPPY GLAD SAFE LOVED SURPRISED PROUD EXCITED PLEASED

X	E	S	A	F	E	P	K	O
M	A	B	C	D	F	G	S	K
H	L	O	V	E	D	J	C	B
K	L	M	N	S	T	U	V	H
E	X	C	I	T	E	D	I	N
F	H	L	K	T	D	B	D	E
Z	H	A	P	P	Y	W	O	Y
X	X	T	I	I	U	M	Z	A
P	R	O	U	D	R	X	J	E
A	G	C	W	E	F	G	B	C
S	U	R	P	R	I	S	E	D
H	J	I	A	B	D	D	E	O
F	P	L	E	A	S	E	D	W
G	L	A	D	J	G	N	C	Y

Can you find the *sour pickle words*?

MAD UPSET SAD LONELY SCARED WORRIED ANGRY CONFUSED

O	S	A	D	X	N	B	Y	L
Y	Z	W	C	D	W	L	E	A
F	G	I	M	N	O	K	R	U
P	S	C	A	R	E	D	B	C
E	F	G	H	I	J	K	Z	A
U	P	S	E	T	W	X	M	I
V	W	X	Y	Z	F	O	A	Q
T	A	W	O	R	R	I	E	D
E	X	T	O	E	U	M	O	S
R	L	O	N	E	L	Y	B	Z
C	D	E	F	G	Z	I	O	E
C	O	N	F	U	S	E	D	S
Z	U	B	X	X	C	I	R	W
M	A	D	M	A	N	G	R	Y
X	A	B	C	P	Y	Q	O	L

Name ______________________________

WORD SEARCH CHALLENGE

Find the hidden *sweet* and *sour pickle words*. The words are hidden across, down, and diagonally. Circle each word you find.

ZANY
YUCKY
PATIENT
KIND
CHEERY
JUMPY
QUIET
NEEDED
RESPECTFUL
LONELY
COOPERATIVE
PROUD
MAD

			A	P	I	
		E	Z	K	L	
	C	P	R	O	U	D
I	O	X	E	Y	Q	B
C	O	O	S	D	U	G
L	P	N	P	J	I	L
O	E	N	E	S	E	W
N	R	X	C	H	T	X
E	A	M	T	N	Y	M
L	T	D	F	M	O	Y
Y	I	J	U	M	P	Y
N	V	C	L	D	K	I
E	E	F	G	H	I	J
C	H	E	E	R	Y	B
M	Z	N	D	R	Q	P
P	A	T	I	E	N	T
X	N	A	Z	W	D	C
W	Y	U	C	K	Y	D
	K	I	N	D	F	G
		M	V	D	A	R
		T	A	W	N	
			K	D		

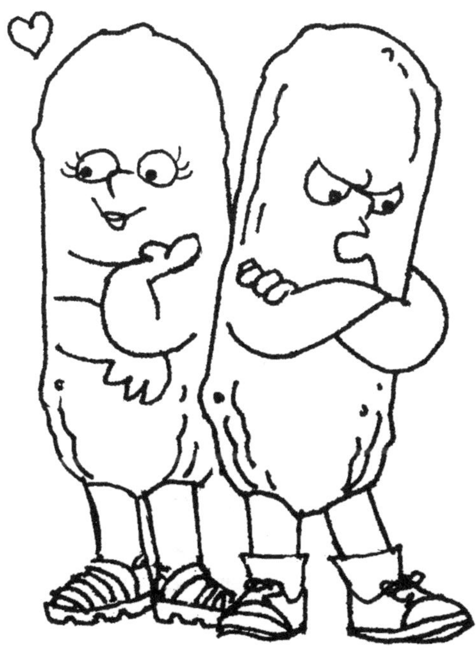

Name ______________________________

PICKLE PUZZLES

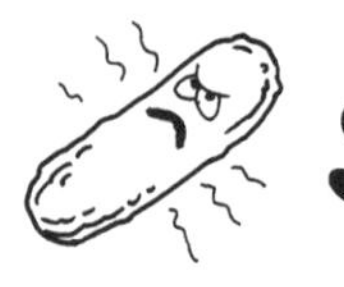

SOUR	SWEET
I am sad when ...	I am thankful when ...
I am scared when ...	I am happy when ...
I am mad when ...	I feel loved when ...
I am worried when ...	I am excited when ...

Name ______________________________

SONNY'S BIRTHDAY

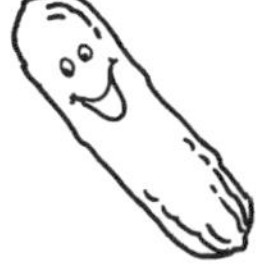 **SWEET PICKLE**

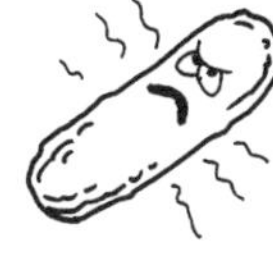 **SOUR PICKLE**

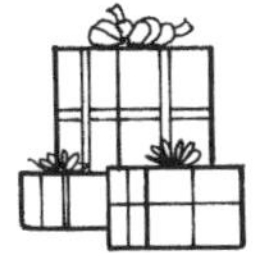 **PRESENTS**

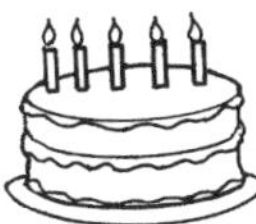 **BIRTHDAY**

 **BIKE**

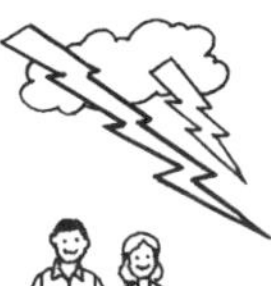 **LIGHTNING**

 **RAINBOW**

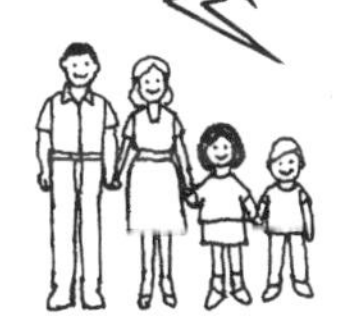 **FAMILY**

 **SUN**

It was Sonny's 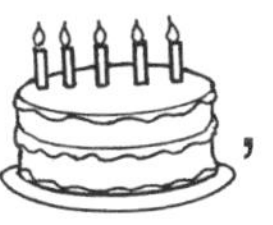, but the  was not shining. It was a 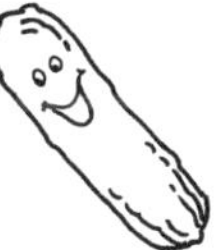 day when his 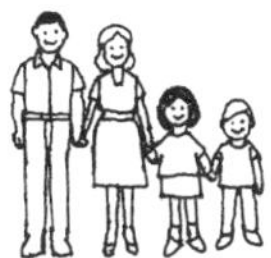 gave him a new . He had a 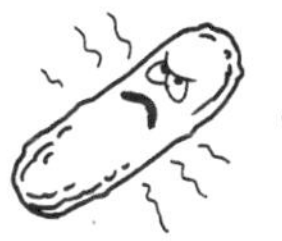 feeling when he saw the  outside. He opened his other 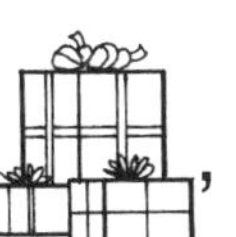, using good manners. Then the 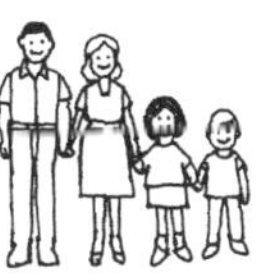 ate  cake and had a 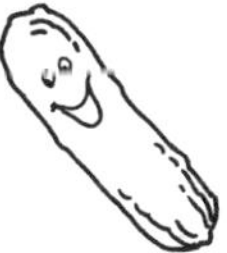 time. When Sonny looked outside, the  was gone. The  was shining. When he went out with his , he was surprised to find he also got a  for his .

Name ______________________________

KATE'S CAT

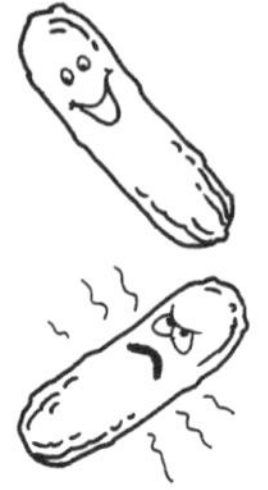 **SWEET PICKLE**

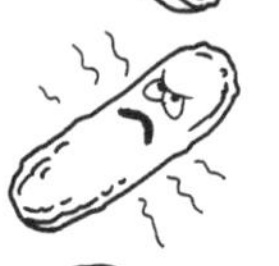 **SOUR PICKLE**

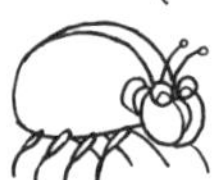 **BUG**

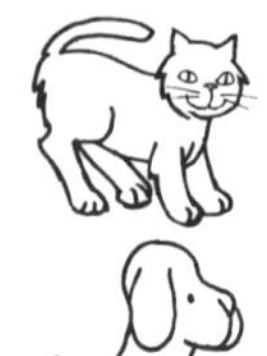 **CAT**

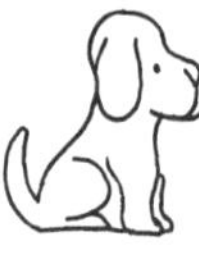 **DOG**

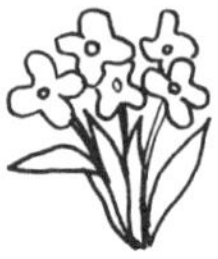

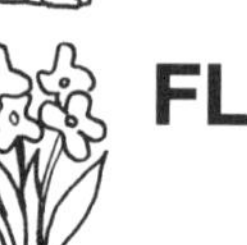 **FLOWERS**

 **NIGHT**

 **DAY**

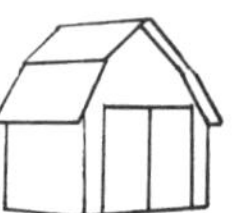 **SHED**

One 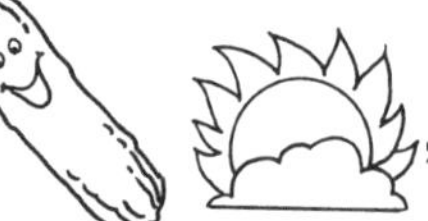, Kate played with her 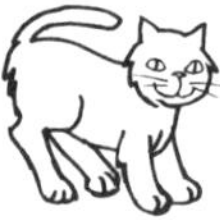 while her mom planted 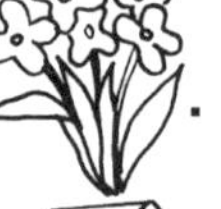. The followed when Mom went to get tools out of the little 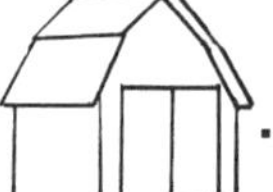. The chased a 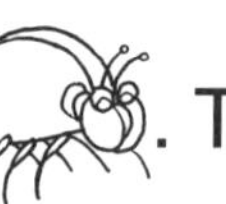. The 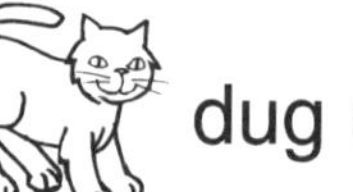 dug up the  Mom had just planted. Mom had a feeling, but it didn't last long. When the 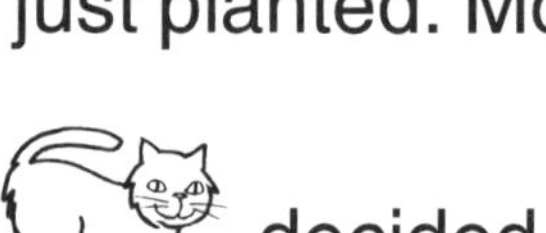 decided to chase the 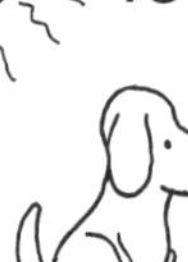, Mom and Kate laughed. After supper, they could not find the 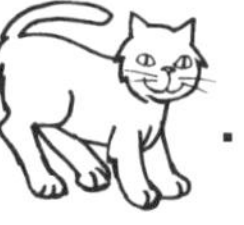. They looked until it got dark. It was a 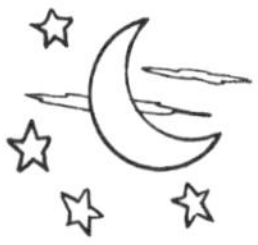 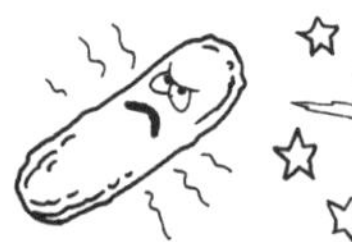 for Kate. The next , they still could not find the . It was almost 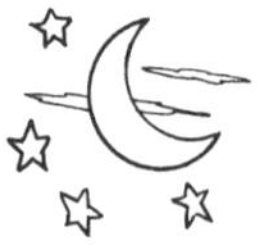 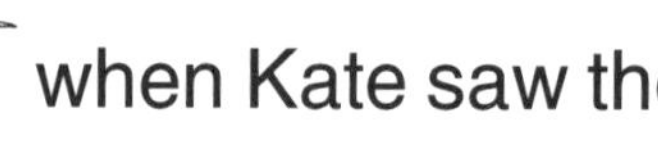 when Kate saw the 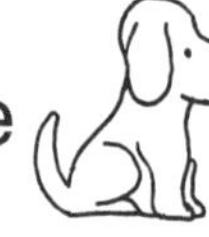 barking at the 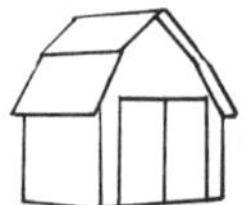. She opened the door to the 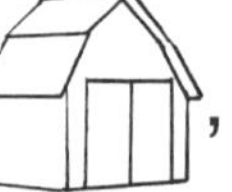, and out ran the 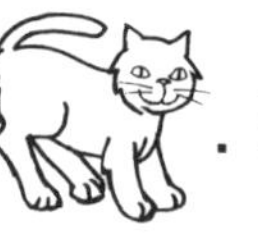. He was playing hide and seek and the 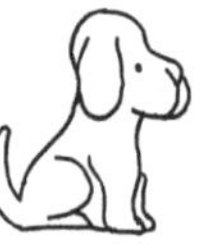 had found him. Now it was a 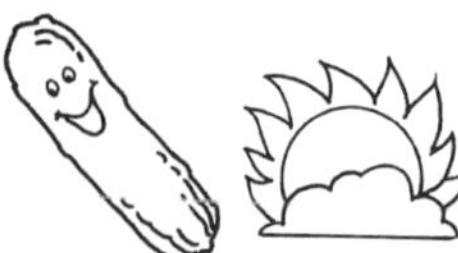 for Kate and the 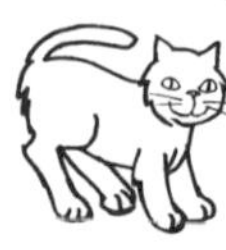 and the 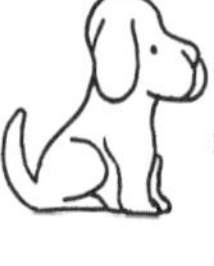, who got a bone.

Name ______________________________

SWEET PICKLES

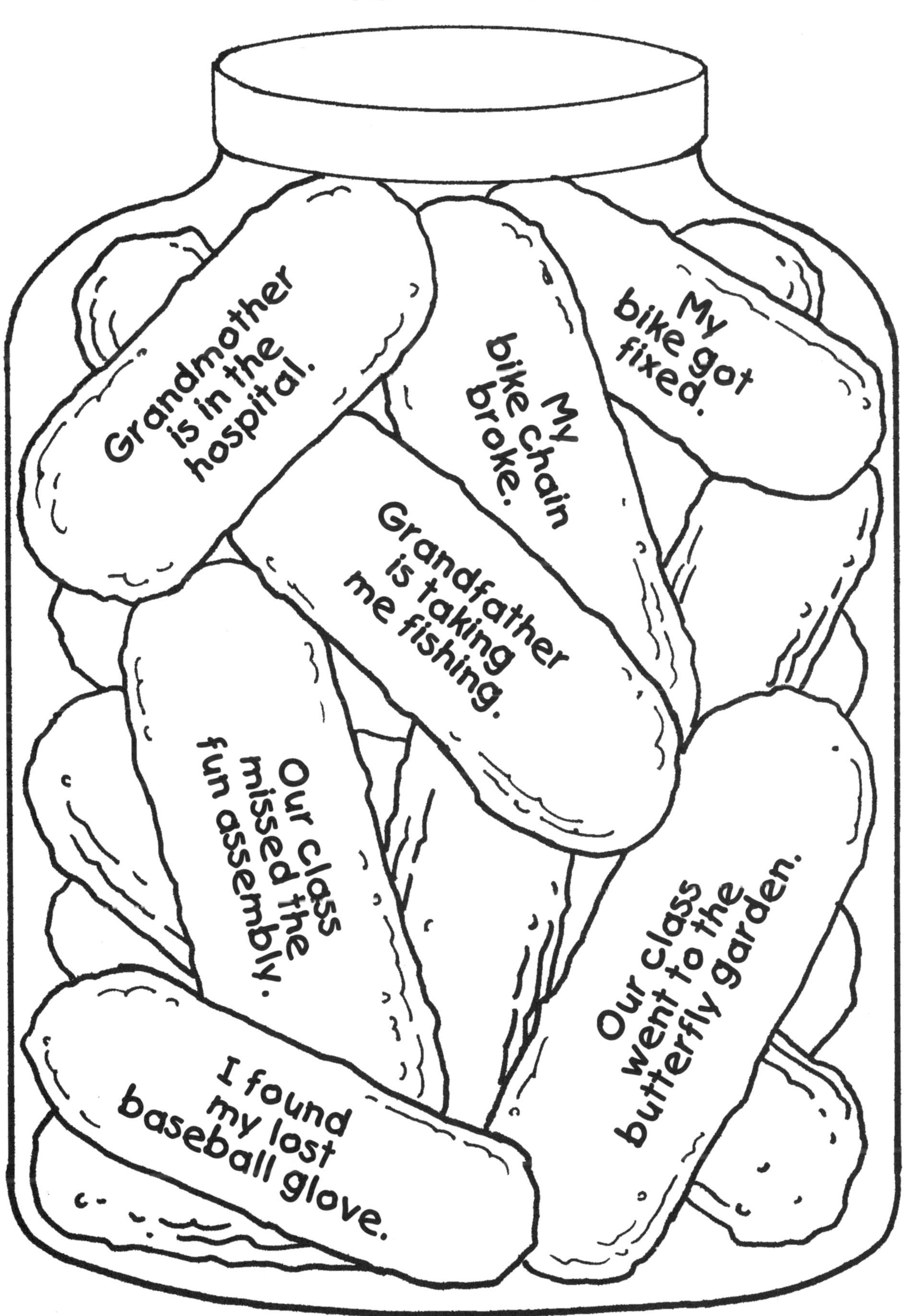

Name ____________________________

SOUR PICKLES

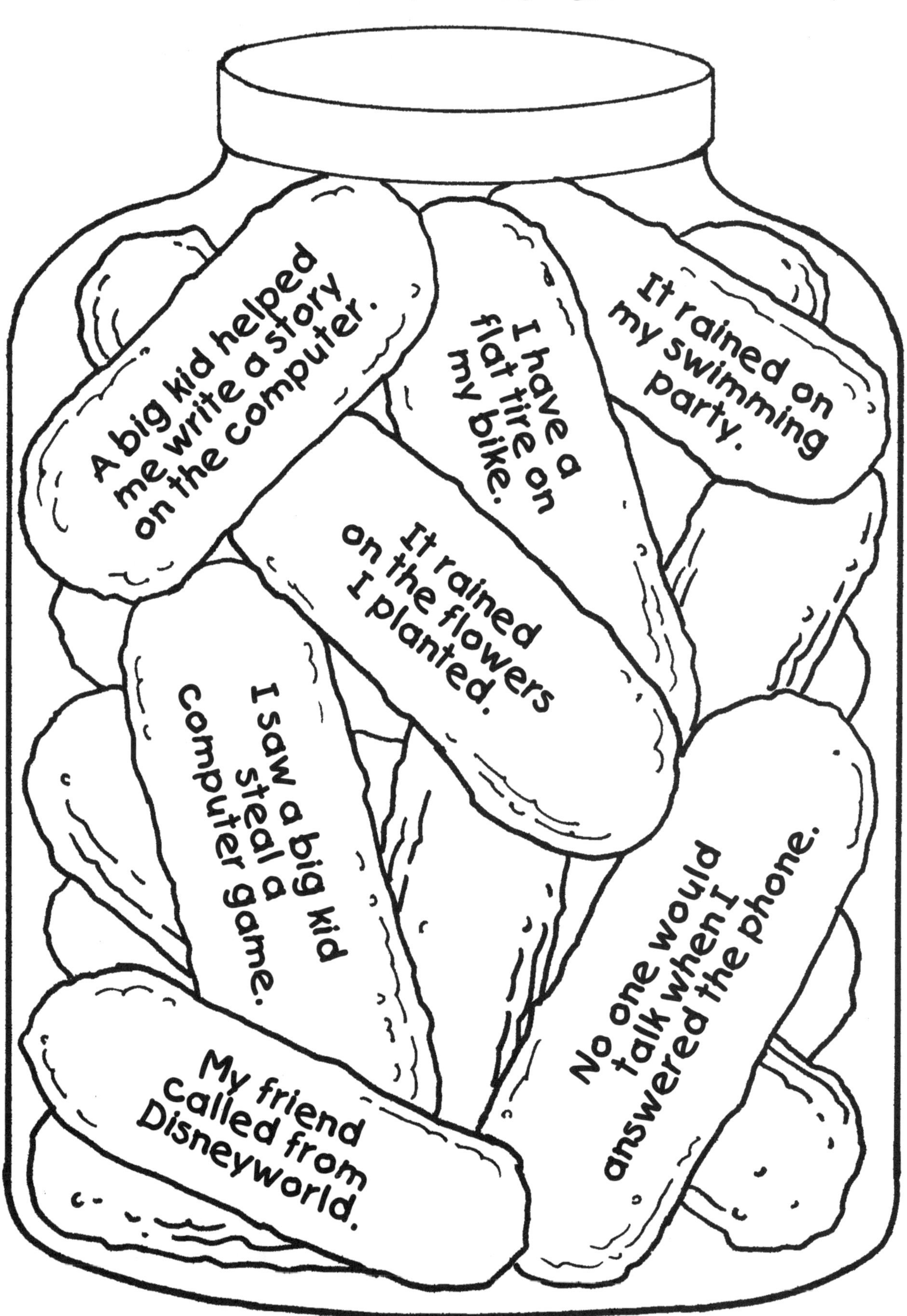

Name ______________________________

WHAT ARE BREAD AND BUTTER PICKLES?

Have you ever wondered how *bread and butter pickles* got their name? Do you think you would put them on bread with butter? Do you think they taste like either bread or butter? Do you think they are made with either bread or butter? It is a strange name for a pickle that isn't very sweet or very sour, just sort of in-between.

They got their name from Mrs. Fanning's popular pickles. She made her pickles not very sweet and not very sour, just sort of in-between and she traded them for bread and butter. People liked her pickles. Soon they were asking for Mrs. Fanning's bread and butter pickles.

Sometimes things in life are like Mrs. Fanning's pickles: Not very sweet and not very sour. Just sort of in-between.

Read the two sentences on each of the lines below. Underline the one that is neither good nor bad by itself, but just sort of in-between. Since people do not all think alike, you and your friend may not have the same answers.

1. It's raining. — It rained on my skates.
2. We're moving. — We're moving to a small apartment.
3. Mom has supper ready. — Mom burned the pizza.

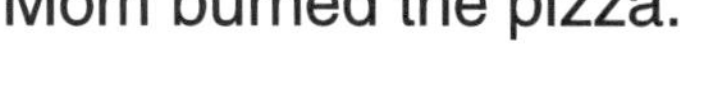

4. I missed school today. — I missed school today to get a tooth pulled.

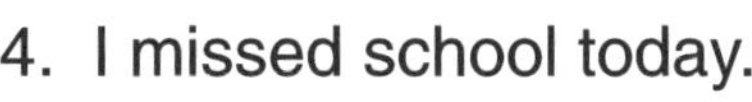
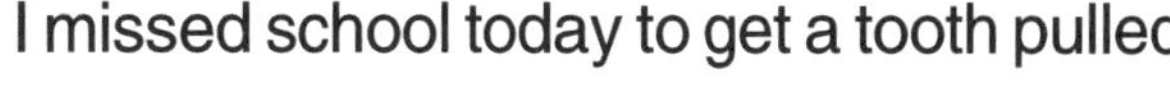

5. My new shoes hurt my feet. — I had to get new shoes.

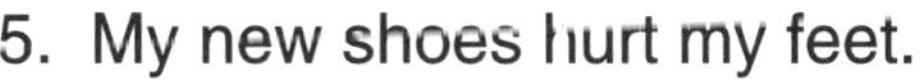

6. The pickle jar broke. — The pickle jar is sticky.

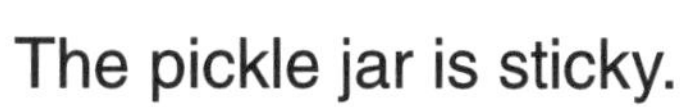
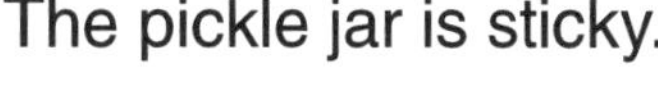

7. The shirt has a big rip. — The shirt has a big wrinkle.
8. The phone rang. — The phone rang and woke the baby.

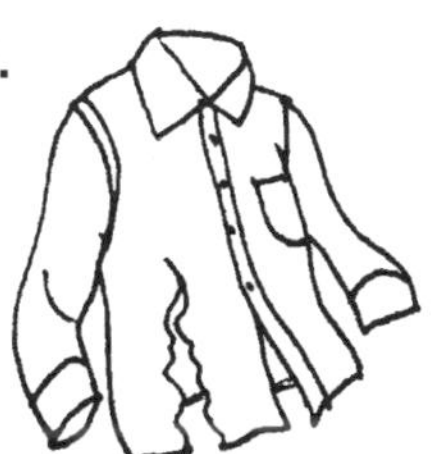
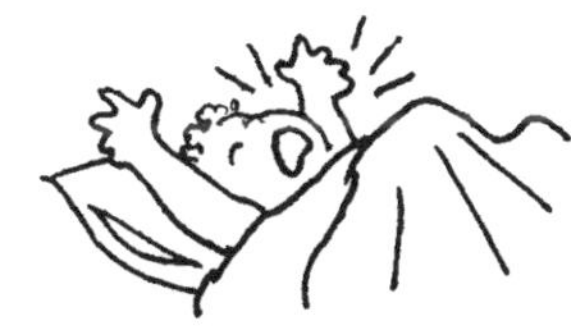

*Mrs. Fanning's Pickles are distributed by GFA Brands, Inc., P. O. Box 397, Cresskill, New Jersey 07626-0397

Name ______________________________

BREAD AND BUTTER CHOICES

Sometimes bread and butter pickle days become sour pickle days because of the way we think. Remember, bread and butter pickles are neither sweet nor sour, but just in-between. Look at each pickle below. Read the statement printed next to each pickle and the two thoughts below it. Then draw a star beside the thought that would make you feel better and have a better day.

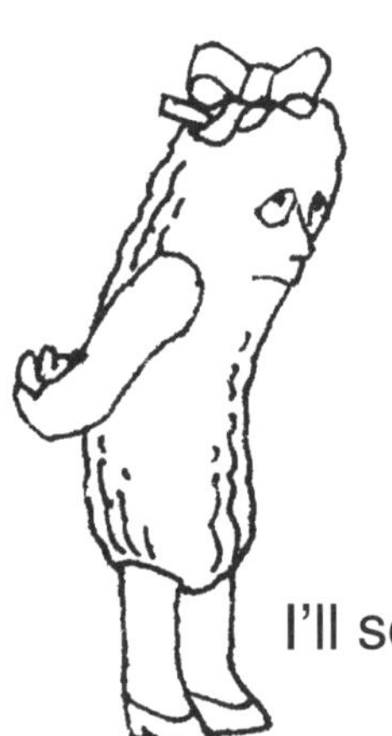

I didn't get to sit next to my friend on the bus.

I'll see my friend at recess.

What a lousy day!

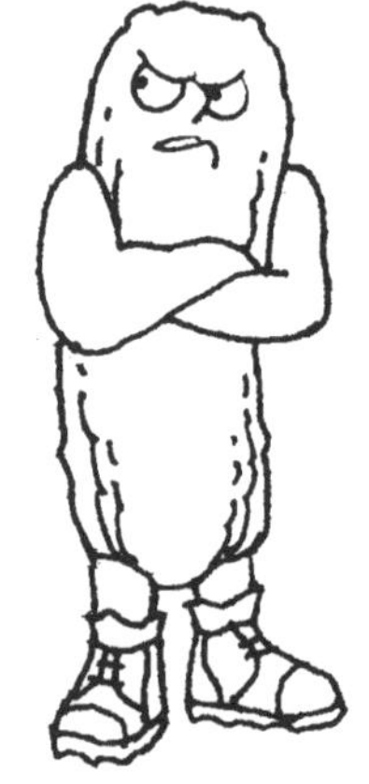

We got tacos, but I wanted pizza.

Oh, well! Next week, I get to choose.

I never get what I want.

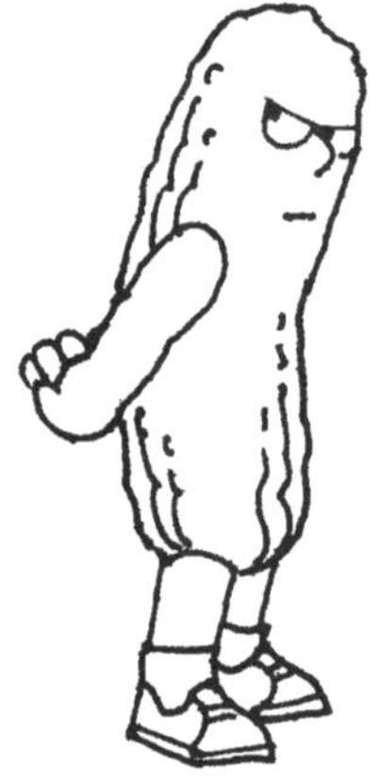

I missed three words on my spelling test.

I never do anything right.

I got seven answers right!

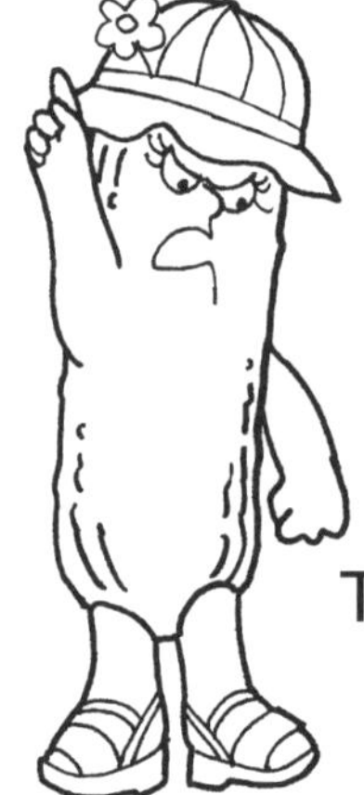

We lost the ball game.

They were a good team, and we did okay.

We're lousy.

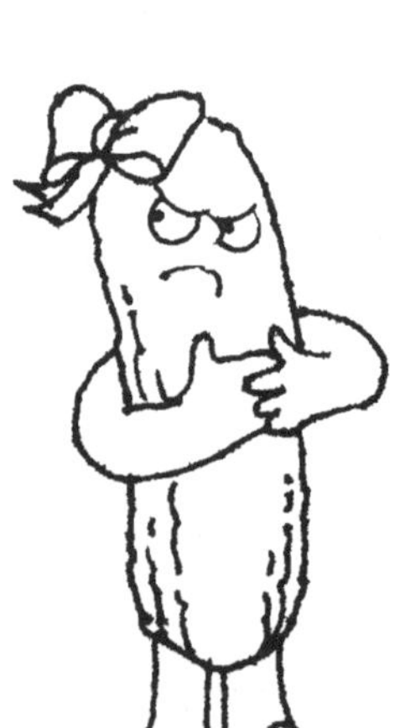

I didn't get picked for a part in the school play.

Nobody likes me.

I had a part in the school play last year.

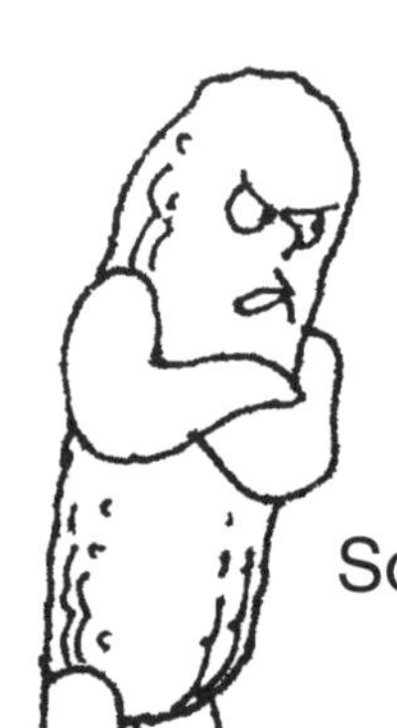

Mom won't give me the money for a new shirt.

Sometimes Mom doesn't have extra money.

Mom never lets me buy anything.

Name ______________________________

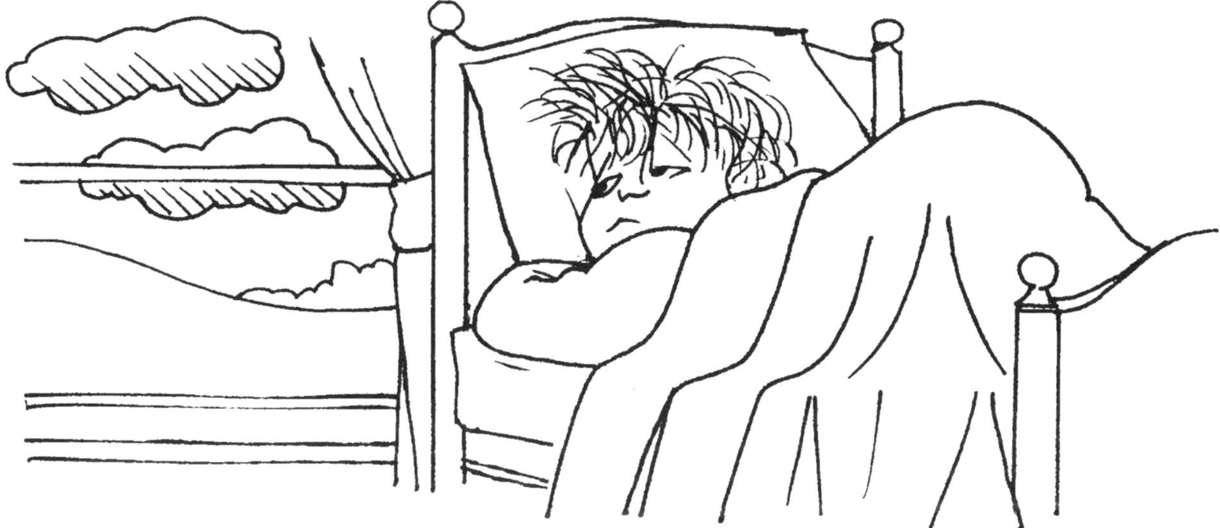

When I wake up in the morning,
And the sun's not shining bright.
I tell myself that it's okay,
The day will be all right.

This day may not be perfect,
Things may not go my way.
But if I look for good things,
This day will be okay!

Name ______________________________

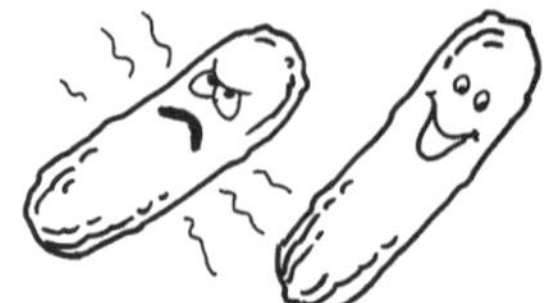

SECRET CODE #1

A B C D E F G

H I J K L M N

O P Q R S T U

V W X Y Z CLAWED HAND .

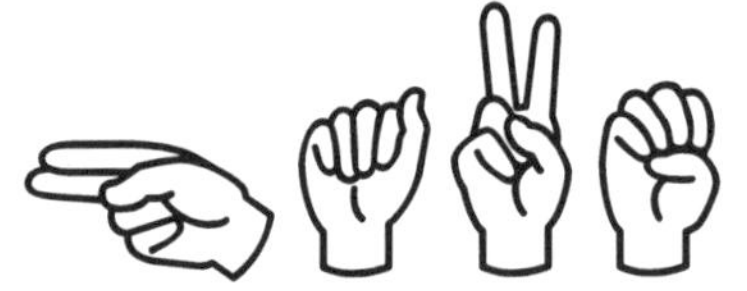 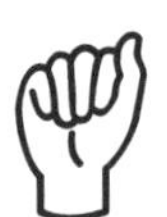 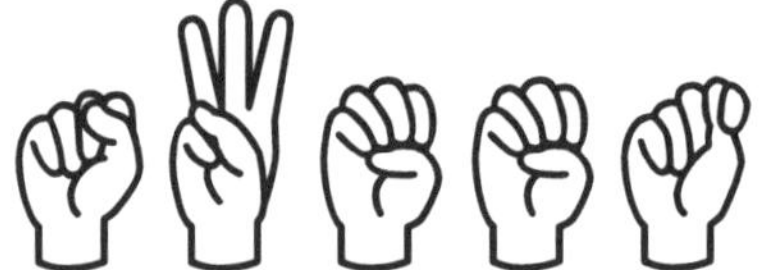

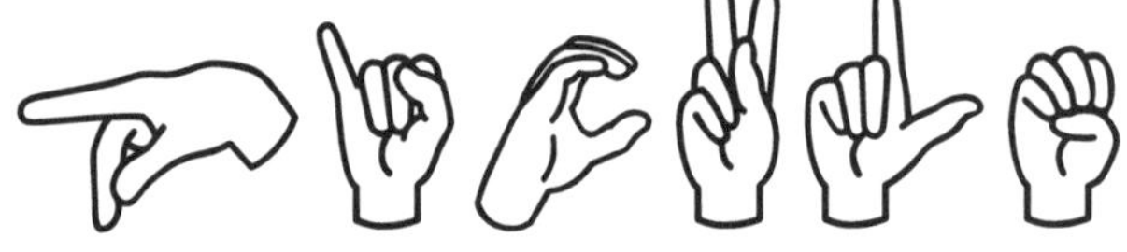 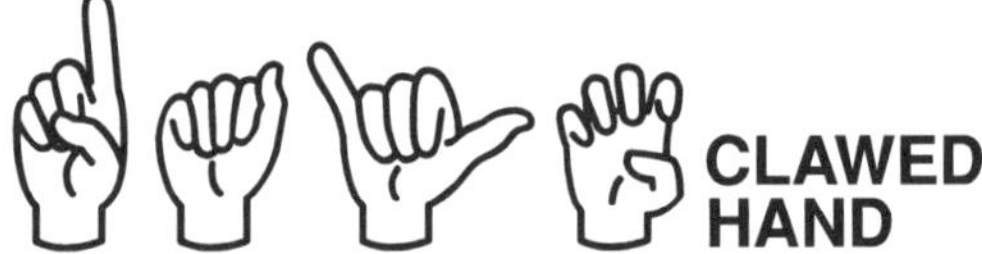

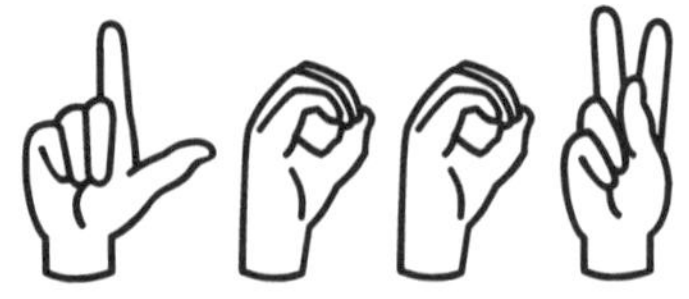 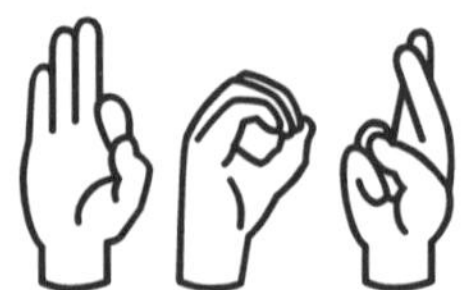 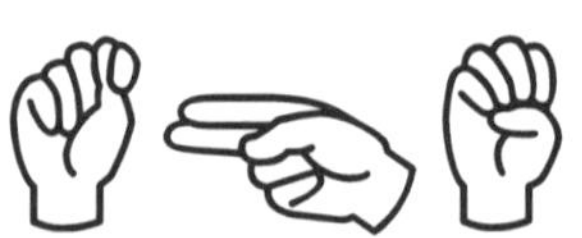

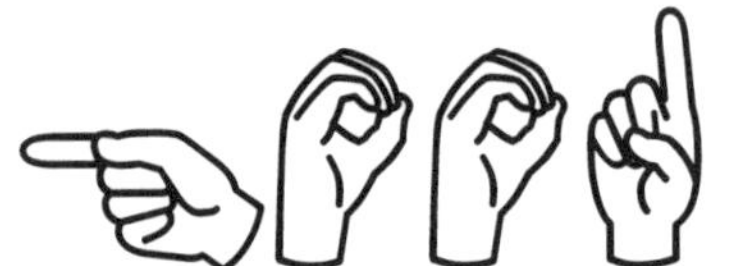 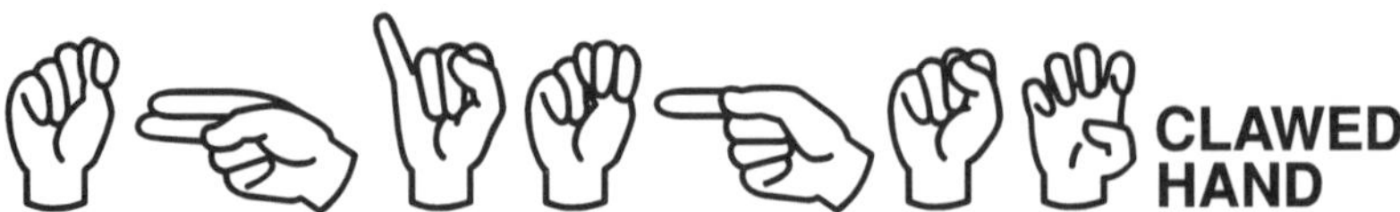

Name ______________________________

SECRET CODE #2

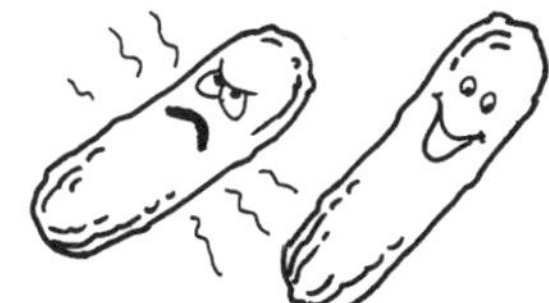

A B C D E F G

H I J K L M N

O P Q R S T U

V W X Y Z CLAWED HAND .

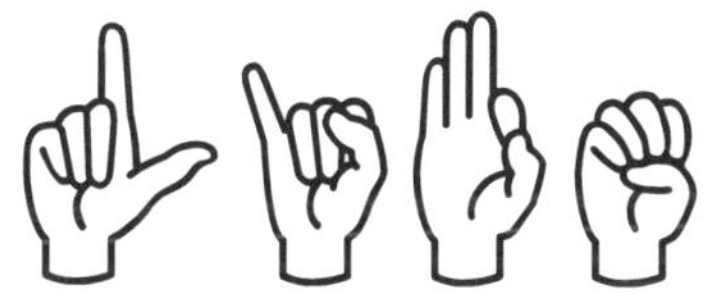 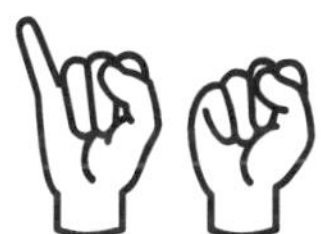 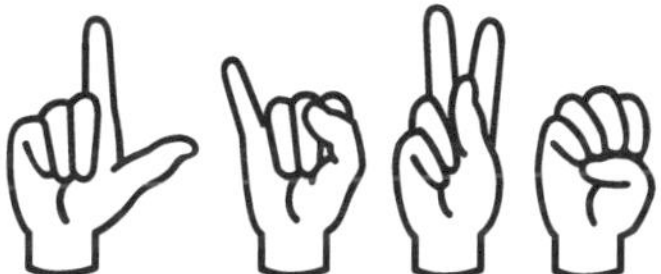

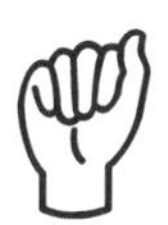 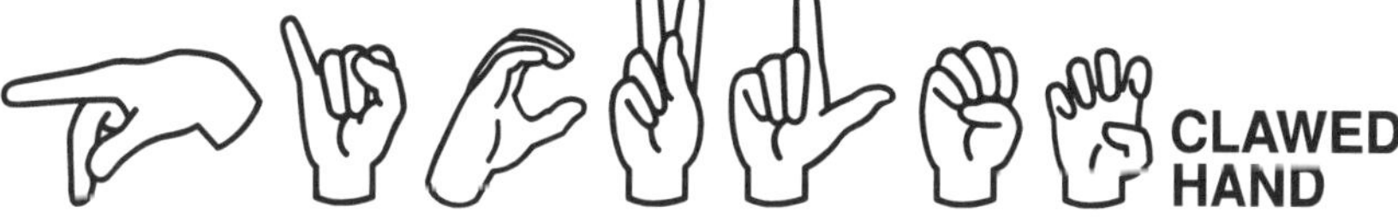

CLAWED HAND

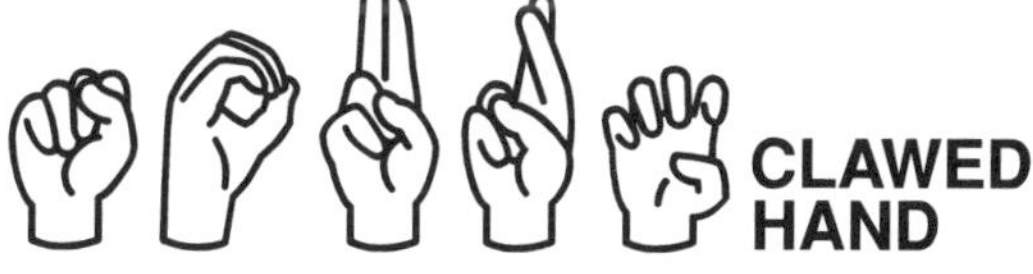

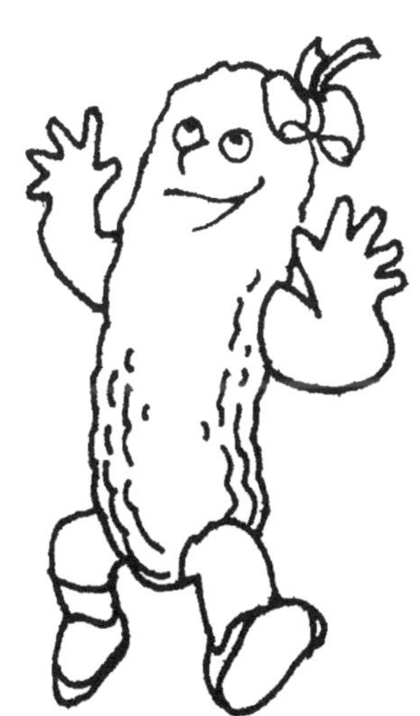

Name ______________________________

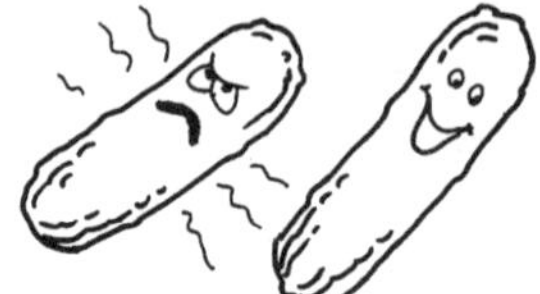

SECRET CODE #3

A B C D E F G

H I J K L M N

O P Q R S T U

V W X Y Z CLAWED HAND .

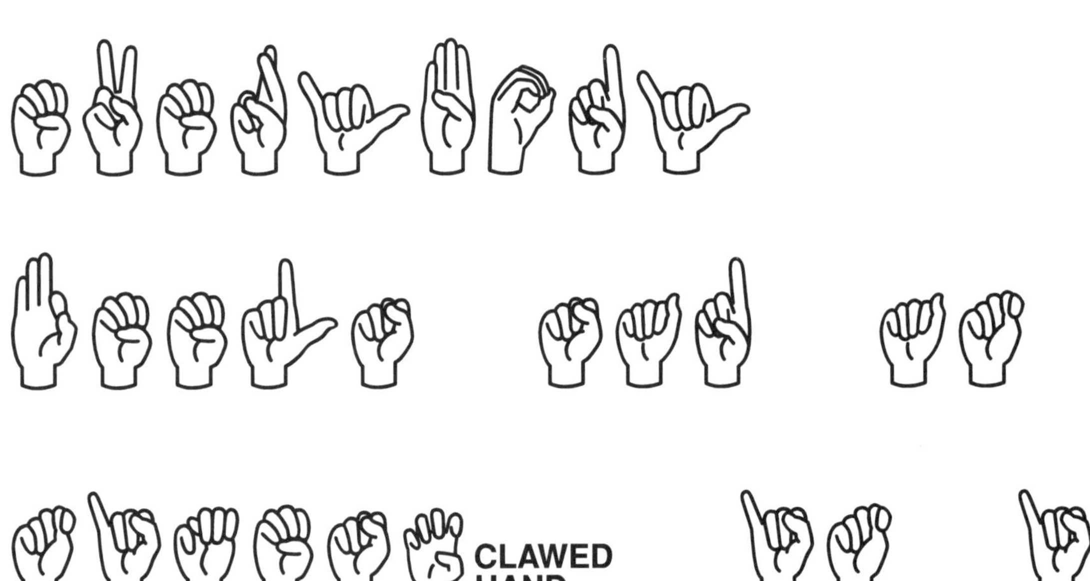

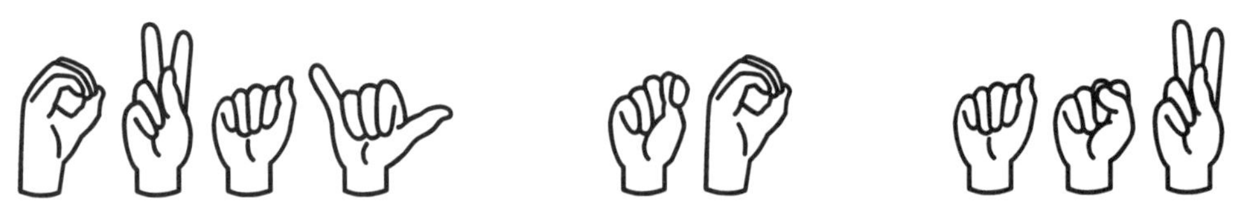

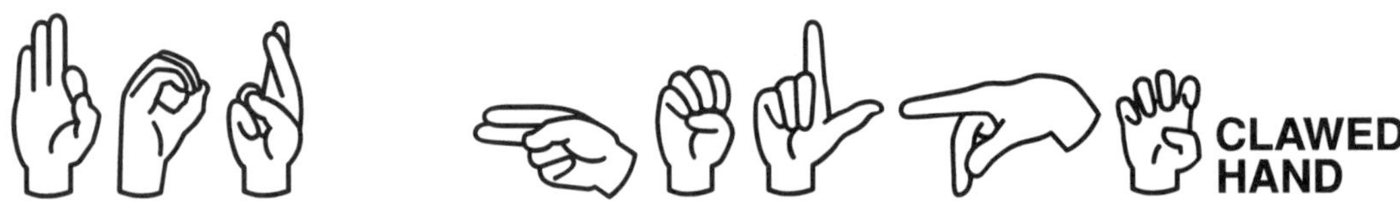

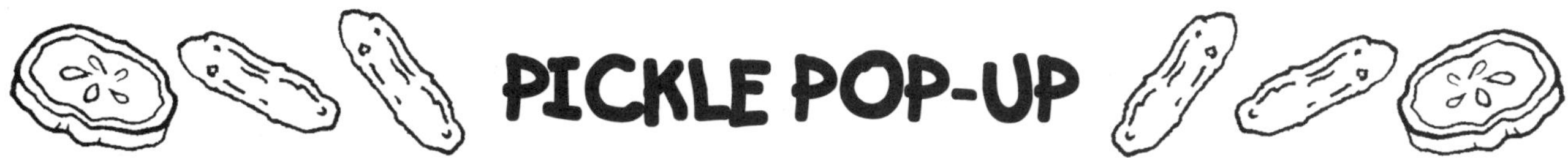

This is a *listening*, as well as a *doing*, activity that lends itself to the discussion of *feelings*. The students are directed to stand when they hear the words *sweet pickle* and sit when they hear the words *sour pickle*. If the students stand, they are to remain standing until they hear the words *sour pickle*. If seated, they should remain seated until they hear the words *sweet pickle*. There are some sample stories below, but you can make up you own to fit your school. The last story was made up during a classroom lesson, with the help of first-grade students.

Story #1 (Begin with the students standing.)
A dog chased a cat. Sour pickle for the cat. The cat ran up a tree. Sweet pickle for the cat. The dog went away. Sweet pickle for the cat. The cat didn't know how to get down from the tree. Sour pickle for the cat. Then a car parked under the tree. Sweet pickle for the cat. The cat jumped down onto the car. Sweet pickle for the cat. Oh, no! Here comes the dog again. Sour pickle for the cat.

Story #2 (Begin with the students sitting. This story is also useful for discussing adaptability.)
John wanted ice cream. Mom said, "OK." Sweet pickle. John went to the freezer. His brother had eaten all the ice cream! Sour pickle. Mom took John to the store to buy ice cream. Sweet pickle. He chose vanilla ice cream. Sweet pickle. On the way home, they had to wait behind a car accident. Sour pickle. Almost all the ice cream melted. Sour pickle. When John finally got home, he poured his mushy ice cream into a glass, added chocolate syrup, and had a milkshake. Sweet pickle for John.

Story #3 (Begin with the participants sitting. This story can be used to add a little movement and humor at a teacher in-service.)
It was a sweet pickle morning when the red bird sang outside the window. The clock struck nine. School had started an hour ago. Sour pickle. It was still a sour pickle day when she heard the message on the answering machine ask, "Where are you?" She made a phone call, and it was a sweet pickle day again. She gathered up her homework. Oops! Muddy dog prints were on the homework. Sour pickle. The weather was beautiful, and she could walk to school. Sweet pickle. She locked the door behind her without taking the keys. Sour pickle. Finally, she was at school two hours late, locked out of the house, with muddy homework. She was embarrassed as she walked into the room. She didn't even have a note from her mother. Sour pickle. The teacher did not fuss at her because she *was* the teacher. Sweet pickle.

Story #4 (Begin with the students sitting.)
It was recess time. Sweet pickle. Casey fell down. Sour pickle. Bailey tried to help her up and she fell down, too. Sour pickle. The teacher took them to the nurse. Sweet pickle. They got back outside just as recess ended. Sweet pickle for Casey. Sour pickle for Bailey. Casey likes recess to be over. Bailey does not like recess to be over. Do we all feel the same way about recess?

Name ______________________________

SWEET AND SOUR FEELINGS

My birthday is ______________________________ .

On my last birthday, I turned ______________________________ .

I live with ______________________________ .

Family members who do not live with me are ______________

______________________________ .

I am happy when ______________________________ .

I get angry when ______________________________ .

I am good at ______________________________ .

I am also good at ______________________________ .

I am afraid of ______________________________ .

I feel good when ______________________________ .

I am sorry when ______________________________ .

I worry about ______________________________ .

I get excited when ______________________________ .

I am sad when ______________________________ .

I feel loved when ______________________________ .

I am scared when ______________________________ .

I am proud of ______________________________ .

I am thankful for ______________________________ .

NOTES: ______________________________

____

____

____

____

Name ______________________________

HOW DO YOU FEEL ABOUT SCHOOL?

Many students have both sweet and sour feelings about school. Draw a mouth on each pickle that shows how you feel about what is written below it.

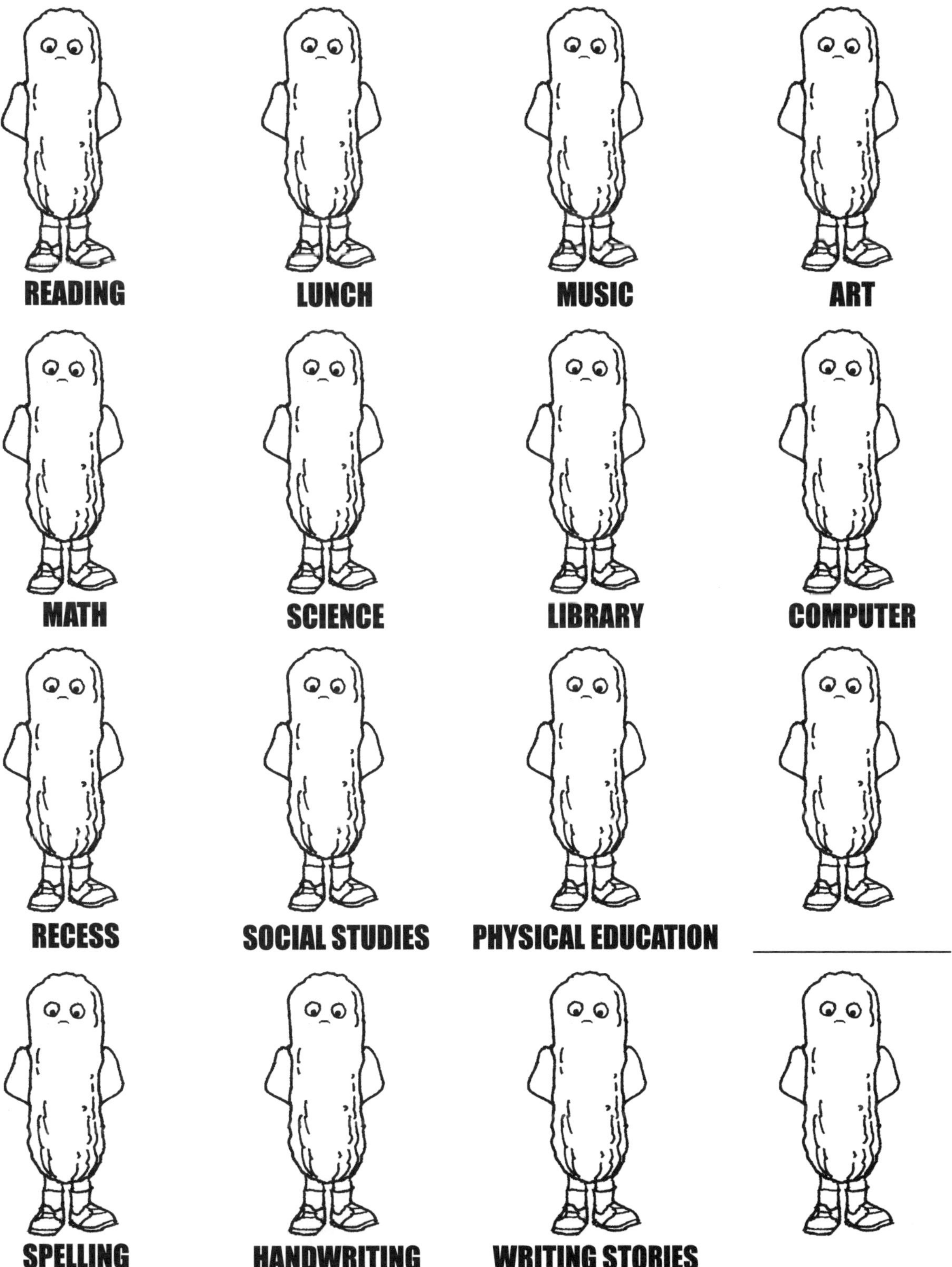

Name ____________________________

JUST THINKING

1. It would be a sweet pickle day if I had a hundred dollars.

   I would ____ .

2. I think a sweet pickle job would be ________________ .

3. Three people who make my life sweet are ________________ ,

   ____________________, and ____________________ .

4. Someone who sometimes makes my life sour is ___________ .

5. Something that can make a sweet pickle day at school is ___

   ____ .

6. Something that can make a sour pickle day at school is ____

   ____ .

7. If I could change one thing about school, it would be _______

   ____ .

8. Something that can make a sour pickle day at home is _____

   ____ .

9. Something that can make a sweet pickle day at home is ____

   ____ .

10. If I could change something at home, it would be __________

    ____ .

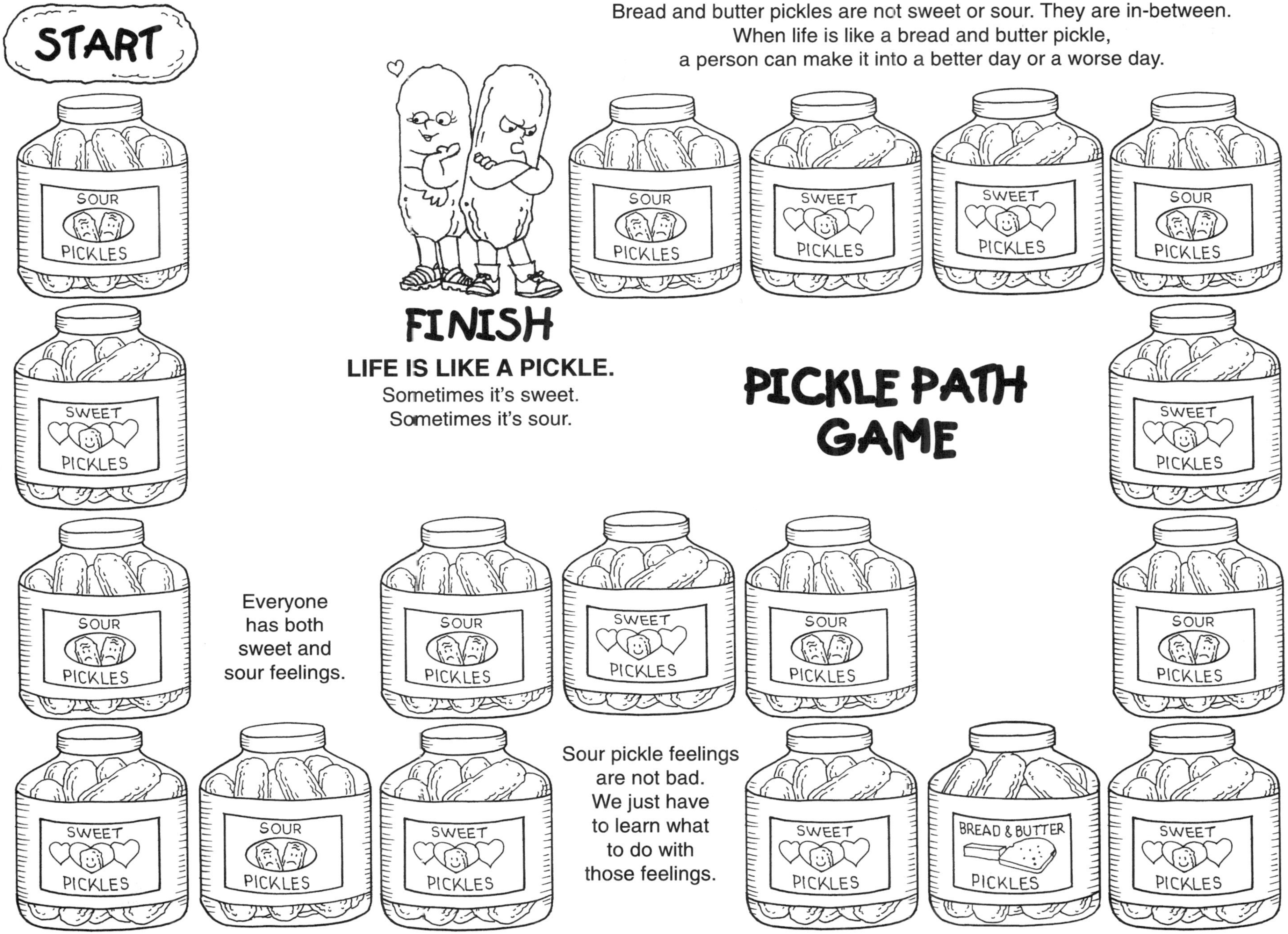
START
Bread and butter pickles are not sweet or sour. They are in-between.
When life is like a bread and butter pickle,
a person can make it into a better day or a worse day.
FINISH
LIFE IS LIKE A PICKLE.
Sometimes it's sweet.
Sometimes it's sour.
PICKLE PATH GAME
Everyone has both sweet and sour feelings.
Sour pickle feelings are not bad. We just have to learn what to do with those feelings.
SOUR PICKLES
SWEET PICKLES
BREAD & BUTTER PICKLES

PICKLE PATH GAME CARDS

Instructions: Cut out the cards below, shuffle them, and put them in a stack with the words face down. Use pieces of wrapped candy for markers. Each player chooses one piece of candy and places it on "Start." Decide who will play first, then continue in a counterclockwise manner. The first player draws a card, follows its directions, then places the card on the bottom of the stack. As each player reaches "Finish," he/she may eat the candy.

You saved money for a new game. Move to the next *Sweet Pickle Space*. *Pickle Packet II © 2004 Mar∗co Products, Inc.*	**You lost your favorite toy. Move to the next *Sour Pickle Space*.** *Pickle Packet II © 2004 Mar∗co Products, Inc.*
You helped make dinner. Move to the next *Sweet Pickle Space*. *Pickle Packet II © 2004 Mar∗co Products, Inc.*	**You lost your library book. Move to the next *Sour Pickle Space*.** *Pickle Packet II © 2004 Mar∗co Products, Inc.*
You talked back to your mother. Move to the next *Sour Pickle Space*. *Pickle Packet II © 2004 Mar∗co Products, Inc.*	**You left your jacket out in the rain. Move to the next *Sour Pickle Space*.** *Pickle Packet II © 2004 Mar∗co Products, Inc.*
You copied from your friend's paper. Move to the next *Sour Pickle Space*. *Pickle Packet II © 2004 Mar∗co Products, Inc.*	**You rescued a kitten from a tree. Move to the next *Sweet Pickle Space*.** *Pickle Packet II © 2004 Mar∗co Products, Inc.*
You lost your homework, so you called a friend and asked for the assignment. Move to the *Bread and Butter Pickle Space.* *Pickle Packet II © 2004 Mar∗co Products, Inc.*	**You did your homework before watching TV. Move to the next *Sweet Pickle Space*.** *Pickle Packet II © 2004 Mar∗co Products, Inc.*
You surprised your dad by raking the leaves. Move to the next *Sweet Pickle Space*. *Pickle Packet II © 2004 Mar∗co Products, Inc.*	**You returned your library book on time. Move to the next *Sweet Pickle Space*.** *Pickle Packet II © 2004 Mar∗co Products, Inc.*

It rained all day, but you found something to do anyway. Move to the *Bread and Butter Pickle Space.*

You made a new friend. Move to the next *Sweet Pickle Space.*

You lost your lunch money. Move to the next *Sour Pickle Space.*

You got ice cream with a friend. Move to the next *Sweet Pickle Space.*

Your grandfather is very sick. Move to the next *Sour Pickle Space.*

You got all your math problems right. Move to the next *Sweet Pickle Space.*

You got a birthday card in the mail. Move to the next *Sweet Pickle Space.*

Someone threw your math paper in the trash. Move to the next *Sour Pickle Space.*

Your cat ran away. Move to the next *Sour Pickle Space.*

You made cookies with a grown-up. Move to the next *Sweet Pickle Space.*

Your best shirt was dirty when you wanted to wear it, but you didn't get mad. Move to the *Bread and Butter Pickle Space.*

A man at the grocery store scared you. Move to the next *Sour Pickle Space.*

You get to go to a birthday party. Move to the next *Sweet Pickle Space.*

You missed recess because you didn't finish your work. Move to the next *Sour Pickle Space.*

PICKLE MEMORY GAME

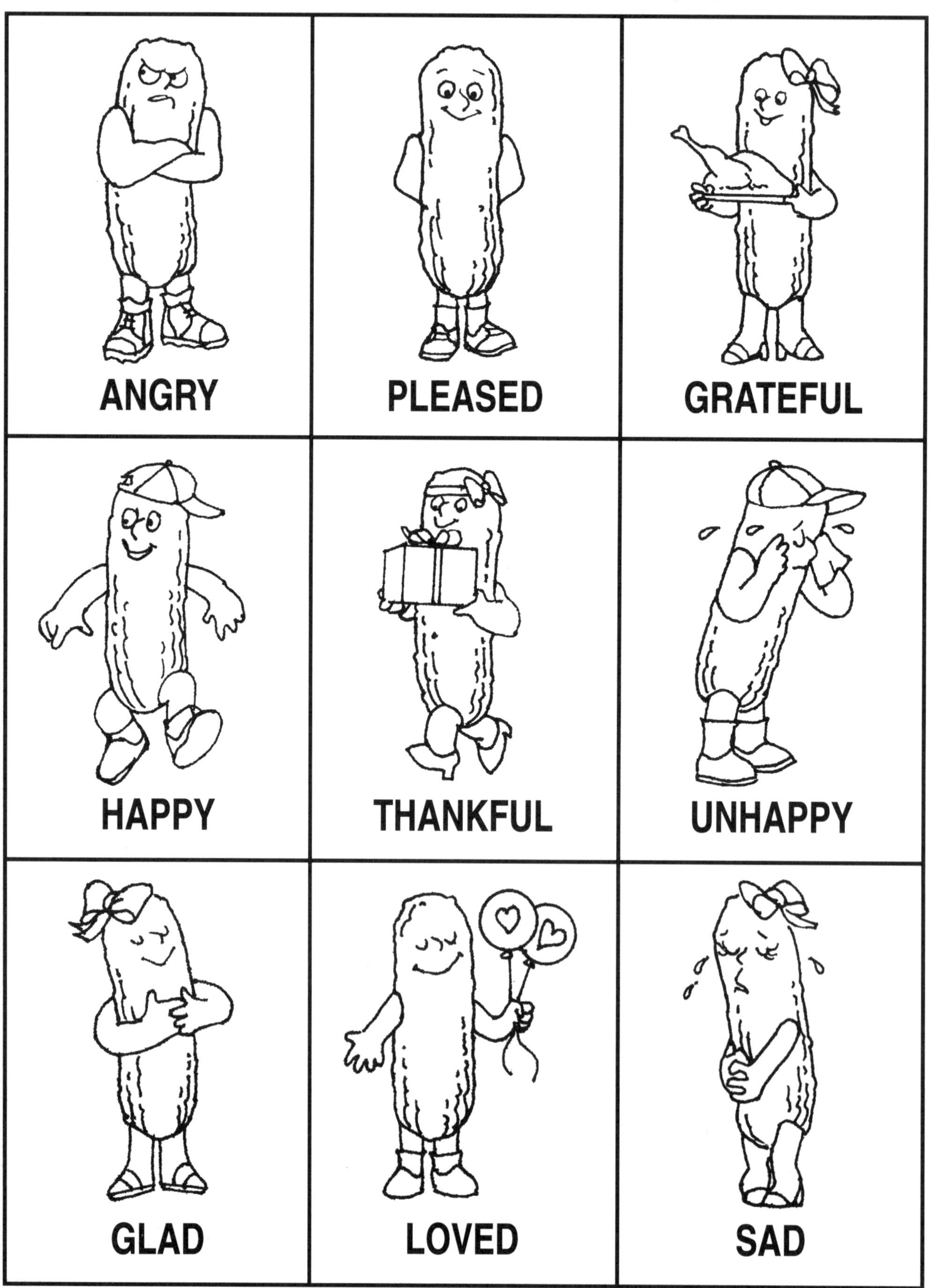

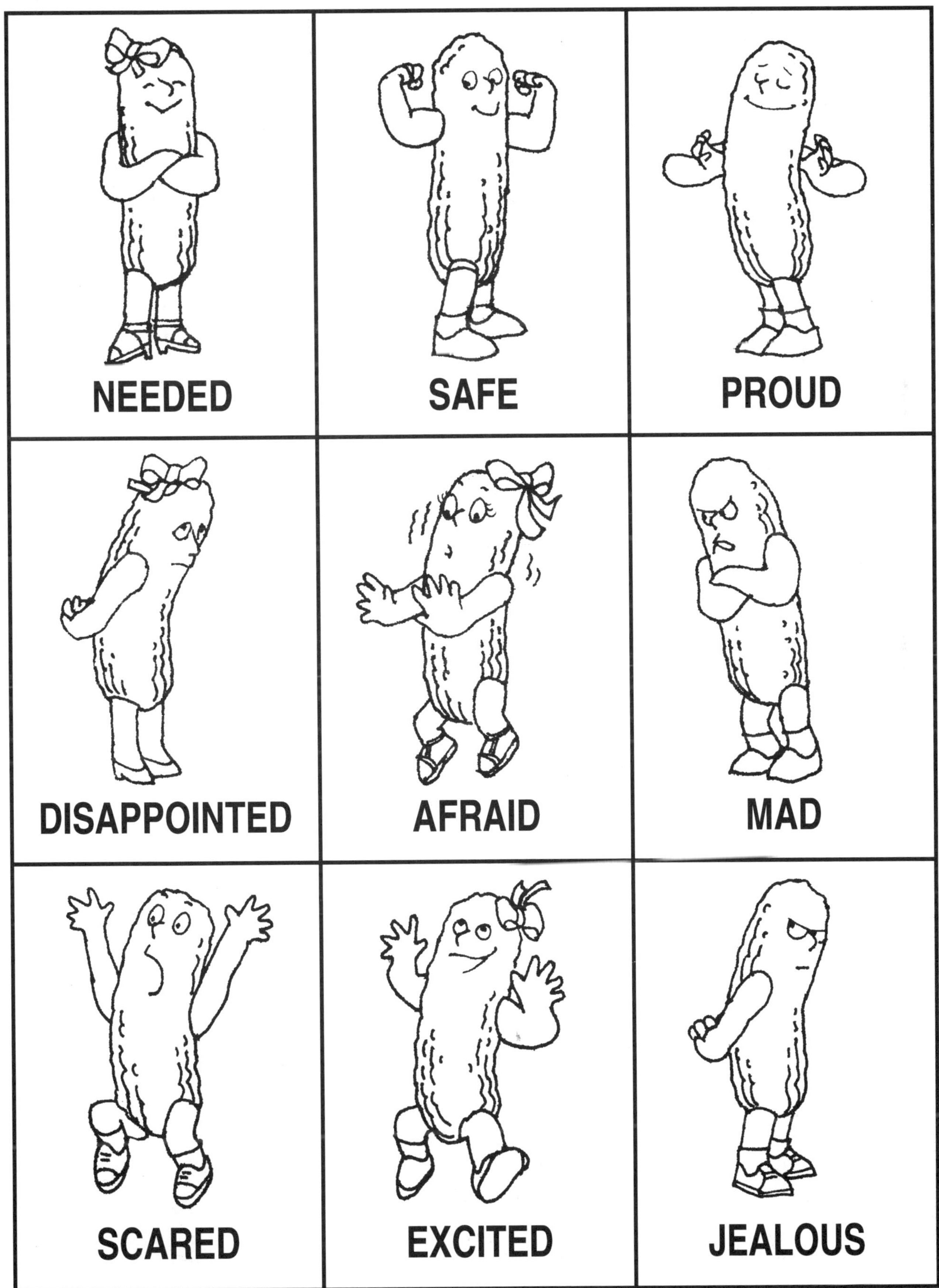
NEEDED
SAFE
PROUD
DISAPPOINTED
AFRAID
MAD
SCARED
EXCITED
JEALOUS

Name ______________________________

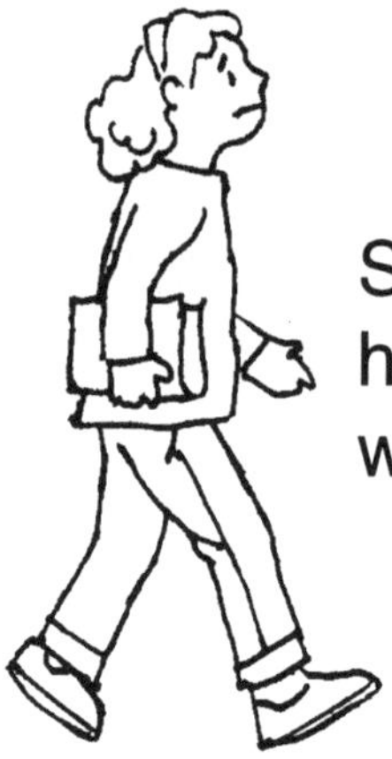

SHERRY'S WALK

Sherry was having a sour pickle day when she lost her library book. Then she found it. Help her find her way from the playground to the library.

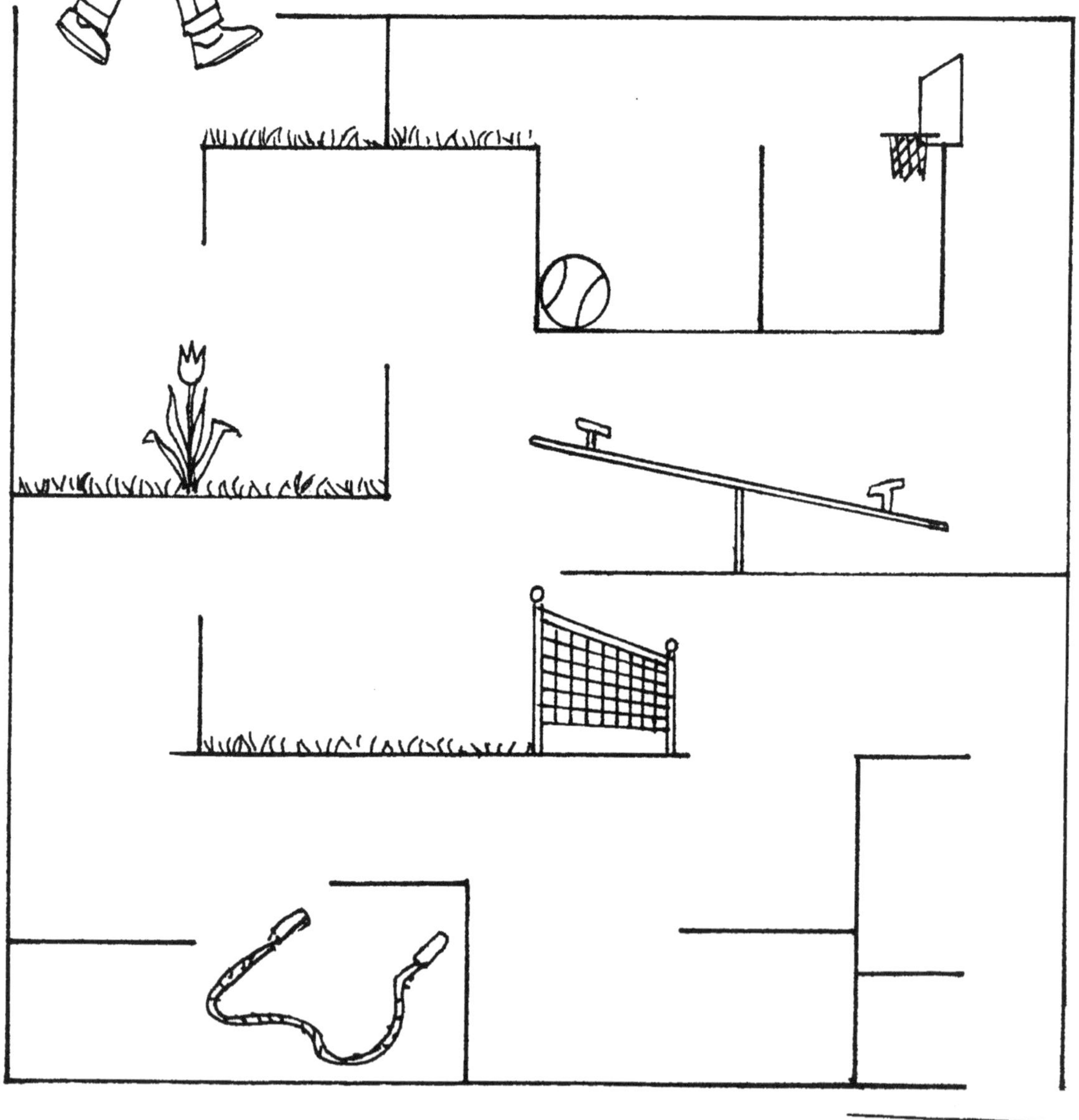

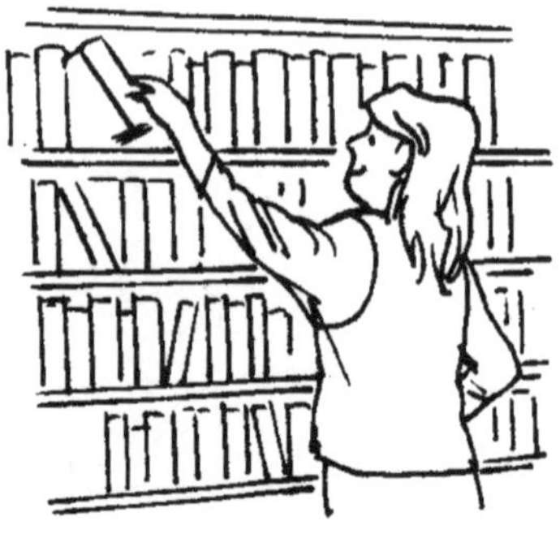

Where do you think Sherry lost her library book? ______________________

Have you ever lost anything? ______________________

Did you need help finding it? ______________________

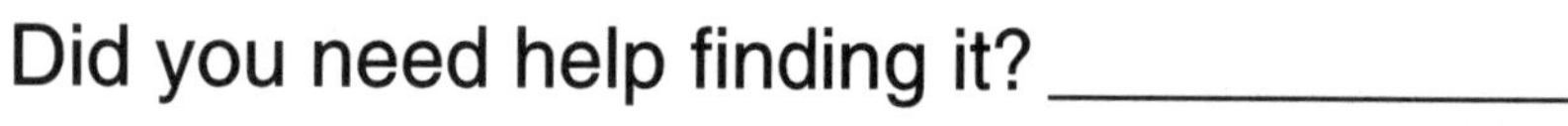

Name ______________________________

"IN A PICKLE" PICTURES

Circle the pictures that show when a child might be "in a pickle."

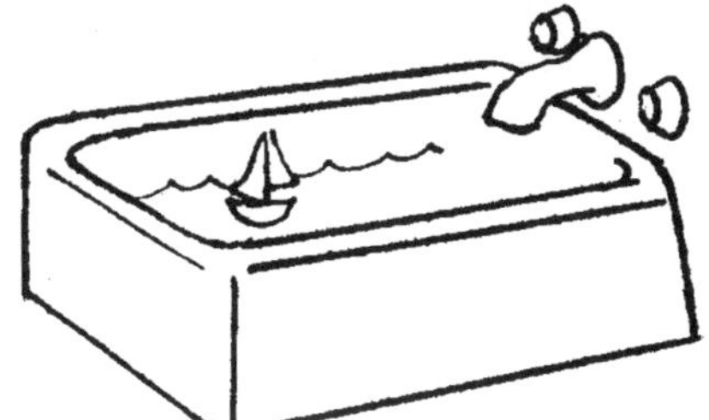

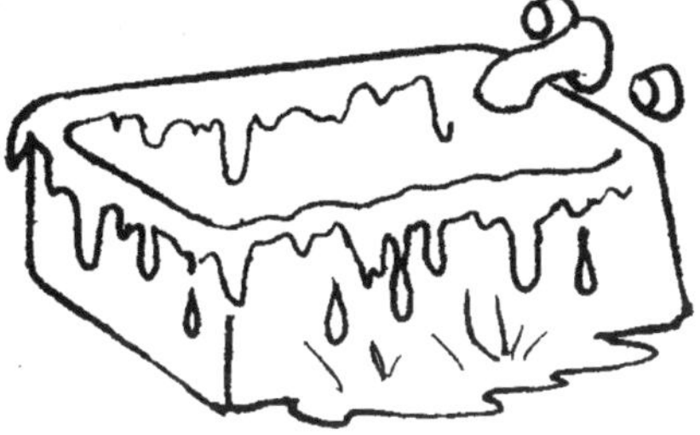

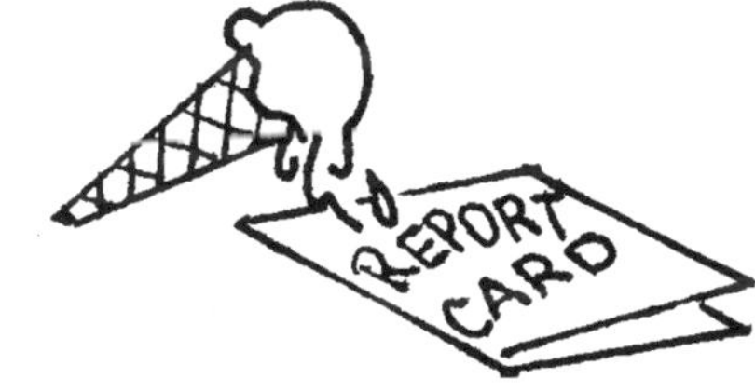

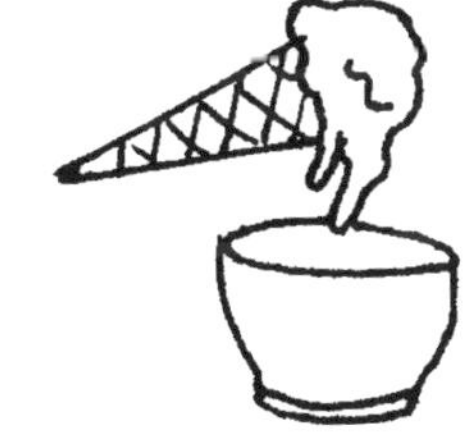

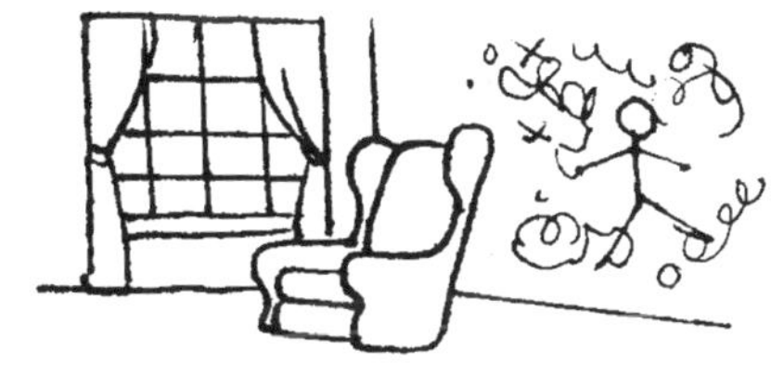

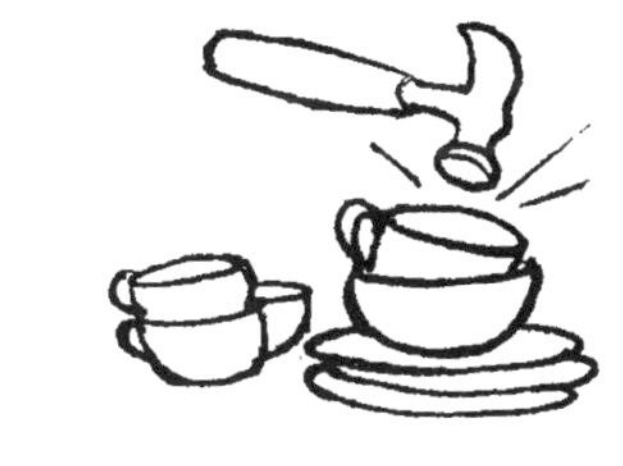

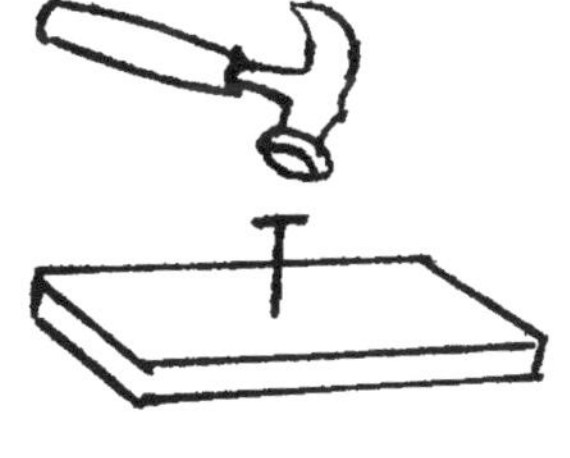

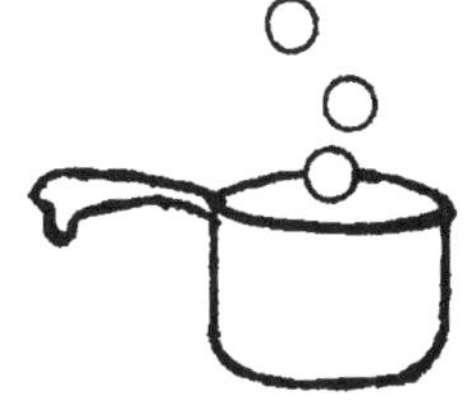

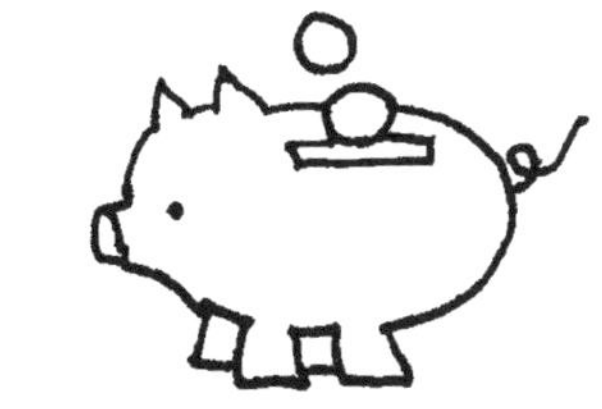

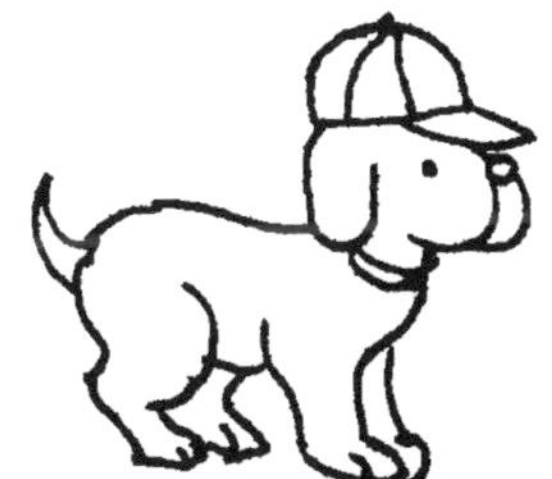

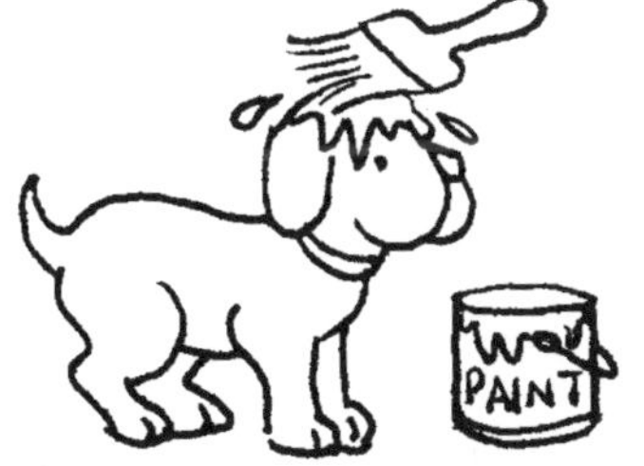

Name ______________________________

"IN A PICKLE" SITUATIONS

When you are "in a pickle," you are asking yourself: "How am I going to get myself out of this problem?" Draw a circle around the sentences in each set that might put you "in a pickle." You might not have the same answers as your friends.

cutting the cake Mom made for school
cutting your candy bar in half to share
cutting your sister's hair

---

getting the only empty swing between two girls
getting on the wrong bus after school
getting in the house before a thunderstorm

---

telling your mom you will vacuum, then doing it
telling two friends you will do two different things at the same time
telling your friend you have half the money for pizza, even though you don't

---

locking your little brother out of the house
locking your keys in the house
locking your yo-yo in the house

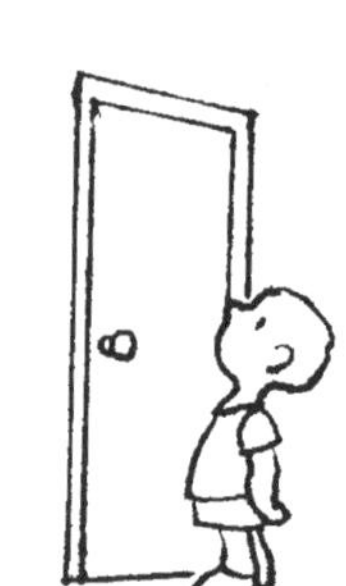

---

taking money from Mom's purse
taking a banana off the kitchen counter
taking a banana from your sister's lunch box

---

leaving your homework at home
leaving your homework on the bus
leaving your homework on the teacher's desk

Name ______________________________

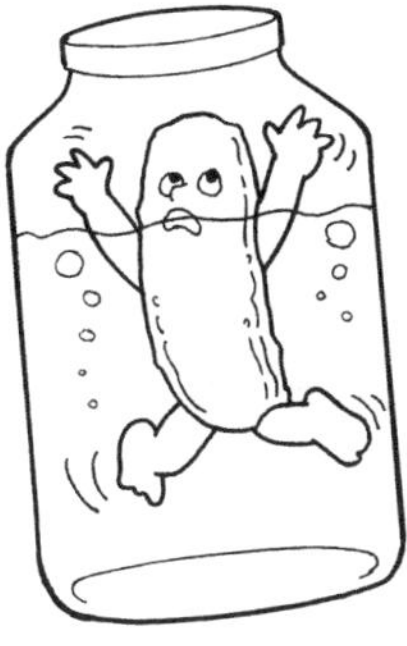

"IN A PICKLE" SENTENCE PUZZLES

We often use words in ways that don't make any sense. Figure out what each of the sentences below *should* say by reading the words and looking at the pictures.

1. She's on 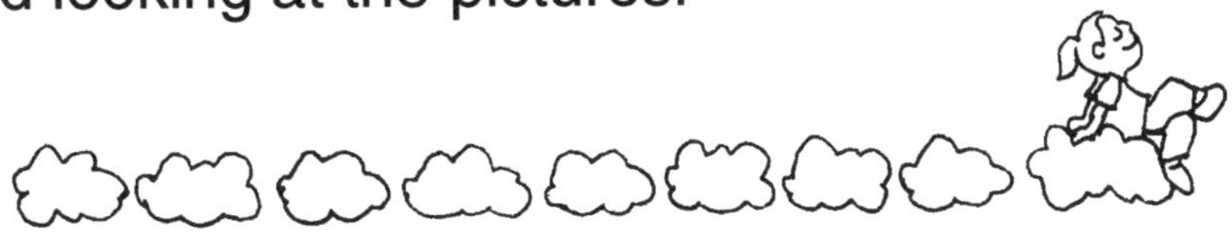 .
2. The 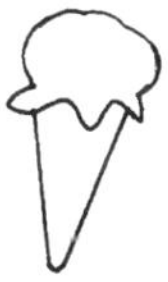 is on the 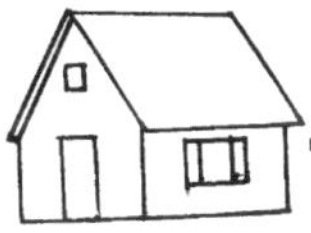 .
3. Don't spill the 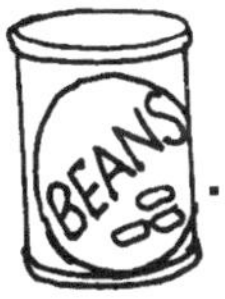 .
4. It's as easy as 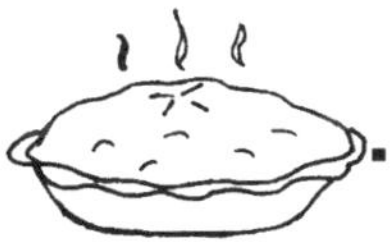 .
5. Don't let the 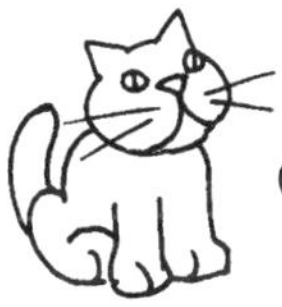 out of the 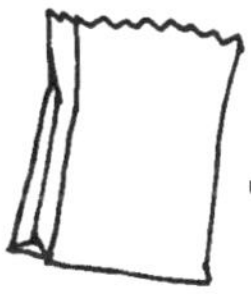 .
6. Don't 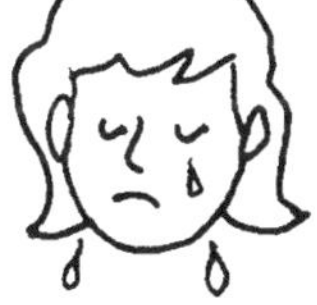 over 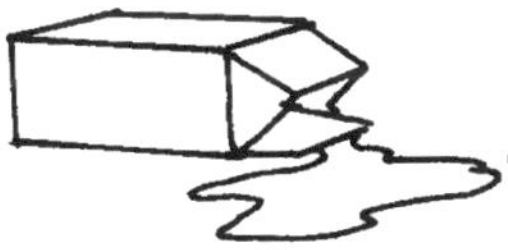 .
7. He's sharp as a 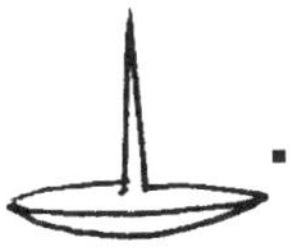 .
8. It's 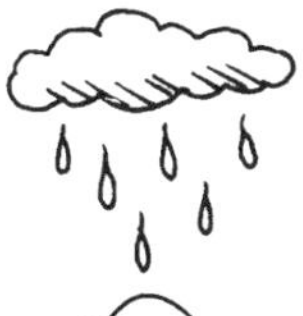 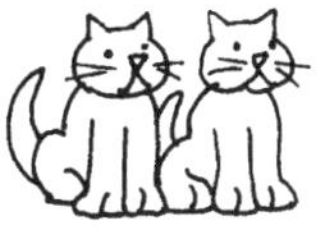 and 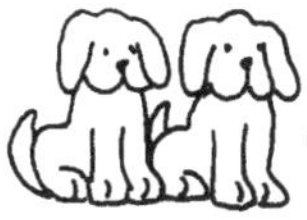 .
9. The 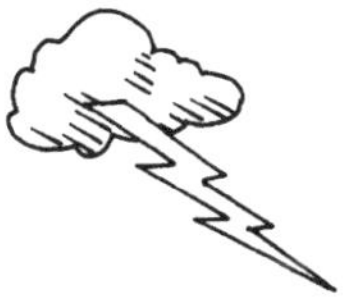 scared his 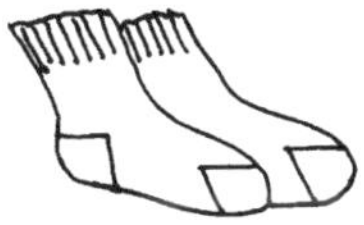 off.
10. The 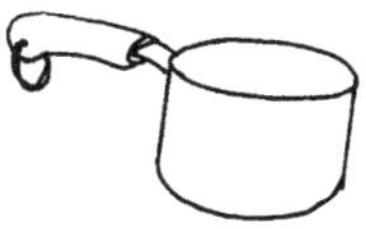 is as clean as a .

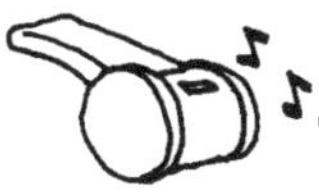

Name ______________________________

"IN A PICKLE" AND OTHER SILLY SAYINGS

Read each sentence in the first column. Then look in the second column for the true meaning of the sentence. Write the letter of the true meaning of the sentence on the blank next to the silly saying.

____ 1. You're in a pickle now.

____ 2. That's a feather in your cap.

____ 3. Hold your horses.

____ 4. You fly off the handle.

____ 5. You hit the nail on the head.

____ 6. Put your nose to the grindstone.

____ 7. Don't make a mountain out of a molehill.

____ 8. You bit off more than you can chew.

____ 9. Don't cry over spilt milk.

____ 10. You have a bone to pick with them.

____ 11. Start your project from scratch.

____ 12. You got cold feet the day before the party.

A. Be patient!

B. Get to work!

C. Don't make a problem bigger than it is.

D. You did something great.

E. You have a problem to get out of.

F. You weren't sure you wanted to go.

G. You got exactly the right answer.

H. You get mad very easily.

I. Don't get upset over something that isn't important.

J. You have a disagreement to discuss.

K. Don't use anything already made.

L. You have more to do than is possible.

Name ______________________________

HOW TO GET OUT OF A PICKLE

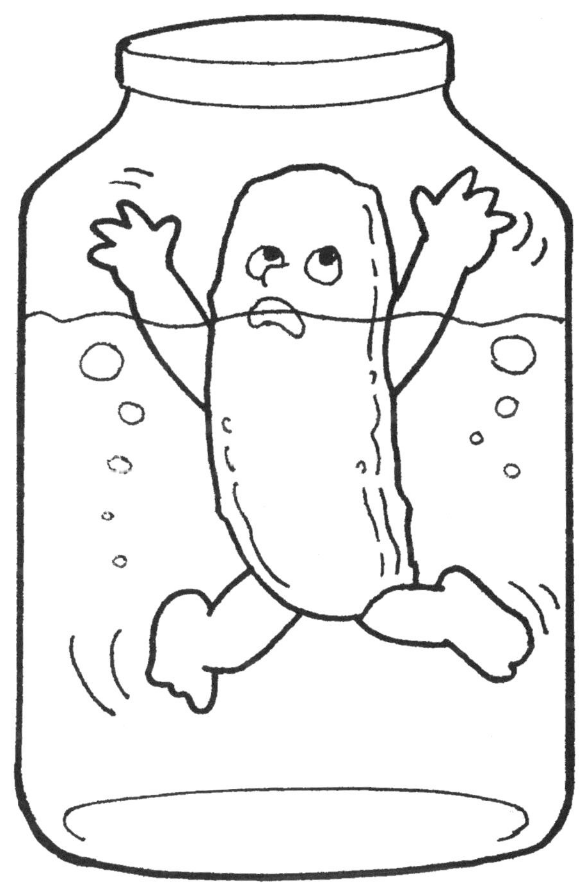

When you are "in a pickle" you need to be able to make good decisions.

Below are four steps you should use when making a decision. Number the steps in the order that would help a person get out of a pickle.

_____ Think of all the possible choices you have.

_____ Think of the consequences of each choice.

_____ Clearly define the problem.

_____ Decide on the best choice.

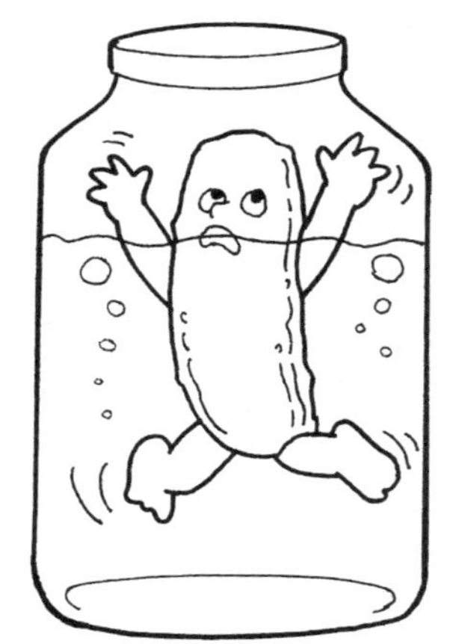
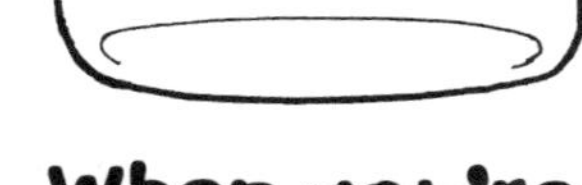

When you're "in a pickle," remember these steps to making a decision.

Clearly define the problem.

Think of all the possible choices you have.

Think of the consequences of each choice.

Decide on the best choice.

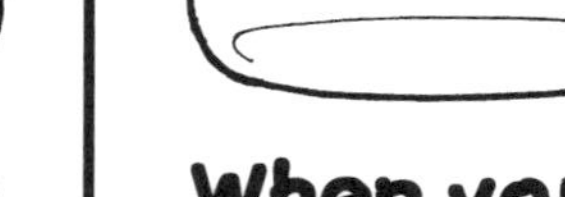

When you're "in a pickle," remember these steps to making a decision.

Clearly define the problem.

Think of all the possible choices you have.

Think of the consequences of each choice.

Decide on the best choice.

When you're "in a pickle," remember these steps to making a decision.

Clearly define the problem.

Think of all the possible choices you have.

Think of the consequences of each choice.

Decide on the best choice.

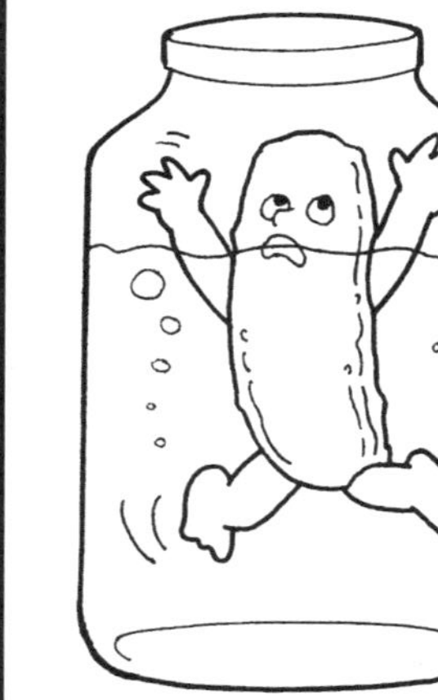

When you're "in a pickle," remember these steps to making a decision.

Clearly define the problem.

Think of all the possible choices you have.

Think of the consequences of each choice.

Decide on the best choice.

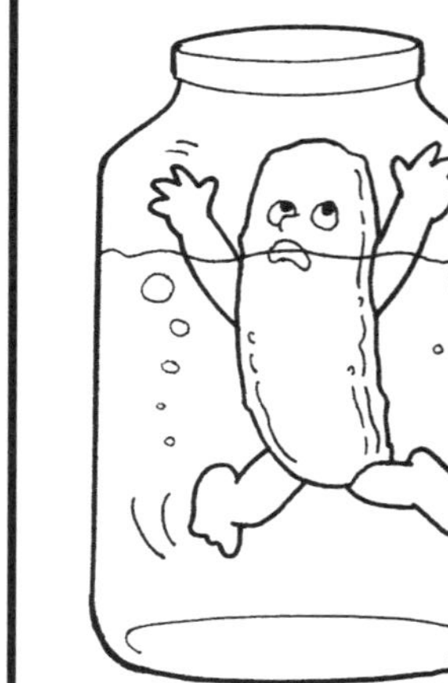

When you're "in a pickle," remember these steps to making a decision.

Clearly define the problem.

Think of all the possible choices you have.

Think of the consequences of each choice.

Decide on the best choice.

CHAPTER 3

PICKLE MOUNTAIN SCHOOL STORIES

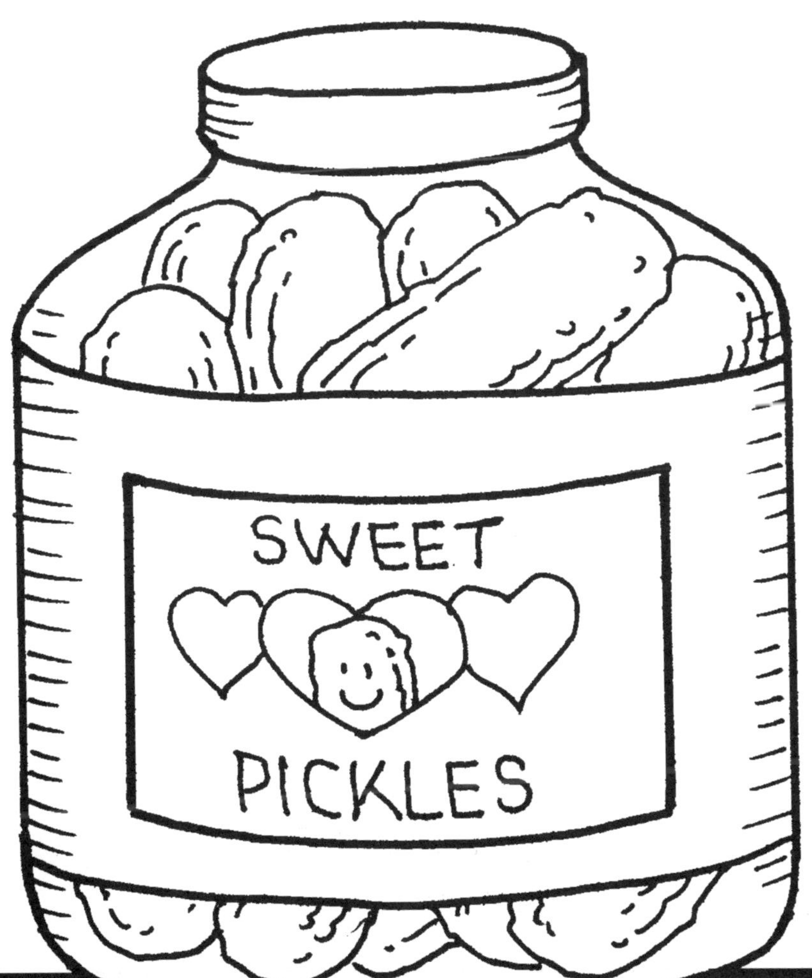

HOW PICKLE MOUNTAIN GOT ITS NAME

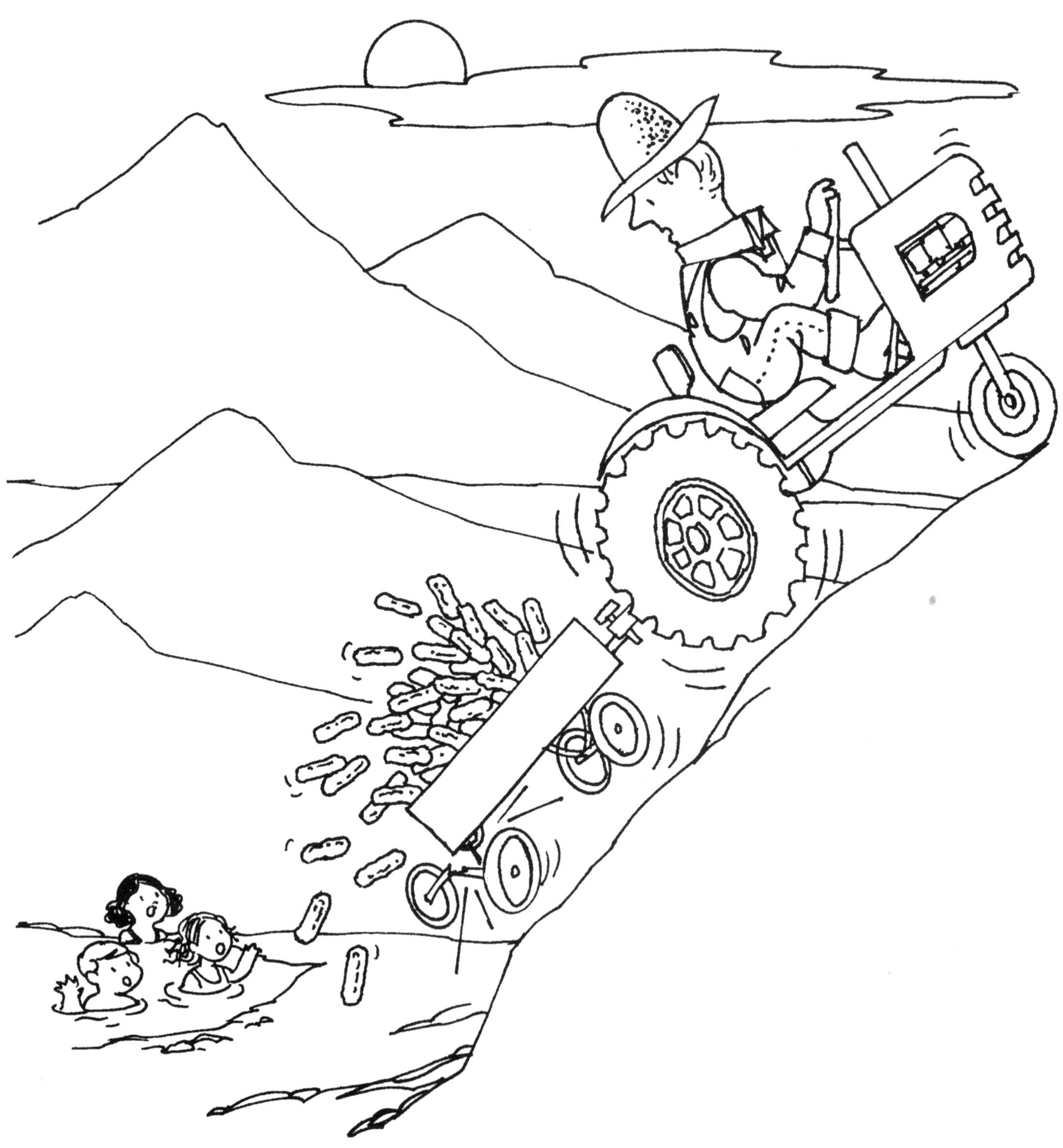

The people of Pickle Mountain do not eat many pickles: maybe two or three a week. Pickles do not grow on Pickle Mountain. Actually, pickles don't grow *anywhere*. *Cucumbers* do. Well, cucumbers do not grow on Pickle Mountain either. How, then, did Pickle Mountain get its name? Listen carefully and I will tell you.

It was near a mountain one summer a long time ago, before there were televisions or air conditioners. The children who lived on the mountain were playing in the creek to stay cool. All of a sudden, they heard a strange sound coming from a nearby road. Curious and a little afraid, they jumped out of the water and ran toward the road. But before they could reach the road, they saw green things rolling down the hill. A man was yelling, "My cucumbers! My cucumbers!"

The man was a farmer on his way to the pickle factory. He had been pulling a wagon full of cucumbers behind his tractor when a back wheel fell off the wagon and the back gate opened. Well, you know what happened next. The cucumbers went rolling out of the wagon and down the hill. As if this weren't enough to upset the farmer, the next thing he found out was that the wheel could not be repaired.

Is it any wonder the farmer was upset? First, he saw his summer's work rolling down the hill. Then his wagon wheel could not be repaired. It seemed that there was no way he could get his cucumbers to the pickle factory.

When the children saw what was happening to the farmer's cucumbers, they immediately started picking them up. Soon, moms and dads and grandpas and grandmas arrived with baskets and helped pick up the cucumbers. Within an hour, they had filled 14 baskets with cucumbers. But the farmer, although thankful, was still upset. Even if he had his cucumbers, there was no way to get them to the factory. It would take two days to get a new wheel for his wagon. The cucumbers would spoil before he could have the wagon repaired and drive it to the factory. Nevertheless, the wagon had to have a new wheel. So the farmer started off to the store to buy one.

The situation seemed hopeless. Then the children came up with a way to show the farmer they cared about him and his dilemma. They asked their parents and grandparents if *they* could make pickles.

Making pickles is not easy, but it still seemed like a good idea. If everyone had a responsibility, they could do it! The children were responsible for washing the cucumbers. Some of the grown-ups were responsible for going to nearby towns to get supplies. Other grown-ups were responsible for going from house to house, collecting jars that had to be very thoroughly cleaned. At one house, some of the grown-ups worked together to make sour pickles. At a second house, some grown-ups made sweet pickles. At a third house, other grown-ups made bread and butter pickles.

When the farmer returned a few days later, he could not believe what he was seeing! The cucumbers were now all pickles in jars. He wouldn't get paid for his cucumbers at the factory, but he was grateful for all of the mountain people's hard work and that the cucumbers wouldn't go to waste. As the farmer was about to leave, the mountain people presented him with another surprise. They weren't, as he had thought, going to *keep* the pickles. They were giving the pickles to him!

This was too much for the farmer. He had never seen such kind and caring people. There was no way he could take all the pickles, so he insisted that they keep half and share them among themselves. After all, without their cooperation and caring, there would only be squashed cucumbers on the road and rotten ones hidden under the bushes.

When the farmer got home with his pickles, he told everyone about the caring people. And when he was asked where these kind and wonderful people lived, he answered, "On Pickle Mountain."

Follow-Up Questions: 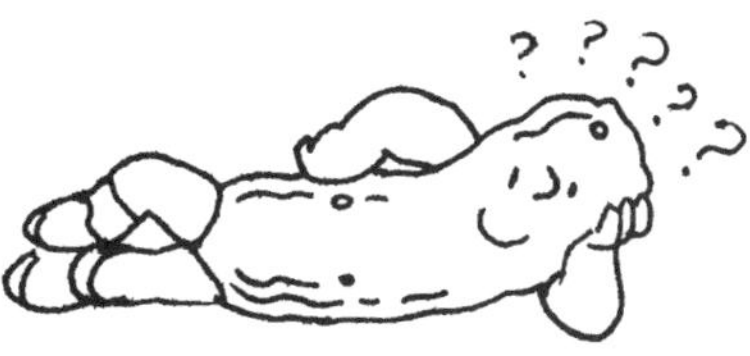

1. What did the mountain children do in the summer to stay cool?

   ____

2. How was the farmer going to make money from his cucumbers?

   ____

3. Who cooperated to help the farmer? ____________________

   ____

4. How many houses were used to make the pickles? ________

5. What responsibility did the children have? ______________

   ____

6. Who was appreciative? ______________________________

7. How did Pickle Mountain get its name? _______________

   ____

8. If the mountain people made 100 jars of pickles, how many did the farmer give them? ______________________________

Answers To Follow-Up Questions:

1. What did the mountain children do in the summer to stay cool? *(They played in the creek.)*
2. How was the farmer going to make money from his cucumbers? *(He was going to sell them to the pickle factory.)*
3. Who cooperated to help the farmer? *(The grown-ups and children who lived on the mountain.)*
4. How many houses were used to make the pickles? *(Three.)*
5. What responsibility did the children have? *(They washed the cucumbers.)*
6. Who was appreciative? *(The farmer.)*
7. How did Pickle Mountain get its name? *(The farmer named it because the people who lived there made pickles out of his cucumbers.)*
8. If the mountain people made 100 jars of pickles, how many did the farmer give them? *(50 jars.)*

TIRED OF STINKY PICKLE

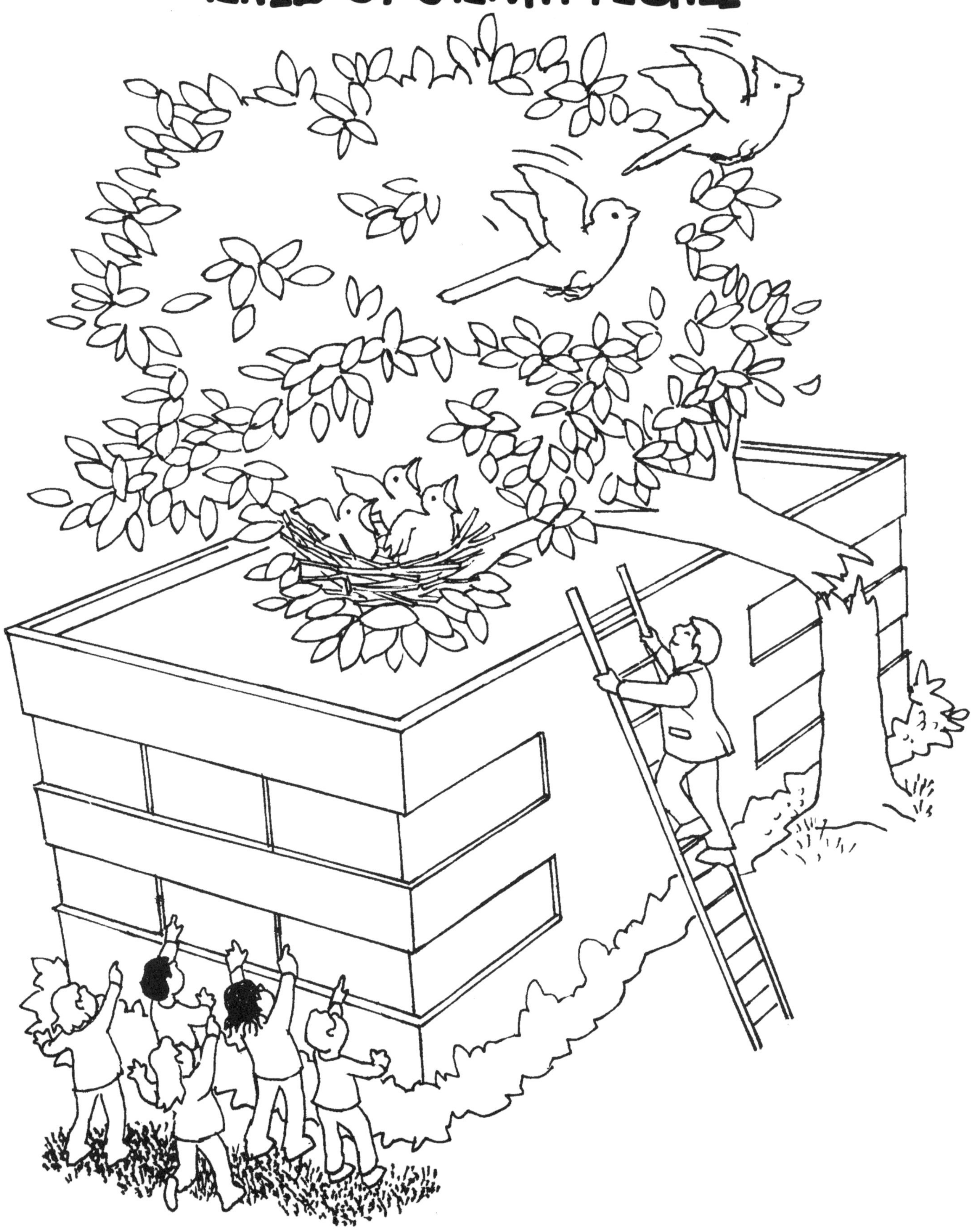

The students of Pickle Mountain School had been dealing with the same problem for years. Every time they met students from another school, they were teased about being *Pickles*. They were called *sour pickle, stinky pickle, bumpy pickle*, and any other unkind name the kids could think of. The students at Pickle Mountain were proud of their school. They were even proud of its name because they had heard the wonderful story about how Pickle Mountain got its name. But they would have liked a mascot that was not a pickle.

The children took their problem to Mrs. Jones, the school counselor. After listening to them, Mrs. Jones thought of an idea. She talked with the principal about her idea of having the children submit names for a school mascot. The principal liked the idea and he and Mrs. Jones agreed that the children's suggestions would be placed in her mailbox.

During the next week, Mrs. Jones' mailbox was filled, not once, not twice, but three times with notes suggesting names for the mascot. With all these suggestions, it was going to be difficult to pick one. The names were put to a vote and seven names received the same number of votes. "This could turn into a disaster," thought Mrs. Jones. "What I need is some time to figure out a fair way we can work this out."

There was a terrible storm one night the next week. When the children arrived at school the next day, they saw a tall tree resting on the roof of the building. Fearful that the tree might go through the roof or damage it in some other way, the principal contacted the man who took care of the school building. Before the man could begin work, one of the youngest students in the school heard a noise coming from the roof. Everyone got quiet, then everyone heard the noise. When they told the principal about it, he took a ladder and climbed up onto the roof to see if he could find out where the noise was coming from.

He found that the noise was coming from a nest that had been protected in the tree. In the nest were three baby birds. The noise was the sound of two adult birds protecting them. As the principal neared the nest, the two adult birds flew out. The children saw them and called out, "Look! They're cardinals!"

About this time, the man in charge of taking care of the school building checked the roof. When he said there was no damage, the principal decided to leave the tree alone. In fact, he even had some ropes tied to the tree to keep it in place. The children were curious to see the baby birds, but they knew they shouldn't go near the nest. Then they discovered that if they sat on the rocks behind the swings, they could see the nest and watch the adult birds take care of their three babies. The children talked about how brave the adult cardinals had been protecting their babies and how much energy it took for them to keep bringing food to the nest. When the adult cardinals flew, they looked powerful, yet graceful.

It wasn't until the next day that a third-grade student shouted, "Cardinals! That's the name we need!" The name sounded right, and the children took their idea to Mrs. Jones. She agreed that it was a good idea, but said they still must vote. When the votes were counted, everyone except one little boy—who wanted the mascot to be a lion because he had a lion costume for Halloween—agreed that the mascot should be the cardinal.

Later, the principal carefully climbed onto the roof and took a picture of the cardinals. Students started drawing pictures of cardinals. The art teacher even made a flag that read *Cardinals* to hang outside the school.

Pickle Mountain School truly was a cardinal school, and the day a little cardinal flew for the first time and sat on top of the pole with the *Cardinals* flag flying in the wind, the children knew they had chosen the best mascot for their school.

Follow-Up Questions: 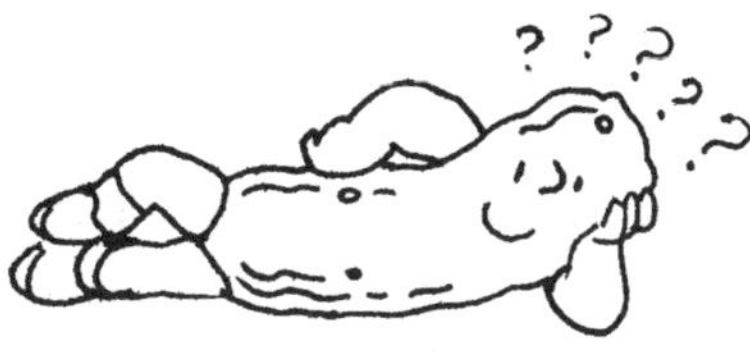

1. Why didn't the students want a pickle for a mascot? _______

   ____

2. How did Mrs. Jones avoid a conflict when the children were choosing a mascot? ________________________

   ____

3. What characteristics of the cardinals did the children notice?

   ____

4. What jobs at the school were mentioned in the story? ______

   ____

   ____

   ____

   Name other work positions at a school. ______________

   ____

5. The children watched the birds for 15 minutes. The mother bird flew in eight times with food. The father bird flew in nine times. How many times altogether did they fly into the nest? ______

Answers To Follow-Up Questions:

1. Why didn't the students want a pickle for a mascot? *(The students didn't want a pickle for a mascot because students from other schools teased them about being pickles.)*
2. How did Mrs. Jones avoid a conflict when the children were choosing a mascot? *(Mrs. Jones had the children vote for the mascot they wanted.)*
3. What characteristics of the cardinals did the children notice? *(The cardinals were brave, energetic, powerful, and graceful.)*
4. What jobs at the school were mentioned in the story? *(The jobs mentioned were counselor, principal, and building maintenance manager.)* Name other work positions at a school. *(Accept any appropriate answers.)*
5. The children watched the birds for 15 minutes. The mother bird flew in eight times with food. The father bird flew in nine times. How many times altogether did they fly into the nest? *(Seventeen times.)*

FIGHT FOR A FROG

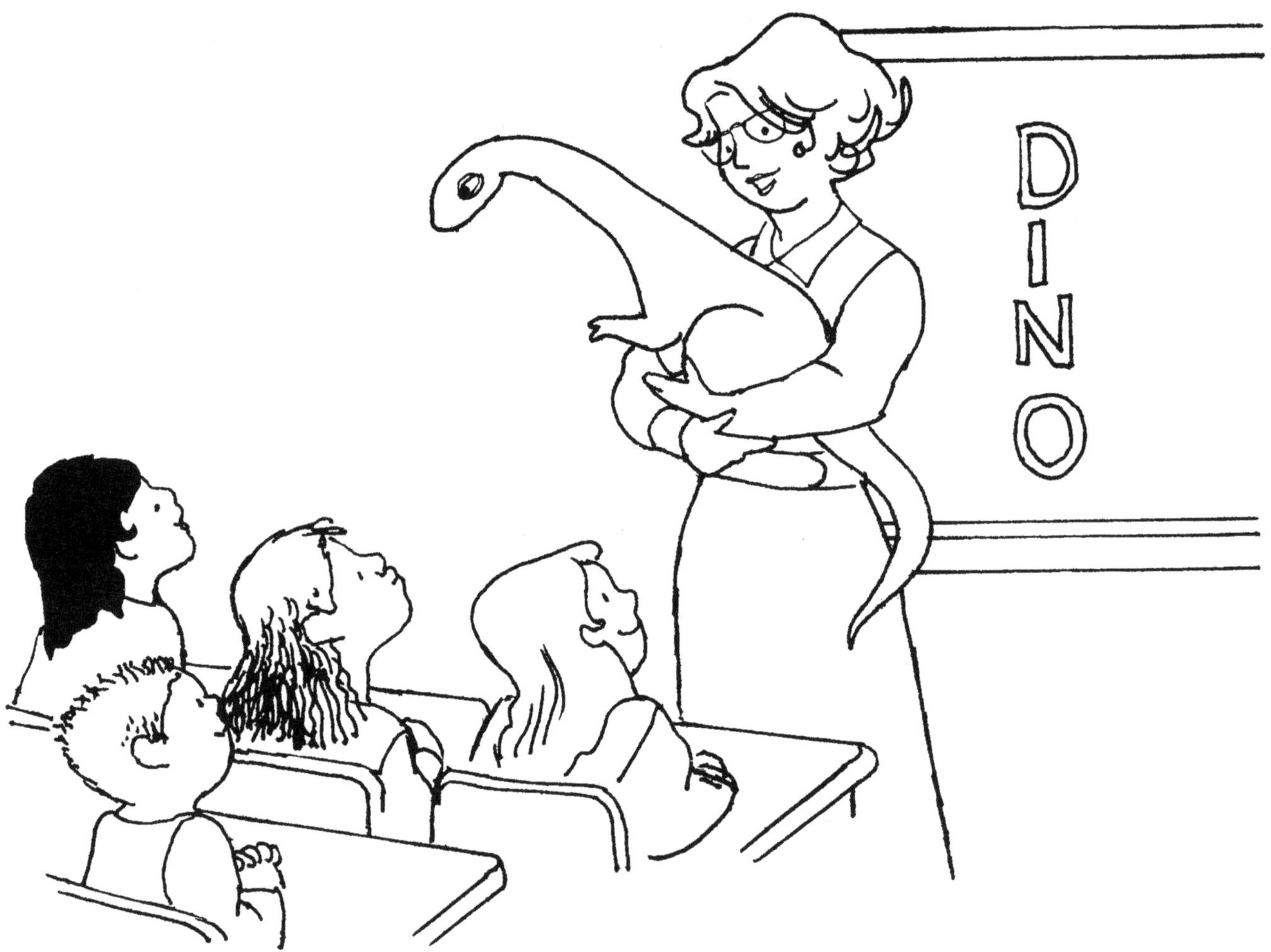

Jerry found it first. Well, maybe he did. Brooke also claimed that she found it first. That frog was causing an uproar in Mrs. Brown's second-grade class at Pickle Mountain School. It was a cute little frog, and both children wanted to take it home. Soon other children decided *they* wanted to take it home. What started out as a simple problem turned into a big one.

As luck would have it, Mrs. Jones, the counselor, was coming to the classroom that day to present a guidance lesson. And as luck would further have it, that lesson was going to be on something called *conflict resolution*. When Mrs. Jones entered the room to begin her lesson, she didn't even know there was an argument going on about who was going to get the frog.

Mrs. Jones came into the room with a bright pink toy dinosaur that she had named *Dinosolve*. Without even mentioning the frog, which she knew nothing about anyway, she began teaching the students four things they needed to do to solve an argument, or a *conflict*, as she called it.

The first thing Mrs. Jones did was go to the chalkboard and write the letters "D," "I," "N," and "O" in a straight column. Then she said, "This is DINO, the name of my dinosaur. It is also the first letter of the words for four things you need to do to solve a conflict."

"The first thing you must do," she said, "is decide if what you are arguing about is important. That's because lots of conflicts are about things that don't really matter." Then she went back to the chalkboard. After the "D," she wrote: *Decide If It Is Important.*

"Next," she continued, "you should look very carefully at the problem. This is called *investigating*, and it means that everyone involved in the argument respects the others enough to listen to them and find out more about the problem." This time she wrote: *Investigate The Problem* after the "I."

Mrs. Jones then went on, "When you have done both of these things, it is time to make a plan that will work for everyone. This is called *negotiating.* When you negotiate, there is a good chance that not everybody will get exactly what they want. But everyone will get *something* that they want." Before she could reach the chalkboard, the children had figured out that she would be writing *Negotiate* after the "N."

"Finally," Mrs. Jones told the children, "you may not be able to work out the problem by yourselves. If you have tried very hard to work out your problem but are getting nowhere, then it is time to ask an adult for help." The children knew the last letter on the chalkboard was "O," but Mrs. Jones didn't give them any clues. So they waited until they saw her write: *Offer To Get Help* after the "O."

When Mrs. Jones had finished teaching the four steps of conflict resolution, she had the children practice using the steps with some problems that usually come up in classrooms. But the frog situation was not one of those problems, because Mrs. Jones still did not know about it. Class ended just in time for recess, and recess rekindled the fight over the frog. The difference this time was that the children remembered Mrs. Jones' lesson and decided to try what she had taught them.

This is what they did:

D They ***DECIDED*** the situation was really important to them.

I They ***INVESTIGATED*** by listening to what each child planned to do with the frog.

N They ***NEGOTIATED*** by suggesting different ideas. Jerry thought that if the frog were a class project, everyone would feel like the frog was theirs. Brooke suggested that the class could study about different kinds of frogs. Then Leo added that when the project was over, they could put the frog in the biggest tree on the playground.

O Although the children liked the idea of the project, it was not something they could make happen without adult permission. So they ***OFFERED*** to take the idea to Mrs. Brown to see if she would agree that this was a good solution.

Do you think the children worked out their conflict?

P.S. It's a good thing they worked out their problem, because the bus driver didn't allow frogs to ride on the Pickle Mountain School bus.

Follow-Up Questions: 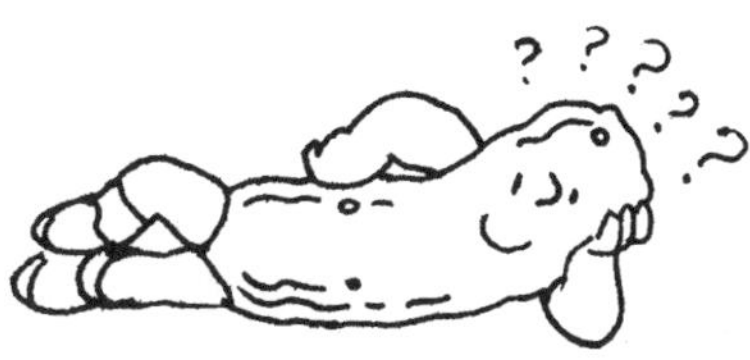

1. Do you think some students would decide the fight for the frog was *not* important and just let it go? ______________________

____

2. Do you think each child got a chance to talk without being interrupted? ______________________________

____

3. Can you think of other ways the problem could have been worked out? __________________________________

____

4. Did the children go to the teacher right away? ___________

____

Answers To Follow-Up Questions:

1. Do you think some students would decide the fight for the frog was *not* important and just let it go? *(Accept any appropriate answers.)*
2. Do you think each child got a chance to talk without being interrupted? *(Accept any appropriate answers.)*
3. Can you think of other ways the problem could have been worked out? *(Accept any appropriate answers.)*
4. Did the children go to the teacher right away? *(No, they worked through the steps of conflict resolution and approached the teacher only when it was necessary.)*

SOLVING CONFLICTS AT PICKLE MOUNTAIN SCHOOL

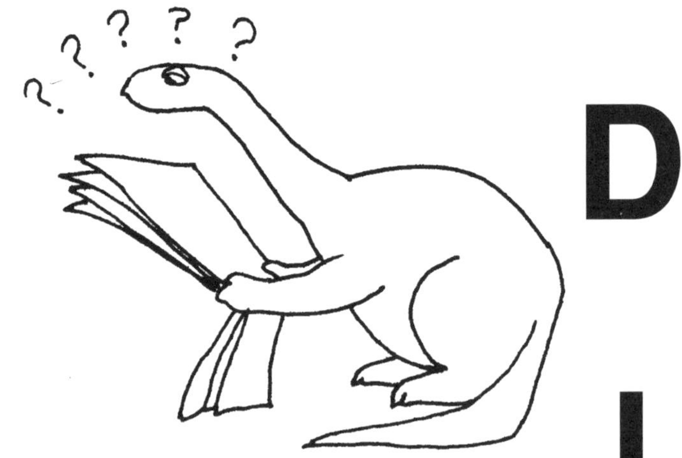

D

DECIDE if the problem is important.

I

INVESTIGATE the problem.
Listen to each other.

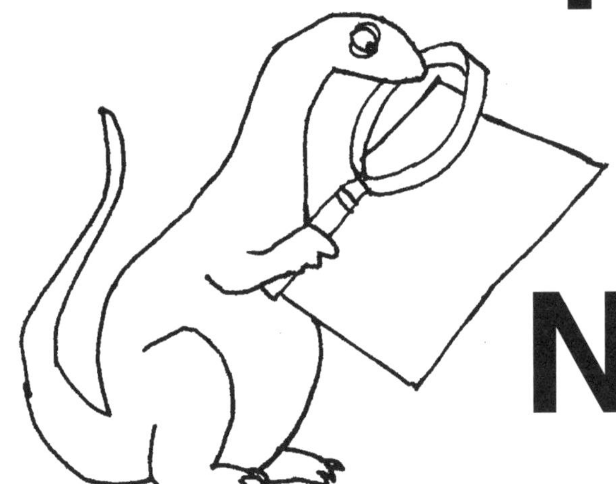

N

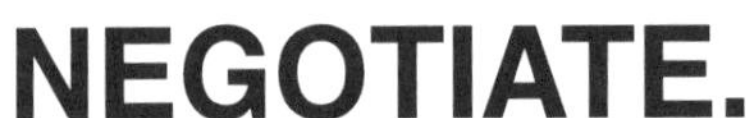

NEGOTIATE.
Make a plan that both sides can accept.

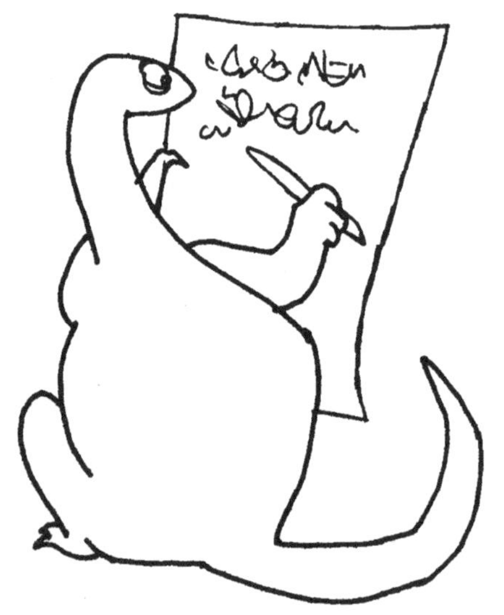

O

OFFER to get help only after you have tried to work it out.

CHARACTER EDUCATION AT PICKLE MOUNTAIN SCHOOL

The principal at Pickle Mountain School was putting together a character-education program. He had a list of about 20 words describing good character traits. The words were all useful words—cooperation, respect, responsibility, integrity, perseverance, compassion, thankfulness, adaptability, self-control, citizenship, courtesy, consideration, efficiency, patriotism, optimism, loyalty, trustworthiness, honesty, courage, contemplation—but the principal wasn't sure they were words that would help the children understand the meaning of character education.

Knowing that the first place he would tell the children to find the meaning of a word was in the dictionary, the principal went to his dictionary and looked up the meaning of *character*. It said that the word means *acting with care*. He looked at the long list of words again. Every one of them fit the definition of acting with care, but he still wasn't satisfied that this was the best way to teach children the meaning of character education. He felt he needed to do something other than present the children with a list of words.

The principal needed something simple. Something that would clearly explain to the children the meaning of *acting with care*. He thought and thought. It had to be something that was not complicated and that the children could easily understand. About that time, he looked at the clock on his wall. It was almost time for lunch, but it wasn't the clock that caught his eye. It was the poster that hung next to the clock. The poster had a simple message. The words were few, and their meaning was easily understood. His question was answered. A poster. That's what he needed! A poster that would explain character education.

After lunch, the principal gathered up the materials he needed to make his poster. When he had completed the poster, it said:

We care about each other.
We care about ourselves.
We care about the earth.

It was simple, yet it said everything that needed to be said. If the children at Pickle Mountain School followed these three simple rules, they would show good character.

Next, he had to find a way to help the children remember the words on the poster. He knew the children liked songs, so he set the words from the poster to the tune of *The Farmer in the Dell*.

We care about each other.
We care about each other.
We put the care in character.
We care about each other.
We care about ourselves.
We care about ourselves.
We put the care in character.
We care about ourselves.
We care about the earth.
We care about the earth.
We put the care in character.
We care about the earth.

The poster and the song gave the principal the beginnings of his character-education program. He shared the poster and the song with all the teachers, who in turn shared them with their students. It wasn't long before the principal heard about children singing the song in the classroom, at recess, and even on the bus.

The students learned the character words on the list, read stories about character education, and played character-education games. All of this was easier because they knew the importance of caring about others, themselves, and the earth.

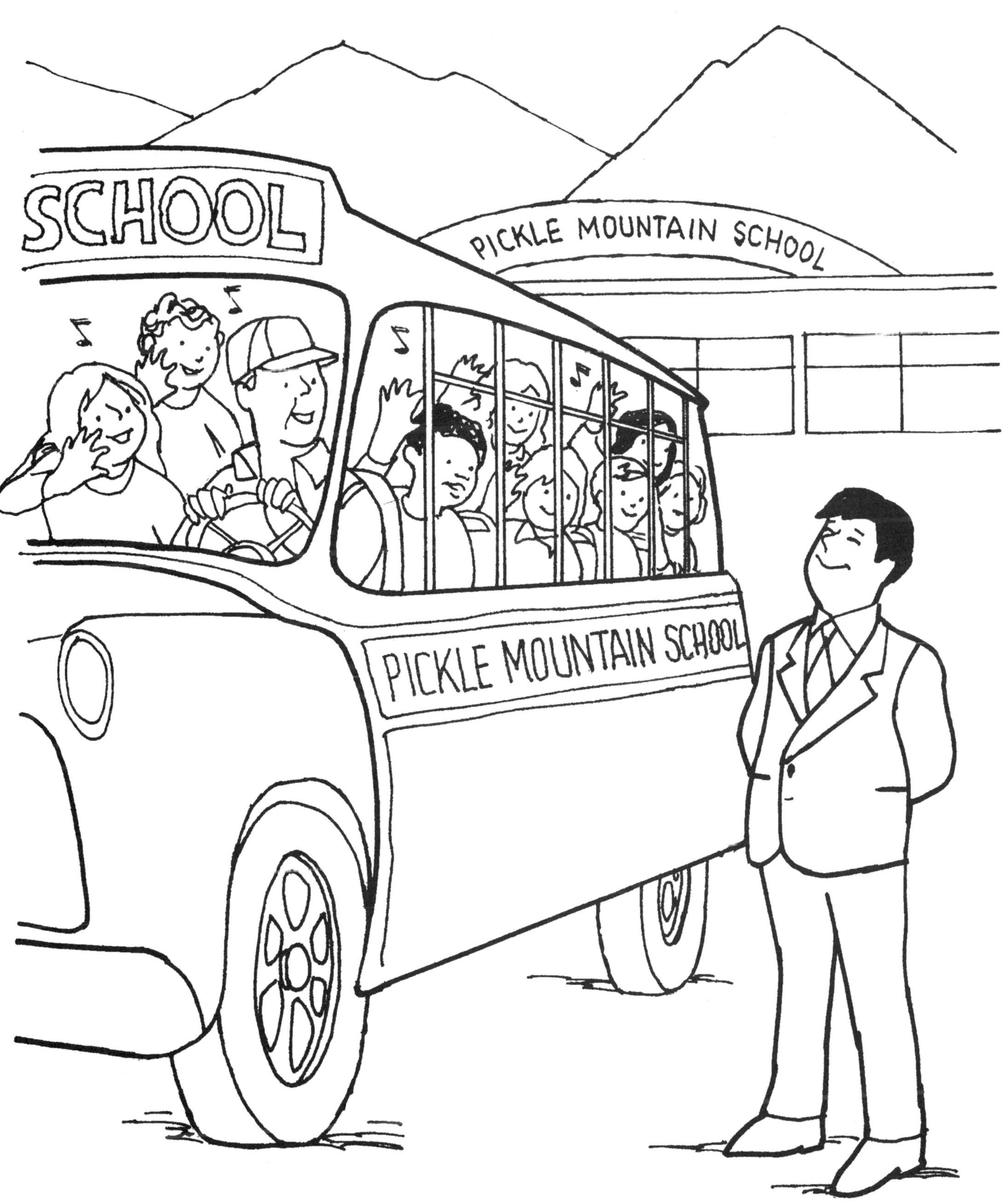
SCHOOL
PICKLE MOUNTAIN SCHOOL
PICKLE MOUNTAIN SCHOOL

Follow-Up Questions: 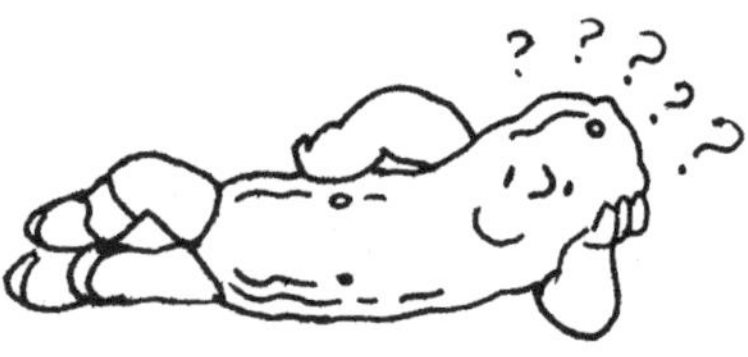

1. Have you learned any character-trait words at your school? Tell about one. ____
____
2. What book did the principal use to help him with his project?
____
3. Have you used a dictionary when it wasn't an assignment? If so, tell about that time. __________________________________
____
4. What did the principal learn the word *character* means? _____
____
5. What are the three things to be treated with care that are listed on the poster? ____________________________________
____
6. What did the principal use to help the students remember the three character behaviors? ___________________________
____

Answers To Follow-Up Questions:

1. Have you learned any character-trait words at your school? Tell about one. *(Accept any appropriate answers.)*
2. What book did the principal use to help him with his project? *(The dictionary.)*
3. Have you used a dictionary when it wasn't an assignment? If so, tell about that time. *(Accept any appropriate answers.)*
4. What did the principal learn the word *character* means? *(Character means* acting with care*.)*
5. What are the three things to be treated with care that are listed on the poster? *(Each other, ourselves, the earth.)*
6. What did the principal use to help the students remember the three character behaviors? *(The principal used the song and the poster.)*

WE CARE ABOUT EACH OTHER.

WE CARE ABOUT OURSELVES.

WE CARE ABOUT THE EARTH.

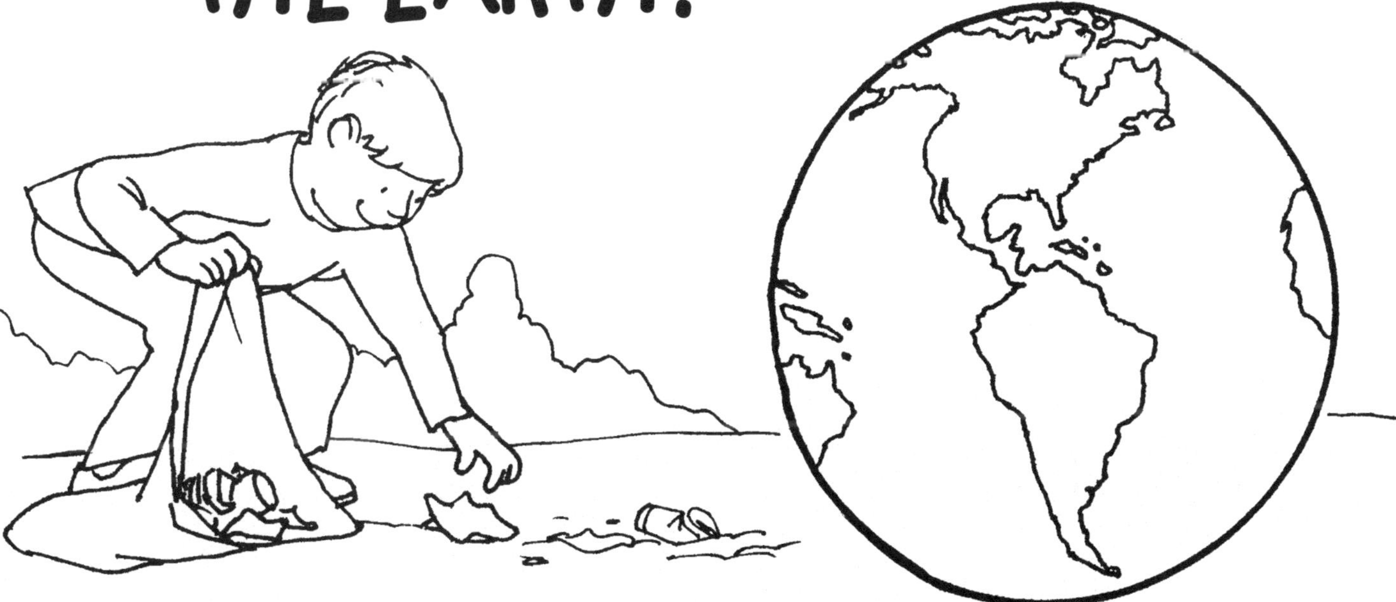

GRATEFUL GARY'S GIFTS

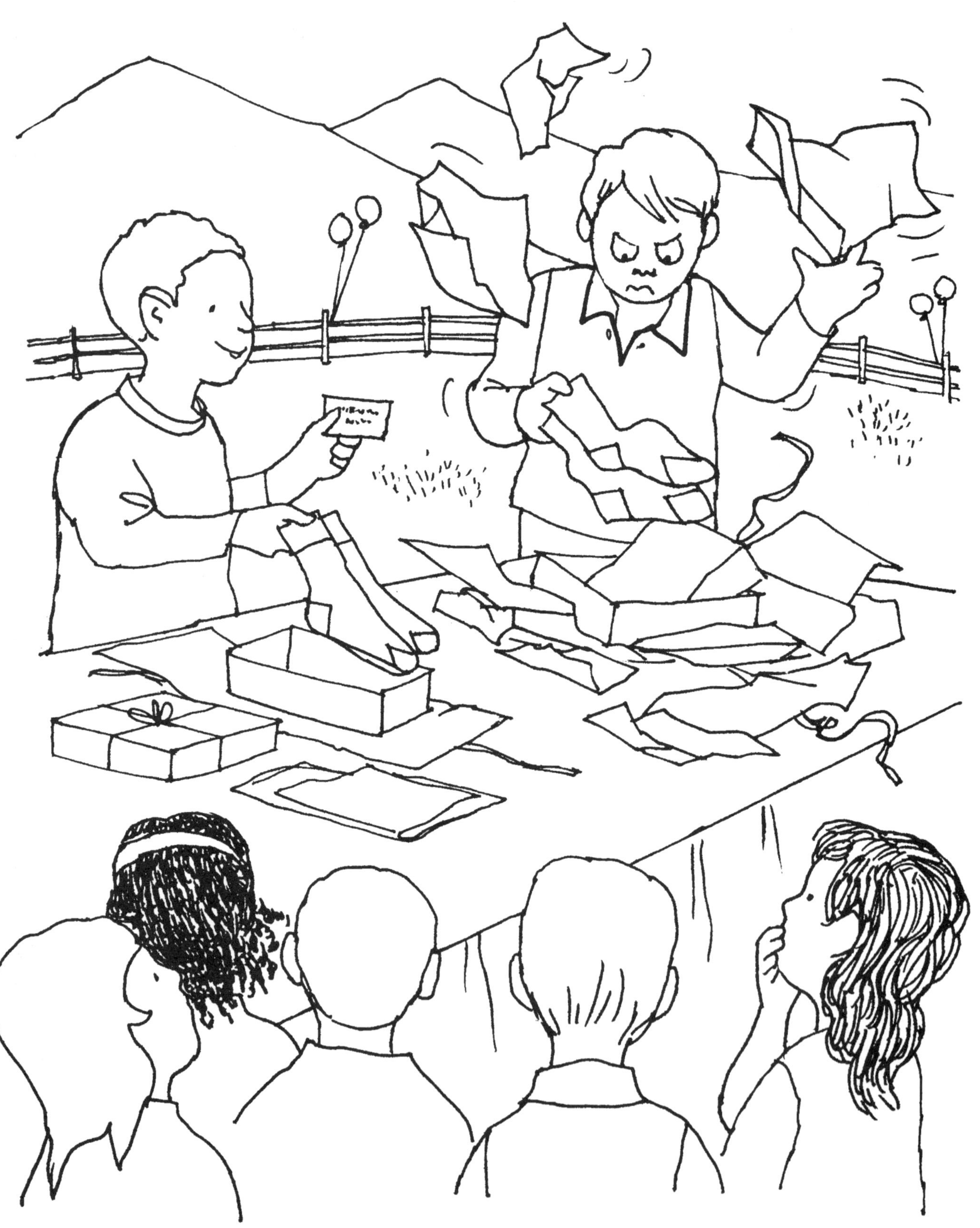

Travis and Gary are cousins and they have the same birthday, July 12. The difference is that Travis is one year older than Gary. Travis used to go to Pickle Mountain School, but moved away when his parents divorced.

It was summertime and Travis came to spend the school vacation at Pickle Mountain with Gary. When it was time for the boys' birthdays, Gary's mom had a party for both boys. Sixteen boys and girls showed up at Gary's house. They played outside and ate cake and ice cream. Travis kept asking when they were going to open presents, but Gary didn't seem to be in any hurry. Gary was having too good a time being with his friends.

However, there is a time at all birthday parties when the gifts are opened. And this party was no exception. Both boys began to open their presents, but they opened them very differently. Travis opened his quickly. Sometimes he didn't even look at the card. If he liked the gift, he made a big deal about it. If he didn't like the gift, he would put it down without saying a word about it. Once, he even said, "I already have one like this." When he didn't see any more gifts for him, Travis asked, "Are there any more for me?"

Gary read each card and found out who the present was from before he opened it. He took the time to open each gift and say something nice about it. He got a pair of funny-colored socks that he didn't particularly like, but he said, "These should be warm when we go out to have snowball fights." When Gary got a gift just like one he already had, he said, "Thanks," in a very friendly way. He knew he and his mom could talk about it later. When Gary had opened all his gifts, he said, "Thanks! This has been a wonderful birthday. Who wants more ice cream?"

Later that day, a package arrived from the boys' grandparents. They sent each boy a birdhouse kit. When their grandmother called, Travis talked with her first, "Grandma," he said, "I already have one and it's still in the box. Can you take this one back and give me the money?" When Gary got on the phone, he thanked his grandmother for the gift. She asked, "Do you already have one?" Gary was honest. He said he had one, but that his tree had room for more than one birdhouse. Then he asked if his grandfather might come soon to help him build it.

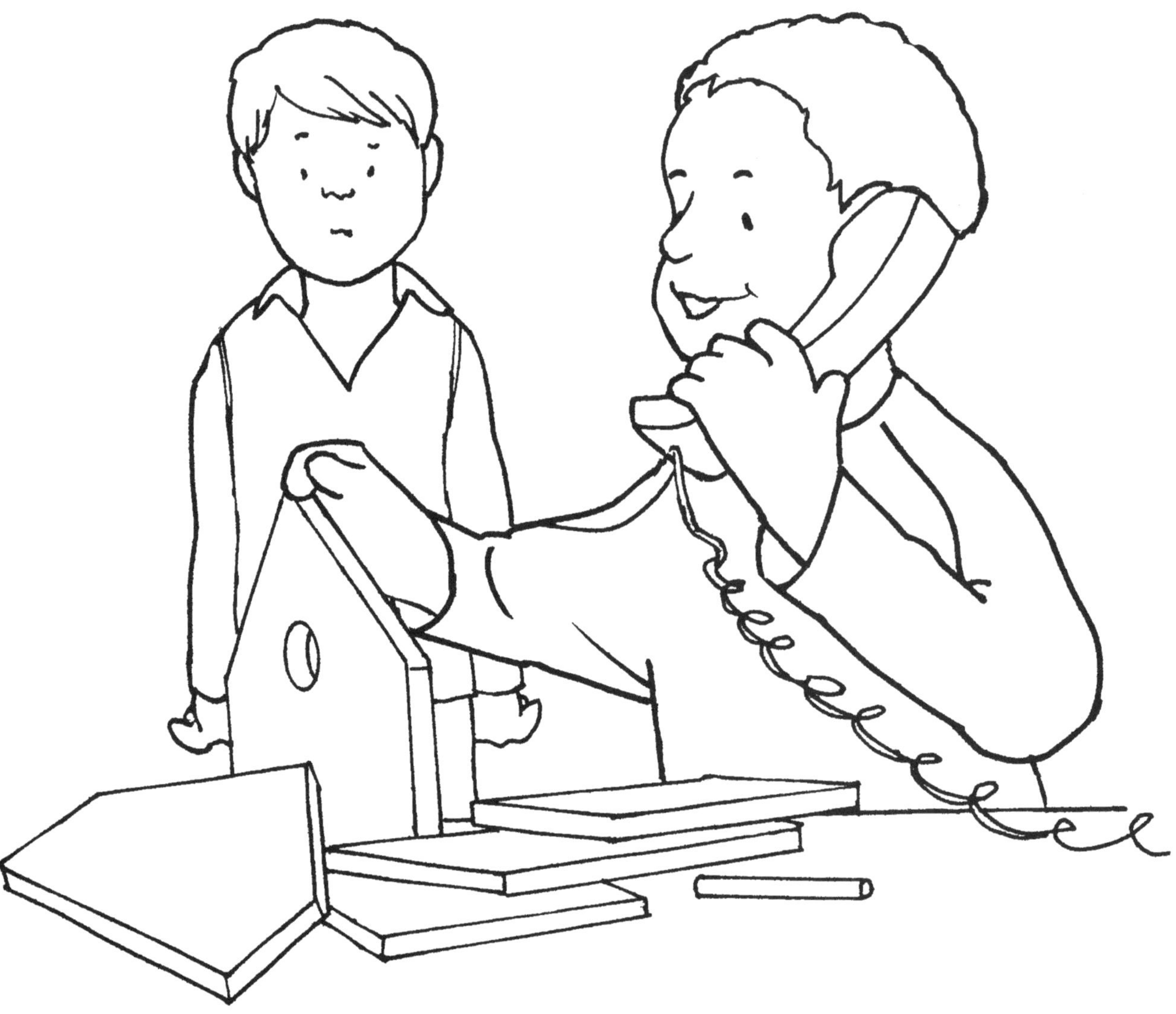

When the day was over, Travis thought his birthday had been okay. Gary thought his birthday had been great. He was grateful for his gifts, his friends, and his family.

Follow-Up Questions: 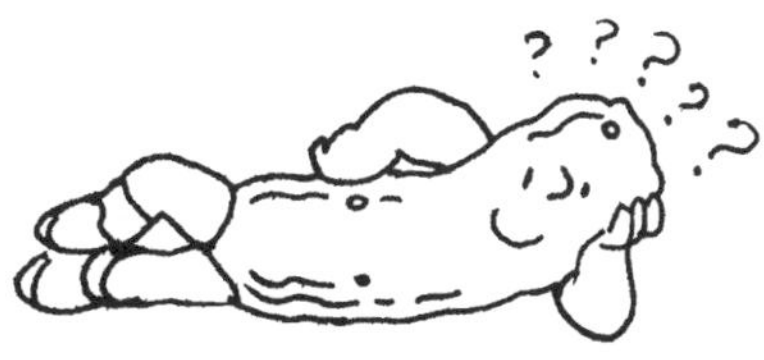

1. Do you think Gary's mother will want to have another party for Travis? Why? ____

____

____

2. What did Gary do before he opened a gift? ______________

____

____

3. There were 16 children at the party. If 9 were boys, how many were girls? ____

4. Travis and Gary each received a birdhouse kit from their grandparents. How did each of them react to the gift? ______

____

____

____

____

Answers To Follow-Up Questions:

1. Do you think Gary's mother will want to have another party for Travis? Why? *(Accept any appropriate answers.)*
2. What did Gary do before he opened a gift? *(He read the card and found out who it was from.)*
3. There were 16 children at the party. If 9 were boys, how many were girls? *(Seven children were girls.)*
4. Travis and Gary each received a birdhouse kit from their grandparents. How did each of them react to the gift? *(Travis said he already had a birdhouse and wondered if they could take it back and give him the money. Gary said he already had a birdhouse, but his tree was big enough for two. He wondered if his grandfather would come over and help him put it together.)*

Name ______________________________

GRANDPA & GRANDMA'S BIRDHOUSE

Travis and Gary's grandparents bought them identical birdhouse kits. Decorate the birdhouse one of the boys built.

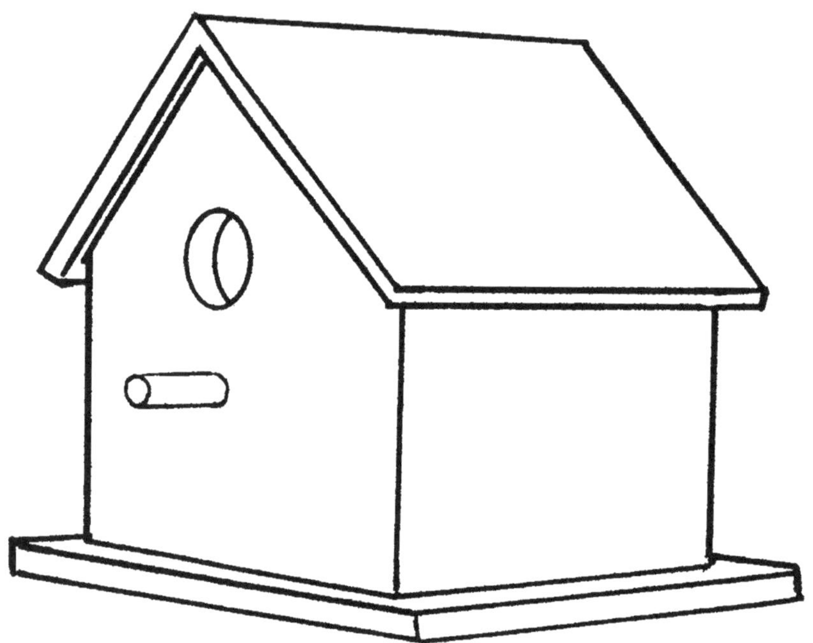

Gary was grateful for his gift. Draw a picture showing how he looked when he got the birdhouse kit from his grandparents.

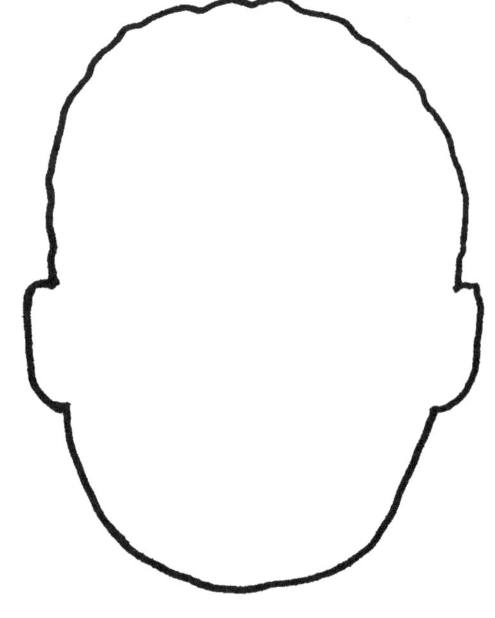

Travis was not polite. He even complained about his gift. Draw a picture showing how Travis looked when he got the birdhouse kit from his grandparents.

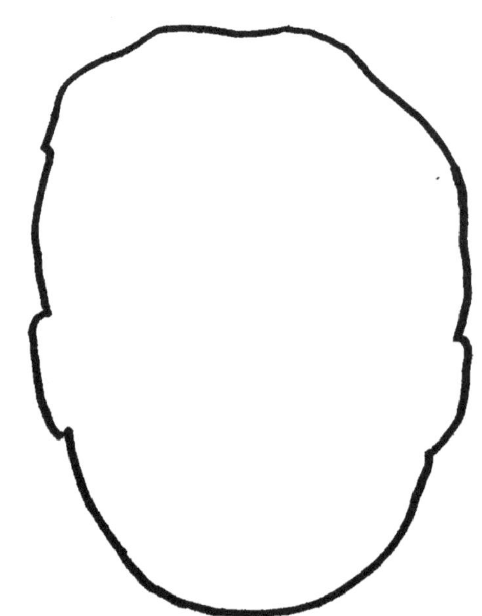

PACKED PICKLE GOES TO THE HOSPITAL

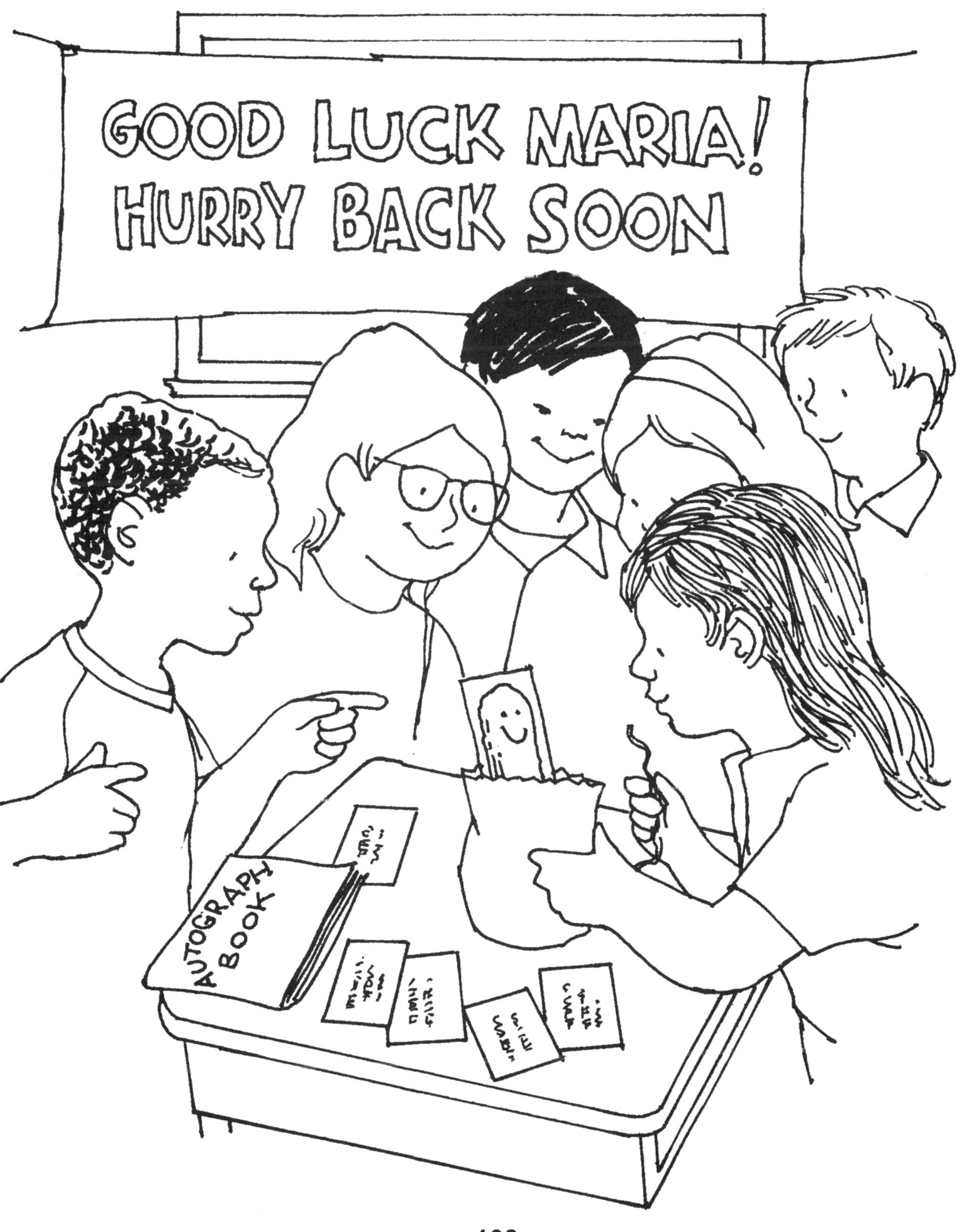

Maria's class at Pickle Mountain School had been hiding something from her all week. Finally, it was Friday. The counselor, Mrs. Jones, had asked Maria to come to her office that afternoon.

In the counselor's office, Mrs. Jones and Maria talked about her going to the hospital. Maria had known since she was seven that she would have surgery when she was nine. She was nervous, but not scared. The doctor had explained everything that was going to happen to her, and her mom, dad, or grandmother would be staying at the hospital all the time.

When Maria returned to her classroom, the room was filled with balloons. A big banner was taped to the wall. The banner said: "Good Luck, Maria! Hurry Back Soon." All the children had drawn pictures and written notes for her. On her desk was a package with a note attached to the ribbon that was tied around it. Maria read the note aloud: "Inside this box is something small. It won't take up much room at all. Take it with you when you go, then bring it back for you to show."

Inside the box was a bag. Packed in the bag was an autograph book and a green bookmark in the shape of a happy-faced pickle. The children had named it *Packed Pickle.* As Maria looked at her book and bookmark, her teacher said, "We want you to put your *Packed Pickle* into your suitcase. At the hospital, get autographs of the different workers you meet. Then when you come back, you'll have stories to tell and something to show the rest of the class."

The autograph book changed Maria's hospital stay from something she thought would be boring into a fun time. She met as many different workers as she could, and she asked them to tell her something about themselves and their jobs, then sign her book. When she was ready to leave the hospital, some of the signatures she had were the:

doctor	nurse	X-ray technician
lab technician	cook	housekeeper
pharmacist	nurse's aid	groundskeeper
gift shop clerk	hospital volunteer	bookkeeper

Maria was excited to go back to school and show the class all the different signatures in her book. She was also excited to tell her class about the people who signed her book and what they did in the hospital. After Maria shared her book with the class, her teacher told her it was hers to keep.

This was the first time anyone in the class had been given a *Packed Pickle*. But the teacher was so pleased with what the students learned, she decided to make more. From that day on, any student who traveled somewhere where he or she could learn about jobs was given a *Packed Pickle.* When Heather flew to visit her grandparents, she took her *Packed Pickle,* and the class learned about jobs at the airport. When Jerome went to Disneyworld, he took his *Packed Pickle*. The class learned about jobs at an amusement park. The idea of the *Packed Pickles* was so successful that soon even children who didn't travel wanted their own. Michael's father was a firefighter and he took a *Packed Pickle* to the firehouse for autographs. Melinda's older brother worked in a grocery store, and she took her *Packed Pickle* and filled it with signatures of the people who worked with him. By the time the school year was over, all the children in the class had their own *Packed Pickles* and everyone in the class knew a lot more about different jobs.

Follow-Up Questions: 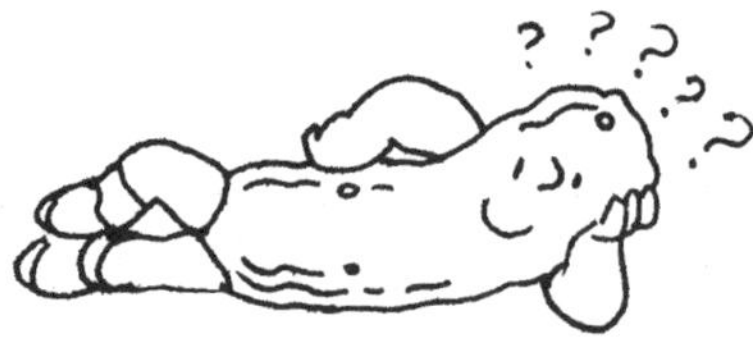

1. Were the students keeping a secret from Maria? ___________

   Was this a sweet secret or a sour secret? _______________

2. How did the children show they felt compassion for Maria?

   ____

3. What did the children give Maria to take with her to the hospital?

   ____

4. How did Maria learn about jobs at the hospital? ___________

   ____

5. Was Maria the only student given a *Packed Pickle?*________

   ____

6. Maria met 12 workers at the hospital. Heather met 10 workers at the airport. Jerome met 14 workers at Disneyworld. How many jobs did the students learn about from Maria, Heather, and Jerome? ______________________________

Answers To Follow-Up Questions:

1. Were the students keeping a secret from Maria? *(Yes.)* Was this a sweet secret or a sour secret? *(It was a sweet secret.)*
2. How did the children show they felt compassion for Maria? *(They gave her a party with balloons and a banner.)*
3. What did the children give Maria to take with her to the hospital? *(Maria got to take a* Packed Pickle *to the hospital.)*
4. How did Maria learn about jobs at the hospital? *(She asked workers about their jobs and had them sign her book.)*
5. Was Maria the only student given a *Packed Pickle? (No. By the end of the year, each of the students had one.)*
6. Maria met 12 workers at the hospital. Heather met 10 workers at the airport. Jerome met 14 workers at Disneyworld. How many jobs did the students learn about from Maria, Heather, and Jerome? *(The students learned about 36 jobs.)*

PACKED PICKLE ACTIVITIES

BOOKMARKS:

Using the pattern (see right), trace four pickles with hats onto 9" x 12" green craft foam, 2mm thick. Cut out the pickles.

Using a brush with a fine tip or paint with a tip on the bottle, decorate the pickles with green glow-in-the-dark paint. *(Tulip™ Glow In The Dark Dimensional Fabric Paint* works well.) When you cut and paint, vary the shapes of the pickles' eyes, smiles, etc. If this is not something you enjoy doing, a creative parent might be enlisted to make the bookmarks.

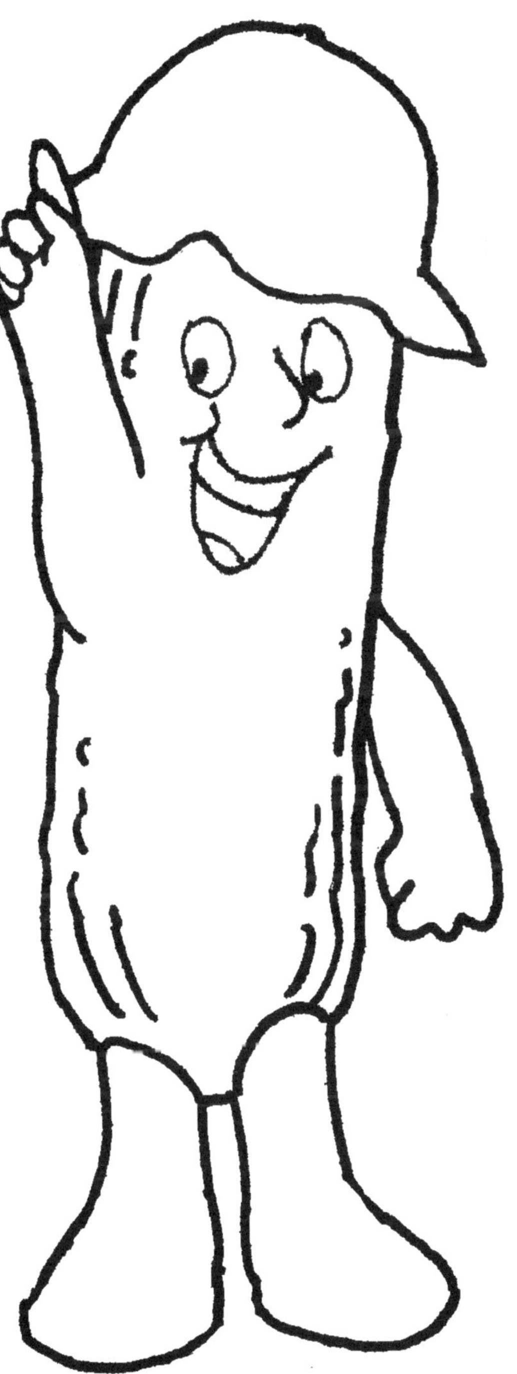

As a Caring Project, bookmarks may be made by the students and given to organizations or put into books.

AUTOGRAPH BOOK:

You may make an autograph book by folding and stapling half-sheets of computer paper, construction paper, etc. Or you may purchase a small notebook, about 3" by 4", with spiral binding. Do not purchase a notebook with a glued-end binding. The pages fall out too easily.

PACKED PICKLE:

The simplest way to make the packs is to pack the pickle bookmark, the autograph book, and one or two markers into a small paper sack. However, a creative parent may wish to make cloth bags.

Packed Pickle is used for career education. It can go to work with a child's parent, to the hospital, on a vacation, etc. You may even have a student take it home for a weekend and get autographs of workers wherever they can be found. Be sure to tell the students to ask the adult to give his/her autograph and also to write the title of his/her job.

THE PICKLE SWEEP

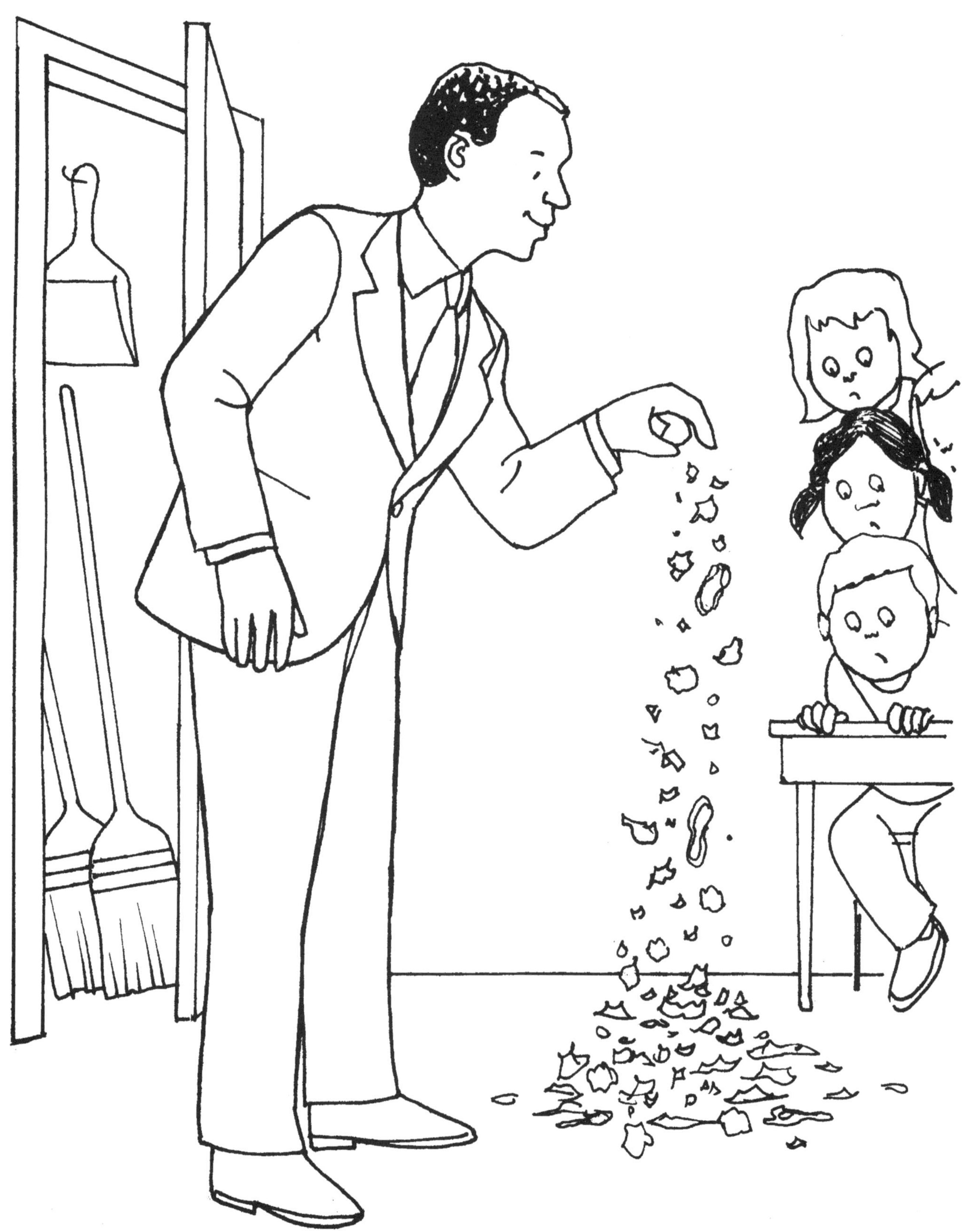

It was autumn, and the leaves were falling from the trees. But faster than the leaves were falling from the trees, the papers were falling to the floor in Mr. Miller's second-grade classroom. The children were cutting out teeny, tiny leaves to put inside kaleidoscopes. Each child was making one to keep for themselves and one to give to a homeless shelter for children's birthday gifts.

The piles of paper were getting bigger and bigger. Mr. Miller asked four students to take the two brooms and dustpans from the closet and sweep up the bits of paper. When the children started to do what Mr. Miller had asked, it very quickly became obvious that two of them had no idea how to use a broom and dustpan. Teaching children to use a broom and dustpan was not in Mr. Miller's lesson plan for the day. But one look at what was going on, and he decided he had better give the class a lesson on how to use a broom and dustpan. Little did he know when he started the lesson that all the children would want a turn. This unplanned lesson took so much time that Mr. Miller breathed a sign of relief when the bell rang for the children to go home.

Mr. Miller knew that he had been rescued for this day only. Tomorrow morning, when the children came to school, he had better have a plan. So he borrowed 10 more brooms and 10 more dustpans, which he hid in the closet. The next day, after the class had settled down for the morning's work, Mr. Miller began throwing bits of paper, cotton balls, and rubber bands on the floor. The children didn't know what to think. They wondered if their teacher had gone crazy.

When he was through throwing things on the floor and the children were staring at him in amazement, Mr. Miller told them that he was going to teach them how to use a broom and dustpan. Mr. Miller then demonstrated how one person can sweep and hold a dustpan at the same time. Looking for a volunteer, Mr. Miller chose Kelly. She had raised her hand, and he believed she could do the job. Kelly found out that the sweeping was easy, but getting everything into the dustpan wasn't.

Then Mr. Miller asked, "How could we make this easier for Kelly?"

"Use two people." "Get a helper." "Cooperation." The students in the class had lots of suggestions.

"That's a great idea," said Mr. Miller, and he told all of the students to get partners. Then he took the brooms and dustpans out of the closet. While the children were working together to get the trash off the floor, they heard the *Hokey Pokey* being played in the music class next door. Kelly started sweeping in time to the music and singing. Mr. Miller watched as Kelly swept up the trash while keeping time with the music.

As Kelly swept away, Mr. Miller got an idea. If this was so much fun for Kelly, then it would also be fun for the rest of the class. But if it was to mean anything, it couldn't just be any song with any words. It had to be special. After the children had swept up the trash and put the brooms and dustpans away, Mr. Miller told the children they were going to write a song to the tune of the *Hokey Pokey.* Then he asked Kelly to write the children's words on the chalkboard as they worked together to write the song. When the children were finished, they titled their song *Pickle Sweep*, because it was written at Pickle Mountain School.

Before class ended, Mr. Miller brought out the brooms and all of the children did the *Pickle Sweep.*

Follow-Up Questions: 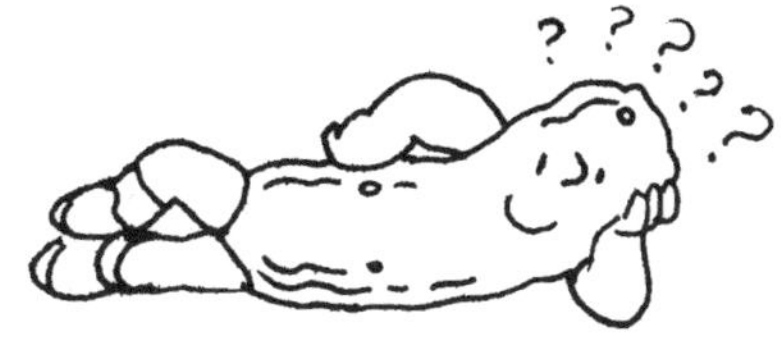

1. What time of year was it? ____________________

2. What were Mr. Miller's students going to do with the kaleidoscopes? ____________________

   ____

3. To what other places could you give something to help children?

   ____

   ____

   ____

4. Would grown-ups in a hospital or retirement home like something made by children? ____________________

5. Do you think Mr. Miller taught the students in a kindly way how to sweep? ____________________

   ____

6. How do you think the children cooperated to make the sweeping easier? ____________________

   ____

7. How could the students use their new skill to be more responsible?

   ____

   ____

8. Mr. Miller had 2 brooms and borrowed 10 more. How many brooms did he have in all? ____________________

9. Did Mr. Miller have the same number of dustpans and brooms?

   ____

Answers To Follow-Up Questions:

1. What time of year was it? *(Autumn.)*
2. What were Mr. Miller's students going to do with the kaleidoscopes? *(They were going to take half to the homeless shelter to be used for children's presents and keep the other half for themselves.)*
3. To what other places could you give something to help children? *(Accept any appropriate answers.)*
4. Would grown-ups in a hospital or retirement home like something made by children? *(Yes.)*
5. Do you think Mr. Miller taught the students in a kindly way how to sweep? *(Yes. He didn't make fun of them. He just showed them how to use the broom and dustpan.)*
6. How do you think the children cooperated to make the sweeping easier? *(Accept any appropriate answers.)*
7. How could the students use their new skill to be more responsible? *(They could help clean the classroom after a messy activity or offer to help sweep up a mess at home. They may also have learned that working together makes everyone more responsible.)*
8. Mr. Miller had 2 brooms and borrowed 10 more. How many brooms did he have in all? *(Mr. Miller had 12 brooms.)*
9. Did Mr. Miller have the same number of dustpans as brooms? *(Yes.)*

THE PICKLE SWEEP SONG

(Sung to the tune of the *Hokey Pokey*)

You put your broom out front.
You put your broom out back.
You put your broom out front
And you sweep it just like that.
You do the Pickle Sweep
And you sweep the bad stuff out.
That's what it's all about.

You put your dustpan up.
You put your dustpan down.
You put your dustpan up,
And then you move it to the ground.
You do the Pickle Sweep
And you sweep the bad stuff out.
That's what it's all about.

You do the Piii-ckle Sweep.
You do the Piii-ckle Sweep.
You do the Piii-ckle Sweep
And you sweep the bad stuff OUT!

BIG AND BIGGER FIELD TRIPS

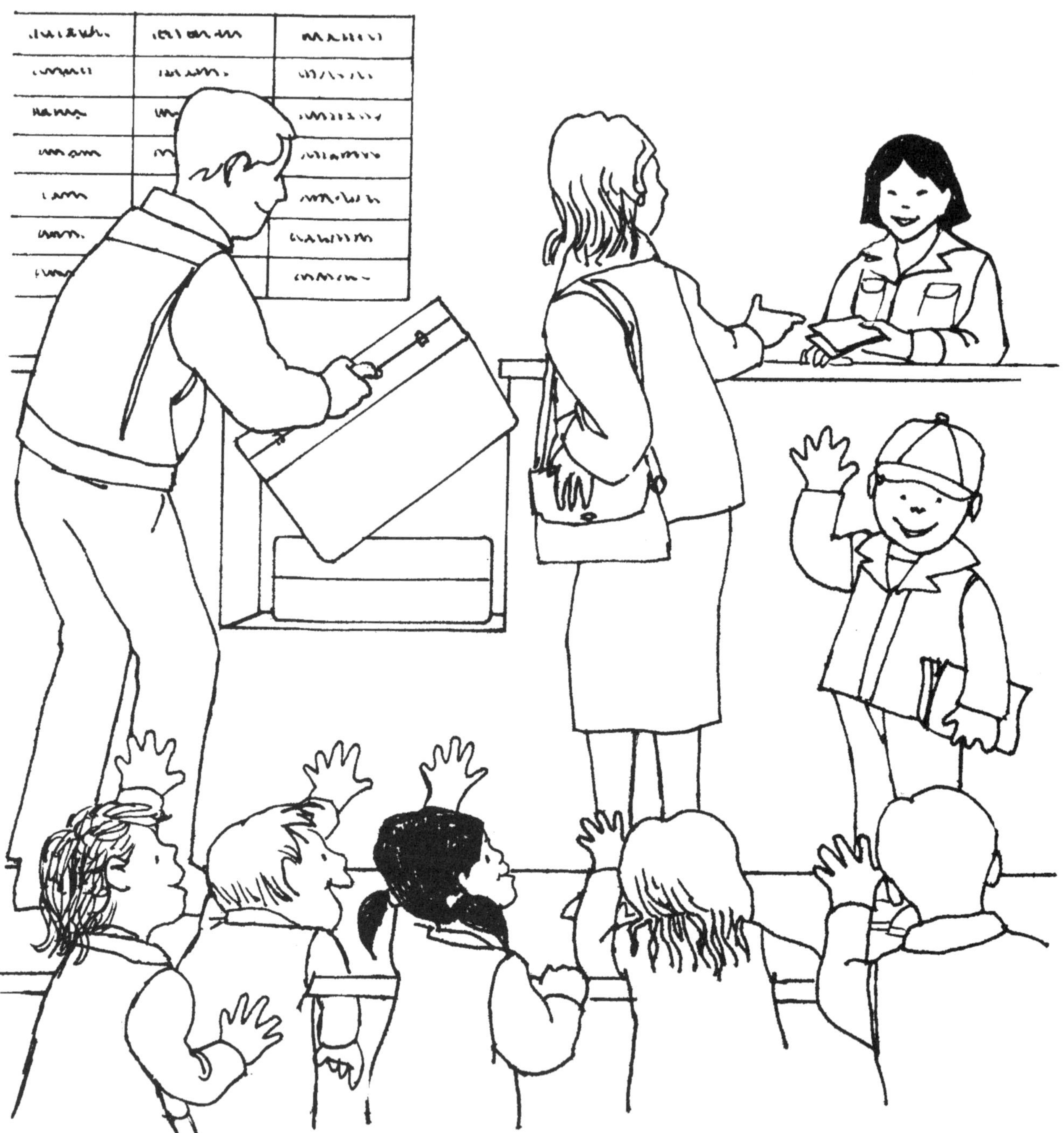

Malcolm's class at Pickle Mountain School was going on a big field trip, but Malcolm was going on an even *bigger* field trip. He had won a trip to watch the launch of a space shuttle in Florida. Even though it was a long drive to the airport in Centerbrook, Malcolm's whole class was going to see him off.

Only three of Malcolm's classmates had ever been to the airport. When the students arrived, they were surprised to see people doing so many different jobs. First, the porter helped Malcolm's mom get the luggage out of the car. Then an airline agent took Malcolm's ticket and checked his luggage. The airport manager came over and welcomed the students, and the school had arranged for flight attendants and a pilot to talk with the students.

When it was time for Malcolm's family to go to their plane's gate, the students in his class gave him a *Packed Pickle* to take to Florida. They told him he was to get autographs of the workers he met on his trip. "Maybe," they said, "he could even get the autograph of an astronaut." Malcolm thanked his classmates for thinking of him and told them he would get all the autographs he could. Then he said good-bye and the security guards screened their luggage and checked his family through the security gate.

After Malcolm's family went to their plane's gate, the students went over to the snack bar and paid the cashier for some cookies. Then the class boarded a bus which took them to the control tower. On the way, they saw groundskeepers mowing the grass on the other side of the runway. They saw mechanics checking out the planes, and a fuel truck operator putting gas into an airplane's tank. When they reached the control tower, they looked up and saw the air traffic controller. They weren't allowed in the tower, because they might distract the air traffic controller who was responsible for helping planes have safe takeoffs and landings. The job was too important to take a chance on that happening. Next to the control tower was the fire station. There they saw the firefighters who stayed at the station in case of an emergency. The students were lucky enough to be given a tour of the fire station.

Finally, it was time for the students to return to the bus that had brought them to the airport. It was time for them to go back home. They had had a big field trip, but Malcolm was flying to Florida on an even *bigger* field trip.

Follow-Up Questions: 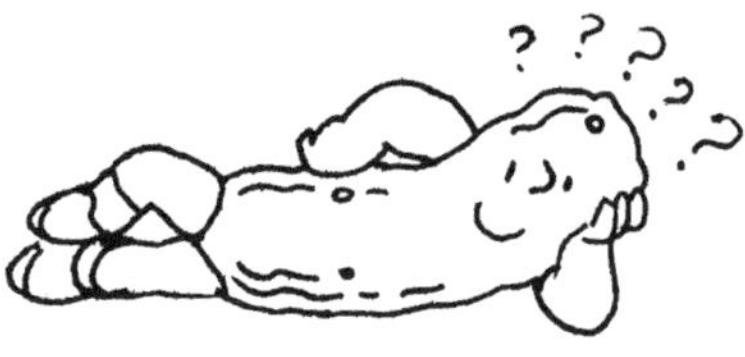

1. What do you think Malcolm will see on his field trip? ________

____

2. Which workers at the airport went with Malcolm on the airplane?

____

3. Do you think the students saw any workers cleaning at the airport?

____

4. Do you think anyone cooks at the airport? ________________

____

5. If the cookies the students bought cost 25¢ a piece, how many could they buy for $1.00? ________________________

6. If Malcolm got on the plane at 11:05 a.m. and the plane took off at 11:30 a.m., how long did Malcolm have to wait? ____________

____

Answers To Follow-Up Questions:

1. What do you think Malcolm will see on his field trip? *(Accept any appropriate answers.)*
2. Which workers at the airport went with Malcolm on the airplane? *(The pilot and the flight attendants went on the airplane.)*
3. Do you think the students saw any workers cleaning at the airport? *(Accept any appropriate answers.)*
4. Do you think anyone cooks at the airport? *(Yes, there are cooks for the restaurants.)*
5. If the cookies the students bought cost 25¢ a piece, how many could they buy for $1.00? *(Four cookies.)*
6. If Malcolm got on the plane at 11:05 a.m. and the plane took off at 11:30 a.m., how long did Malcolm have to wait? *(Malcolm waited 25 minutes.)*

Name ______________________________

THE AIRPORT

Look at the picture below and answer the following questions.

How many vehicles do you see in the picture? ______________

Which vehicle would be the slowest? ______________________

Which vehicle would be the fastest? ______________________

Which vehicle could carry the most passengers at one time?

____

Name some workers who would be needed at this part of the airport. ____

____

Now color your picture.

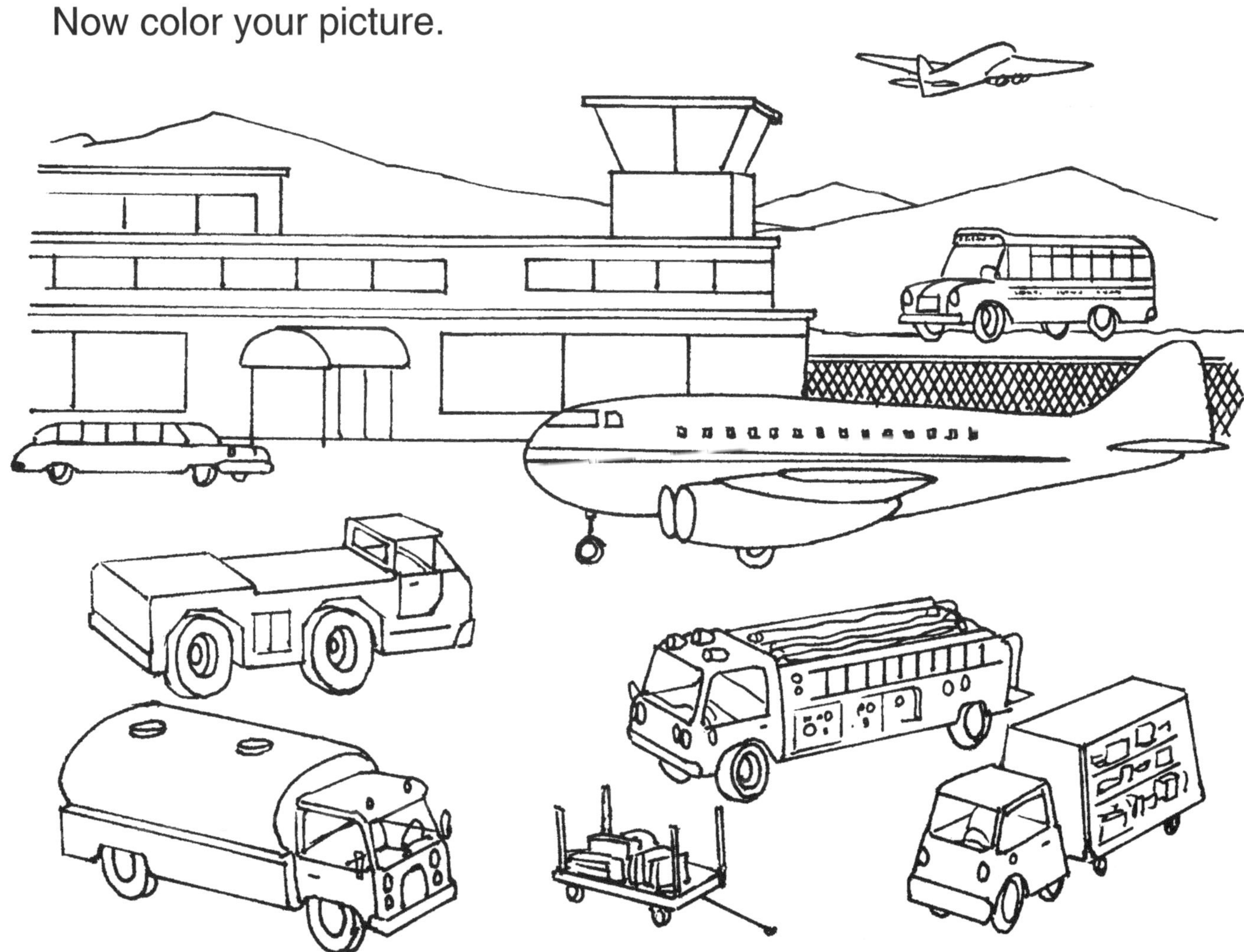

LUNCH FOR SUSAN'S GRANDMOTHER

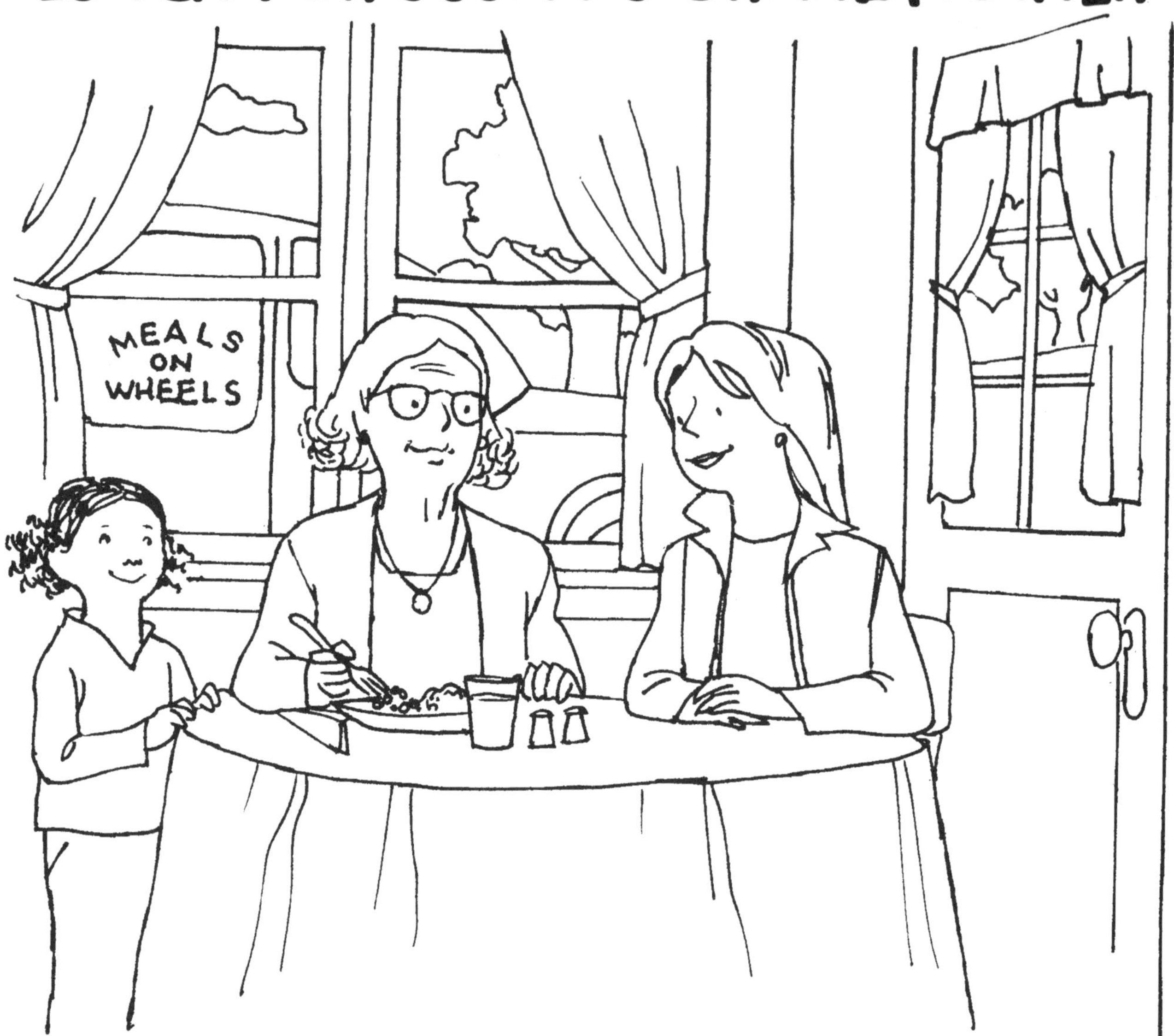

Susan's grandmother lived 12 miles from Pickle Mountain School, in a large stone house on a narrow road. Six months ago, when she was going down some stairs, she slipped and broke her hip. When she first came out of the hospital, she stayed at Susan's house. But after two weeks, she wanted to be at her own house even though she would be alone much of the time.

Susan worried about her grandmother. She talked to her every night on the telephone. On Saturdays, Susan took lunch to her grandmother and spent the night. On Sunday morning, her parents would pick both of them up and take them to Susan's house. Then they would have a big lunch. This was great, but Susan wondered what her grandmother did for lunch when it wasn't Saturday or Sunday. Did she eat lunch on Monday, Tuesday, Thursday?

On the following Wednesday, the teachers were having meetings. Susan didn't have to go to school that day, so she went to spend the day with her grandmother. At 11:15, Susan heard a car coming up the driveway. It stopped outside the house and a lady carrying a box got out. "There's lunch!" exclaimed Grandmother.

The lady brought the food in, sat down, and visited with Susan's grandmother. Susan thought she knew all of her grandmother's neighbors, but she had never seen this woman before. Curious to know who the woman was, Susan asked, "Are you a neighbor of my grandmother's?" The lady told her she wasn't a neighbor, but a volunteer for Meals On Wheels. She explained that she delivered meals to five people who did not leave their homes very often and that there were other volunteers who took food to different homes.

When Susan went home that evening, she thought about her grandmother and the lady from Meals On Wheels. She was glad to know that her grandmother got a good lunch each day while she was at school. She was also glad that such a kind lady cared enough to take time to visit with her grandmother when she brought the food.

A few weeks later, when Susan's class was talking about caring for others and how they could do this in some way, she told them about Meals On Wheels. She told them how the volunteers help others, like her grandmother, not only with food but also by spending a little time with them each day. When she finished, the class decided that this would be their "Caring Project." They would collect pennies and donate the money to Meals On Wheels. They would give their own pennies, ask their parents for some pennies, and carefully watch for any pennies that were on the ground. Collecting the pennies would be the way they would show that they cared about others.

Follow-Up Questions: 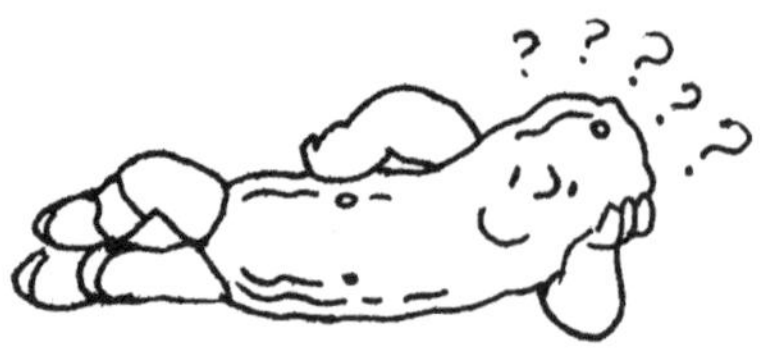

1. What is a volunteer? ______________________________

____

2. How do volunteers show that they are good citizens? ______

____

____

3. Do you think Susan's grandmother was appreciative? ______

4. What did the volunteer do other than just bring food? ______

____

5. If it was a 10-mile round trip to take food to Susan's grandmother, how many miles did the volunteer travel in five days? ______

Answers To Follow-Up Questions:

1. What is a volunteer? *(A volunteer is someone who does something for someone else without receiving any pay.)*
2. How do volunteers show that they are good citizens? *(Volunteers show that they are good citizens by giving their time to help other people.)*
3. Do you think Susan's grandmother was appreciative? *(Yes.)*
4. What did the volunteer do other than just bring food? *(She spent time talking with Susan's grandmother.)*
5. If it was a 10-mile round trip to take food to Susan's grandmother, how many miles did the volunteer travel in five days? *(The volunteer traveled 50 miles.)*

Name ______________________________

MEALS ON WHEELS

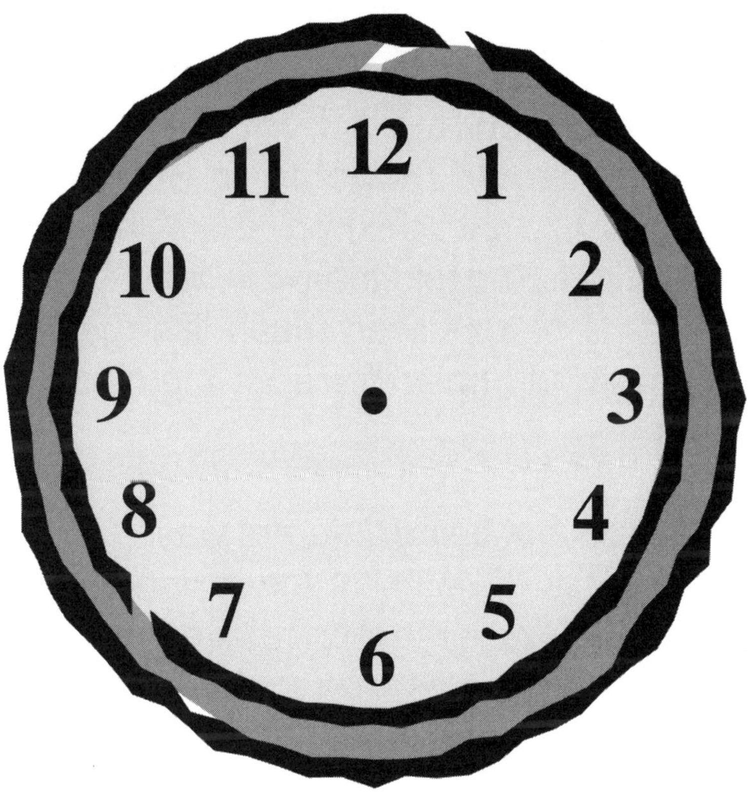

Make the clock show the time that *Meals On Wheels* brought lunch to Susan's grandmother.

Draw pictures of some food the volunteer might bring for Susan's grandmother.

PACKED LIKE PICKLES

When the school year ended and everyone had gone home for summer vacation, the school nurse, Miss Vansen, told the children that she would be going to Honduras, helping in a medical center. She told the children about the people she would meet and how they lived. She told them she would travel through a big city where most of the people lived much like the children of Pickle Mountain. Then she would travel far from the cities to places where life was very different.

Miss Vansen explained that being different wasn't always a problem. It was true that the homes of some of the children in Honduras didn't have electricity and their parents didn't have cars, but they did have families who loved them. It was true that they didn't have fast-food restaurants, but they had food which was grown near their homes. You might think they were sad, but they weren't. They were happy playing games with the other children, swimming in the river, and singing songs.

Then Miss Vansen asked, "How many children at Pickle Mountain School would think a pencil was a wonderful gift?" "What a silly question!" the children thought. Then Miss Vansen told them that the children she would see could not go to school without a pencil, and sometimes they didn't have one. There were also other things that the children in Honduras found exciting, and Miss Vansen told the children as much as she knew.

The children at Pickle Mountain School listened carefully to Miss Vansen. They cared about other people and now, after hearing what Miss Vansen told them, they knew they could also care about children they didn't know. In fact, her words made the children start talking about all kinds of things they could send to the children in Honduras.

"Whoa!" said Miss Vansen. "What you're doing is great, but some of the things you are talking about are large. How would we get big things there? I can't put much in my suitcase, and it is really expensive to mail big packages so far away." Then Miss Vansen held up a jar of sweet gherkins and said, "See how lots of little pickles are packed in this jar? We'd have to pack like pickles to get things to Honduras. The things we send must fit together closely in a small box, and nothing can break or spoil."

"I think what we should do," Miss Vansen continued, "is make a list of little things that would excite the children in Honduras. A *little thing* means that if it wouldn't fit in a toothpaste box, then it is too big." Miss Vansen and the children began to make a list of things they could pack like pickles and send to Honduras. Their list looked like this:

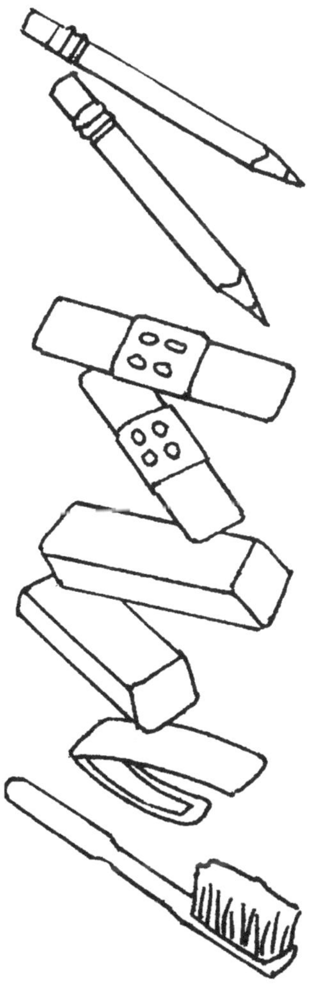

pencils

bandages

small balls

erasers

barrettes

lip balm

little cars

toothbrushes

markers

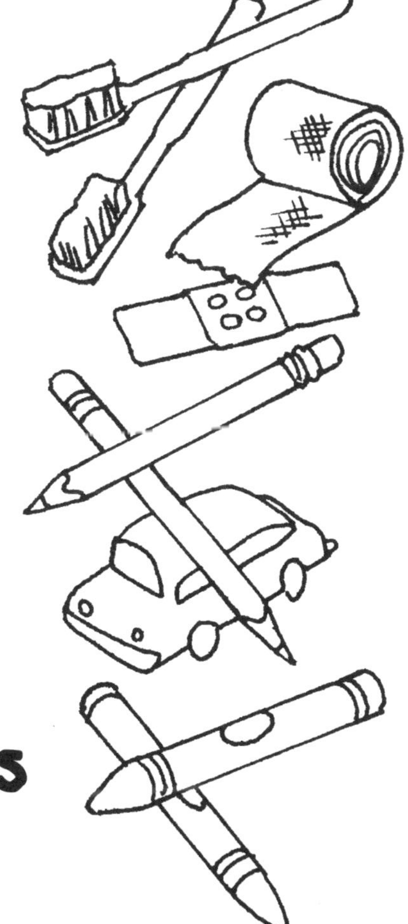

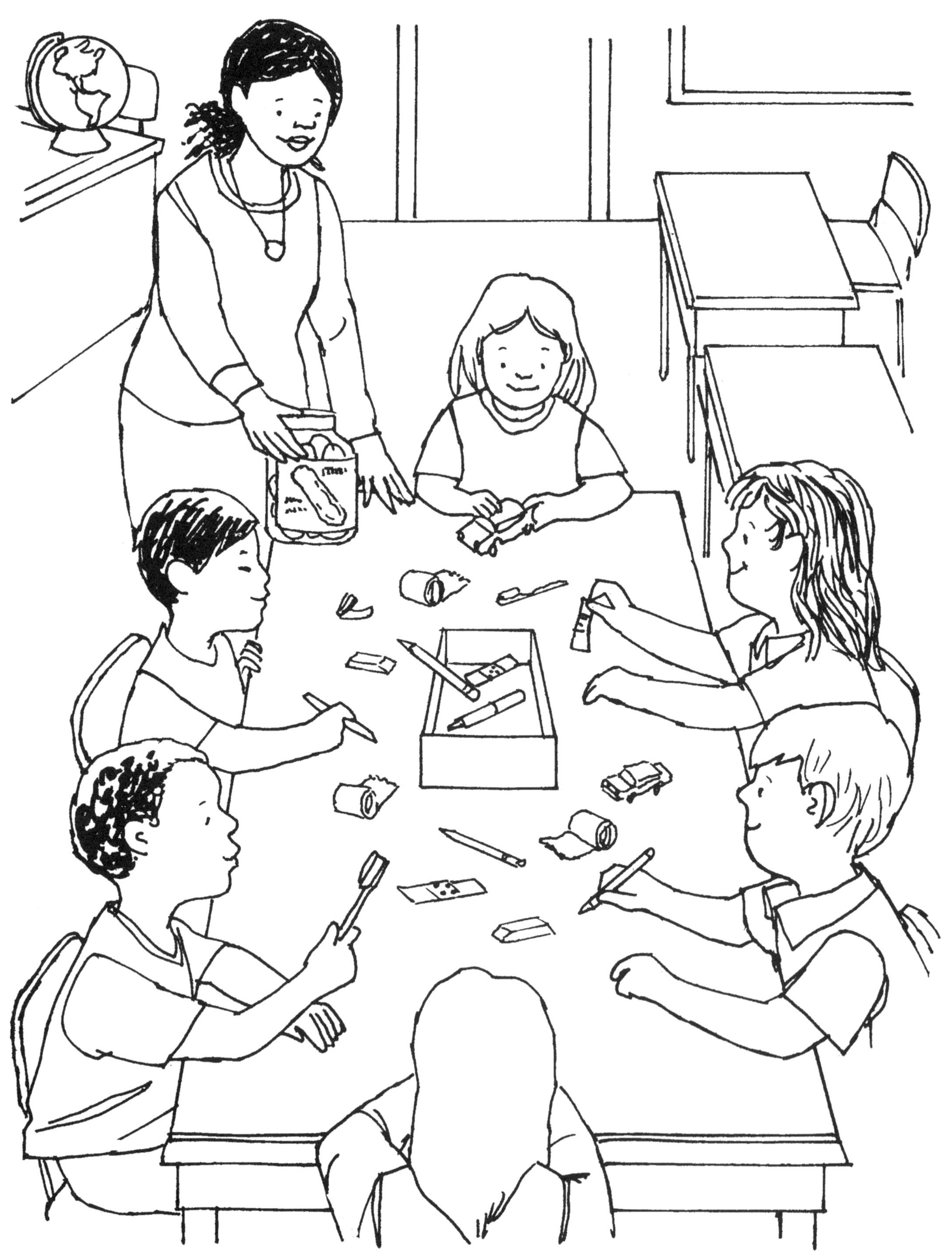

Follow-Up Questions: 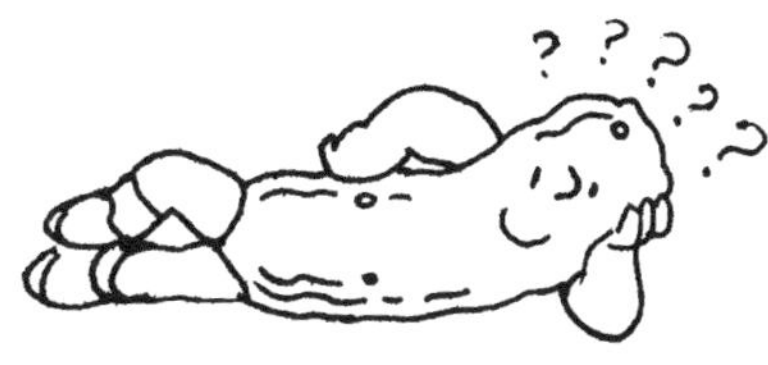

1. Where in the United States would children appreciate little items?

   ____

   ____

2. Is there a place nearby that might need things? ____________

   ____

3. Do you think Miss Vansen will mail the items in pickle jars?

   ____

4. Besides what was on the children's list, what can you think of that would fit in a toothpaste box? ____________________

   ____

   ____

5. What fun things could you do without electricity? ___________

   ____

   ____

6. The children brought empty toothpaste boxes to school. Mrs. Walker's Class brought 15 and Mr. Sanchez's class brought 14. How many boxes did the two classes have? ______________

7. When Miss Vansen shipped all the little boxes in one big box, it cost $25.00. How much change did she get from $30.00?

   ____

Answers To Follow-Up Questions:

1. Where in the United States would children appreciate little items? *(Accept any appropriate answers.)*
2. Is there a place nearby that might need things? *(Accept any appropriate answers.)*
3. Do you think Miss Vansen will mail the items in pickle jars? *(No. They might break.)*
4. Besides what was on the children's list, what can you think of that would fit in a toothpaste box? *(Accept any appropriate answers.)*
5. What fun things could you do without electricity? *(Accept any appropriate answers.)*
6. The children brought empty toothpaste boxes to school. Mrs. Walker's Class brought 15 and Mr. Sanchez's class brought 14. How many boxes did the two classes have? *(The two classes had 29 boxes.)*
7. When Miss Vansen shipped all the little boxes in one big box, it cost $25.00. How much change did she get from $30.00? *(She received $5.00 in change.)*

THE "UNEMPTY" HOUSE

There had been an empty house on Pickle Mountain for nine years. The children made up stories about what was inside the house and why no one lived in it. Once in a while, someone would come to clean the house and make sure everything was all right.

The children were surprised one August day to see carpenters, painters, plumbers, and carpet installers going into and out of the house. Then they saw a big moving van with a houseful of furniture and boxes stop in front of the house. The house that had been empty for nine years wasn't empty any more. It was "unempty."

The children were curious about who would live in the house. They watched it carefully. The next day, they saw a mom, a girl about three, a boy about seven, and a bigger boy who looked like he was about nine years old. They saw their school principal and counselor go to the front door, introduce themselves, and welcome the family to the neighborhood.

As time went on, the children learned that the mother had grown up in the house and had lived there after she had gotten married. When she and her husband were about to have their first baby, they went to stay in Centerville, near the hospital. When the baby was born, they named him Jude. Jude was ill for a very long time and the family couldn't return home. They needed to stay in Centerville to be near the doctors. With good care, Jude recovered from all his problems. Except one. He could not hear. The family needed to stay in Centerville to get help for Jude and to learn sign language.

A few months earlier, when the house was still empty, the children had heard that a man who used to live there had died. The man who died was Jude's father. When he died, Jude's mother decided to return to the house where she had lived as a little girl and a bride.

Jude did not come to school on the first day of school. Jude's teacher knew that Jude would be in his class, but he wanted time to prepare the other children to better understand Jude. The school already had a first-grade girl in a wheelchair and a second-grade boy who could not talk, but they did not have a deaf child. Jude's teacher led the children in different activities that helped them understand disabilities. They learned a few words in sign language, so they would be able to welcome Jude. They also learned how to spell their own names in sign language, so they could introduce themselves to Jude. Then they made simple dictionaries to help them talk with their new friend. They wanted to do everything they could to make Jude feel a part of their class.

Learning sign language was not the first time these students had learned different things to make someone welcome. The year before, the children had learned some Spanish when a new family came to Pickle Mountain. They learned some Japanese when a foreign exchange student had been with them for a year. It was fun to speak a few words in a different language. And now, they were learning a new language—a language that was spoken with their hands. It was an exciting time! And it was all happening because the empty house had become "unempty" when Jude and his family came to live in it.

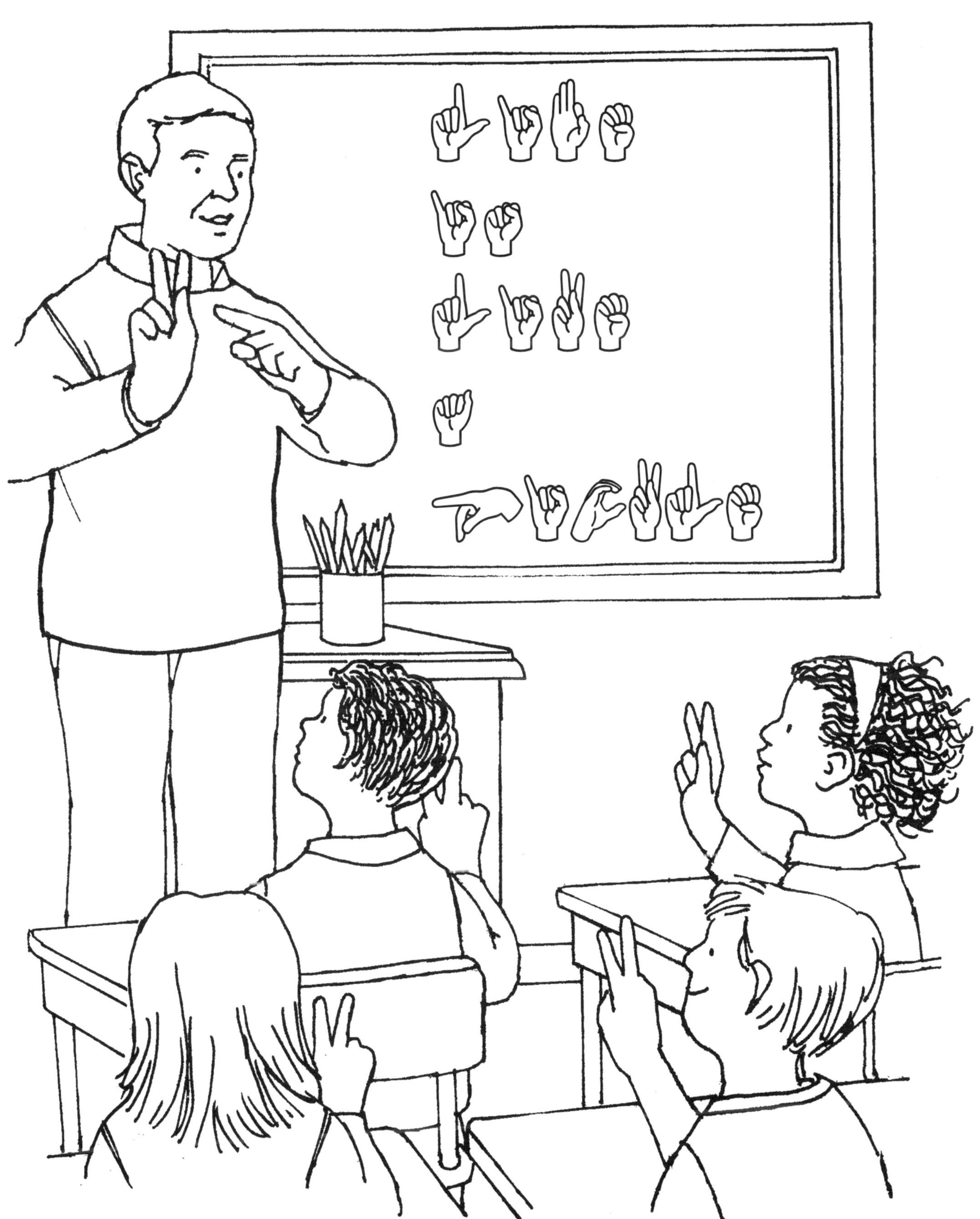

Follow-Up Questions: 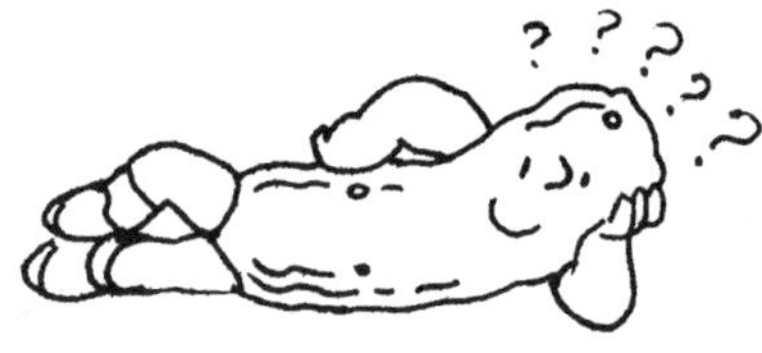

1. What workers prepared the house before the family moved in?
____

2. Why had the family moved to Centerville? _______________
____

3. Why had the family moved back to Pickle Mountain? ________
____

4. What disabilities have you learned about in your school?
____
____

5. What are ways that we are all different from each other? _____
____
____
____

6. How do you show respect for people who are different from you?
____
____

7. If a carpet layer earned $8.00 and hour and worked four hours, how much money did he earn? _______________________

Answers To Follow-Up Questions:

1. What workers prepared the house before the family moved in? *(The workers included: carpenters, painters, plumbers, carpet installers, and movers.)*
2. Why had the family moved to Centerville? *(The family went to Centerville to await the birth of their first baby.)*
3. Why had the family moved back to Pickle Mountain? *(The family moved back to Pickle Mountain because the father had died and the mother wanted to return to the house where she had previously lived.)*
4. What disabilities have you learned about in your school? *(Accept any appropriate answers.)*
5. What are ways that we are all different from each other? *(Accept any appropriate answers.)*
6. How do you show respect for people who are different from you? *(Accept any appropriate answers.)*
7. If a carpet layer earned $8.00 and hour and worked four hours, how much money did he earn? *(He earned $32.00.)*

PENNY PAUSES

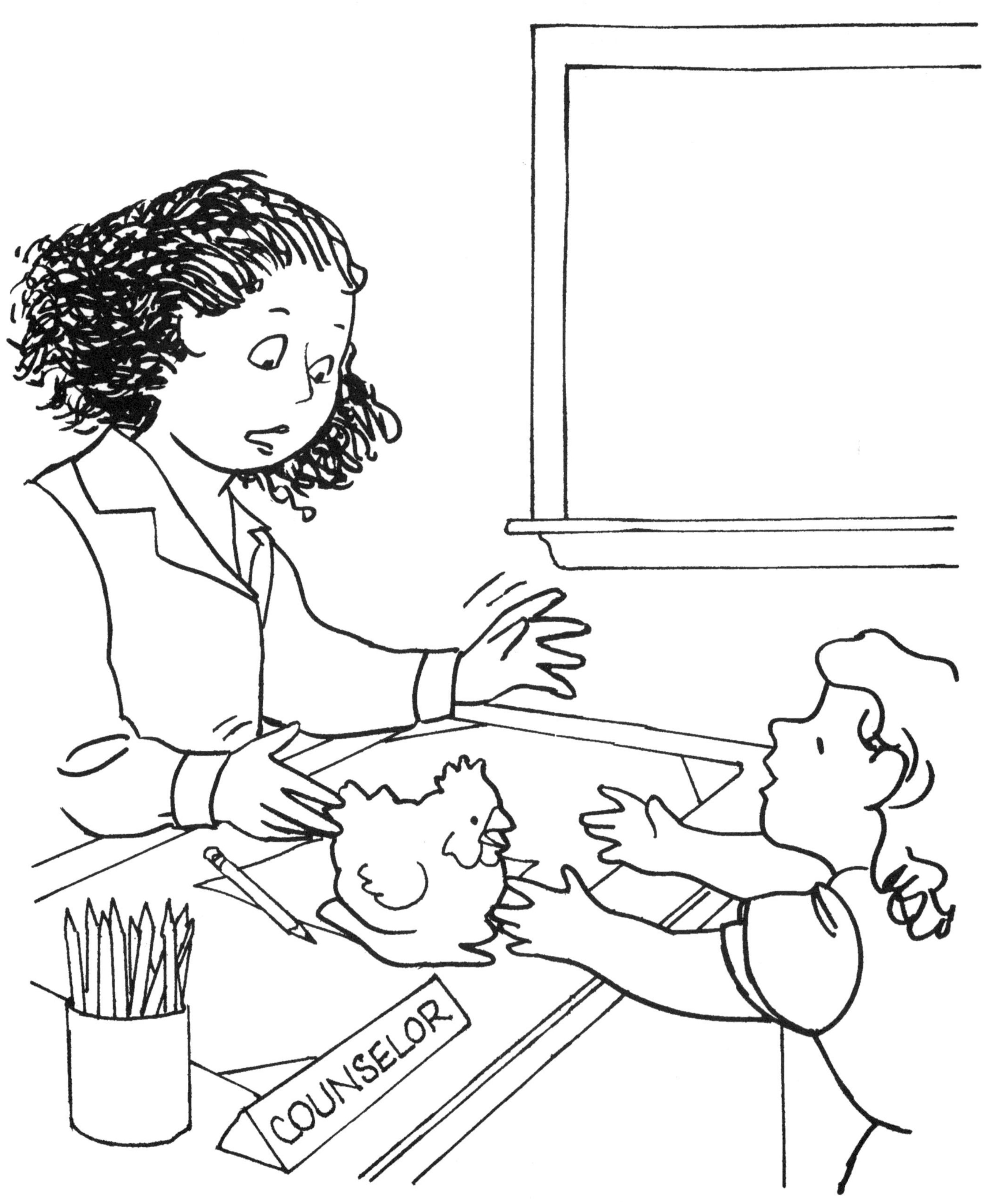

This is the story of a girl named Penny. Everywhere she went, she asked if people would give her things. Have you ever known anyone like Penny? Just listen to the things she asked for in just one morning at Pickle Mountain School.

Penny asked the bus driver is she could have the fancy red cup he used for his coffee.

Penny asked Randy if she could have his new marker.

She asked the teacher for a piece of tape for her paper.

She asked the teacher for the whole bottle of lotion that was on her desk.

A police officer visited the school with a bucket of safety stickers. Penny asked if she could have the bucket.

At lunch, Penny asked Paul for his birthday cupcake.

She asked the lunchroom helper for the carton of milk another student didn't want.

One day, Penny was in the counselor's office. She asked for one of the puppets Mrs. Jones used in her guidance lessons. Mrs. Jones looked at Penny and said, "Penny, that puppet cost me $5.00. I have 500 students. Do you know how much money I would need to give each of my students a puppet?"

Penny thought for a moment. She was good at math, and she quickly answered "$2,500.00. I guess you don't have that much money."

Mrs. Jones knew that Penny was always asking for things, and she wanted to help her to know *when* to ask for things. Mrs. Jones took out a 3" x 5" card and sat down next to Penny. Then she said, "Let's write down some ideas on this card that will help you to know when it is the right time to ask for something." Mrs. Jones took out her pen and began to write:

Before you ask for something, ask yourself these questions:

> Does it cost a lot?
>
> Is there enough for lots of children?
>
> Does it look like it was meant to be given away?

Then Mrs. Jones said, "When you ask yourself these questions, if the answers are *yes,* it does cost a lot and *no,* there isn't enough for lots of children; and *no,* it doesn't look like it was meant to be given away, then you will know not to ask for it."

Mrs. Jones gave the card to Penny and told her to put it in a safe place. Then she smiled and patted Penny on the back. Penny smiled back and left the office.

It wasn't long before Penny saw Lori writing in her new tablet. Penny opened her mouth to ask for the tablet, but then she remembered what was written on her card. She asked herself the three questions. Her answers were: Yes, it did cost a lot. No, there wasn't enough for lots of children. No, it wasn't meant to be given away. Penny walked away without asking for the tablet.

As the days went by, Penny learned to think about her three questions before asking for something. What she didn't realize was that everyone noticed the change in her. Everyone noticed that Penny was much more polite, and they liked her much better.

Follow-Up Questions: 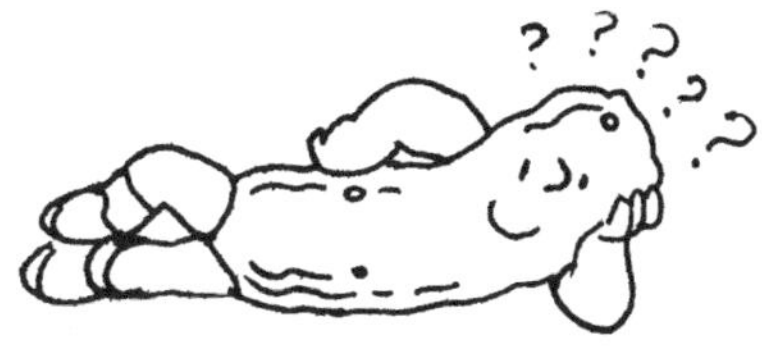

1. Do you think the bus driver gave his coffee cup away every day?

   ____

   If the cup costs $2.00, how much money would he need to buy cups for the school week? ____________________________

2. Did Randy bring new markers for all the children? __________

3. Do you think the teacher has tape to share with students?

   ____

4. How do you think the police officer felt when Penny asked for the bucket? ______________________________________

5. When Penny asked the lunchroom worker for milk someone had put back, was she taking it away from someone? ___________

6. Do you think Mrs. Jones was angry at Penny? _____________

7. How did Mrs. Jones show that she cared about Penny? _____

   ____

Answers To Follow-Up Questions:

1. Do you think the bus driver gave his coffee cup away every day? *(No.)* If the cup costs $2.00, how much money would he need to buy cups for the school week? *(He would need $10.00.)*
2. Did Randy bring new markers for all the children? *(No.)*
3. Do you think the teacher has tape to share with students? *(Yes or no. Either answer could be justified.)*
4. How do you think the police officer felt when Penny asked for the bucket? *(Accept all appropriate answers.)*
5. When Penny asked the lunchroom worker for milk someone had put back, was she taking it away from someone? *(Yes or no. Either answer could be justified.)*
6. Do you think Mrs. Jones was angry at Penny? *(No.)*
7. How did Mrs. Jones show that she cared about Penny? *(Mrs. Jones helped Penny solve her problem.)*

LAUGHING LEAVES

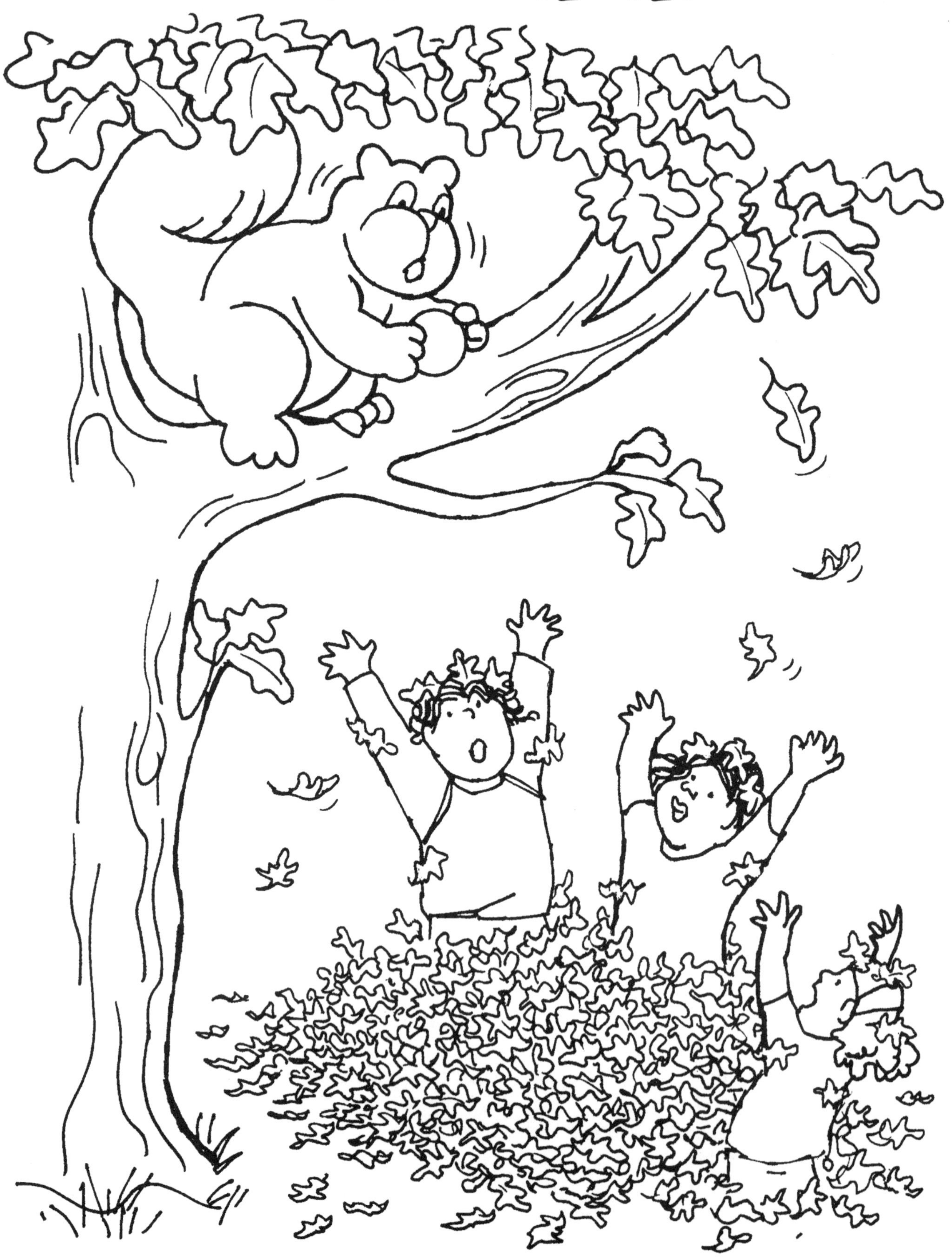

Outside Pickle Mountain School, the leaves swirled as they fell from the trees. It was autumn, and the wind threw the leaves up in the air like colorful fireworks. Recess turned the leaves into musical instruments, and the children romped through them, making joyful noises. The leaves seemed happy as they crunched and crumbled under the children's feet. It was almost as if the leaves were laughing. Lisa and her friends were jumping and kicking the leaves when a leaf landed in Lisa's hair. The leaf was so light that Lisa didn't know it was there until one of her friends yelled, "Lisa, you have something in your hair!" Lisa felt the leaf and said, "Look at me! I'm a tree. I'm growing leaves." She laughed, and her friends laughed with her. Then each girl put three leaves in her own hair.

The counselor sat nearby reading to a child. When the wind blew leaves onto her back and her legs, she laughed. Then the children piled more leaves on themselves, and they all laughed together.

While some children were giggling and digging through the leaves like they were looking for treasure, Tina was not laughing. She was searching for the ball to her new jacks set. It had come from her grandfather in a special leather bag. When the children looked at Tina's face, they knew this was a time *not* to laugh. Laughing would only make her feel worse. The best thing they could do was to help her search for the ball.

The children began digging through the leaves, searching for the ball, but nobody could find it. It just wasn't there. Tina said it *had* to be, because this is where she had lost it. As the children continued their search, they heard a strange sound on a tree branch above them. Looking up, they saw a squirrel. But they also saw something else. The squirrel had Tina's ball! "Hey, give us back Tina's ball!" yelled one of the children. The frightened squirrel dropped the ball. Down it came, landing right on Lisa's head. The squirrel scurried off, and Lisa gave Tina her ball. All the children laughed to think that a squirrel would take a tiny rubber ball. The more they thought about it, the harder they laughed. They all laughed and laughed among the laughing leaves.

Follow-Up Questions: 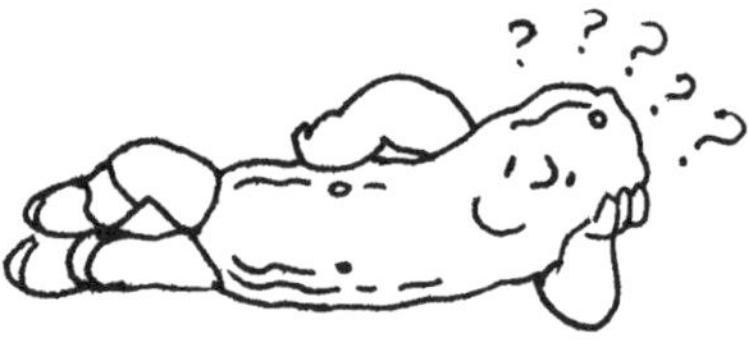

1. Should you *always* laugh when something you think is funny happens to someone else? ______________________________

2. Did the counselor get upset because her story was interrupted by the blowing leaves? ______________________________

   How do you know? ______________________________

   What is it called when a person does not get upset when something non-hurtful happens unexpectedly? ____________

3. How did the children know they shouldn't laugh at Tina? _____

   ____

4. How did the children show they cared about Tina? __________

   ____

   What is another word for caring? ____________________

5. Lisa was playing with three friends, who each put three leaves in their hair. How may leaves did the three girls have in their hair?

   ____

   ____

   How many leaves would there be if you added Lisa's one leaf?

   ____

Answers To Follow-Up Questions:

1. Should you *always* laugh when something you think is funny happens to someone else? *(No.)*
2. Did the counselor get upset because her story was interrupted by the blowing leaves? *(No.)* How do you know? *(She laughed.)* What is it called when a person does not get upset when something non-hurtful happens unexpectedly? *(Adaptability.)*
3. How did the children know they shouldn't laugh at Tina? *(They could tell by the look on her face that she was serious.)*
4. How did the children show they cared about Tina? *(They all helped her look for her ball.)* What is another word for caring? *(Compassion.)*
5. Lisa was playing with three friends, who each put three leaves in their hair. How may leaves did the three girls have in their hair? *(Nine leaves.)* How many leaves would there be if you added Lisa's one leaf? *(There would be ten leaves.)*

SNOW DAYS SECRETS

It was Carlos' first day at Pickle Mountain School. It was November, and soon it would snow. This was exciting for Carlos, who had come from Florida and had only seen snow on television.

Even on his first day, Carlos had fun with the children in his class. Mark showed him the "secret" place on the playground where they could find the most four-leaf clovers. Fay showed him the "secret" envelope where they were saving change to buy their teacher a present.

Just before it was time to go home, the teacher told the children she had some news, but they had to keep it a secret, even from the principal. A few weeks earlier, the class had written letters to a pickle company. They had told the story about how Pickle Mountain got its name and had drawn pictures to go with the story. The company president was so pleased with the children's effort that she decided to send a truck with jars of pickles and balloons for all the classes. She had notified the newspaper, and a photographer was coming to take pictures. All of this would happen on Monday, but it was a secret until then.

What a great first day for Carlos! He couldn't wait to go back to school!

That night, the weather changed. The next morning, Carlos woke up to what he had never seen before—snow. It kept snowing the next day and the next. On Monday, it was still snowing. The buses couldn't make it up the mountain to the school, and Carlos had another new experience—school cancelled because of snow.

By the time school reopened, the children had missed a whole week of classes. They were excited to be back in school. All except Carlos, who was very quiet and looked like he might cry. When the teacher asked what was wrong, Carlos wouldn't even look at her. He went to recess with Mark, but when Mark asked what was wrong, Carlos said, "It's a secret. I can't tell. Something happened at home and I'm not supposed to tell. But I'm worried about my little sister. I'm afraid she might get hurt while I'm at school."

Mark knew this was a secret that should be told. He went to Mrs. Jones, the counselor, and told her that something was bothering the new boy, Carlos. That afternoon Mrs. Jones asked Carlos to come to her office. Carlos had never been to a counselor before and he had never seen a room at school with so many toys and even a rocking chair. Mrs. Jones began to talk with Carlos. She didn't say anything about his secret, only that he seemed sad or maybe scared. As they began to talk, Carlos felt more and more safe. Finally, he felt safe enough to talk with her. His was a sour secret, and Mrs. Jones was glad he shared it with her. She made him feel even better when she said she would find a way to help.

Both Mrs. Jones and Carlos felt better, and as Carlos was getting ready to go back to class, they heard lots of happy noises outside her door. Mrs. Jones couldn't imagine what was going on. As she opened the door, Carlos remembered the secret the teacher had told them more than a week ago. This was a sweet secret, but it wasn't a secret any more.

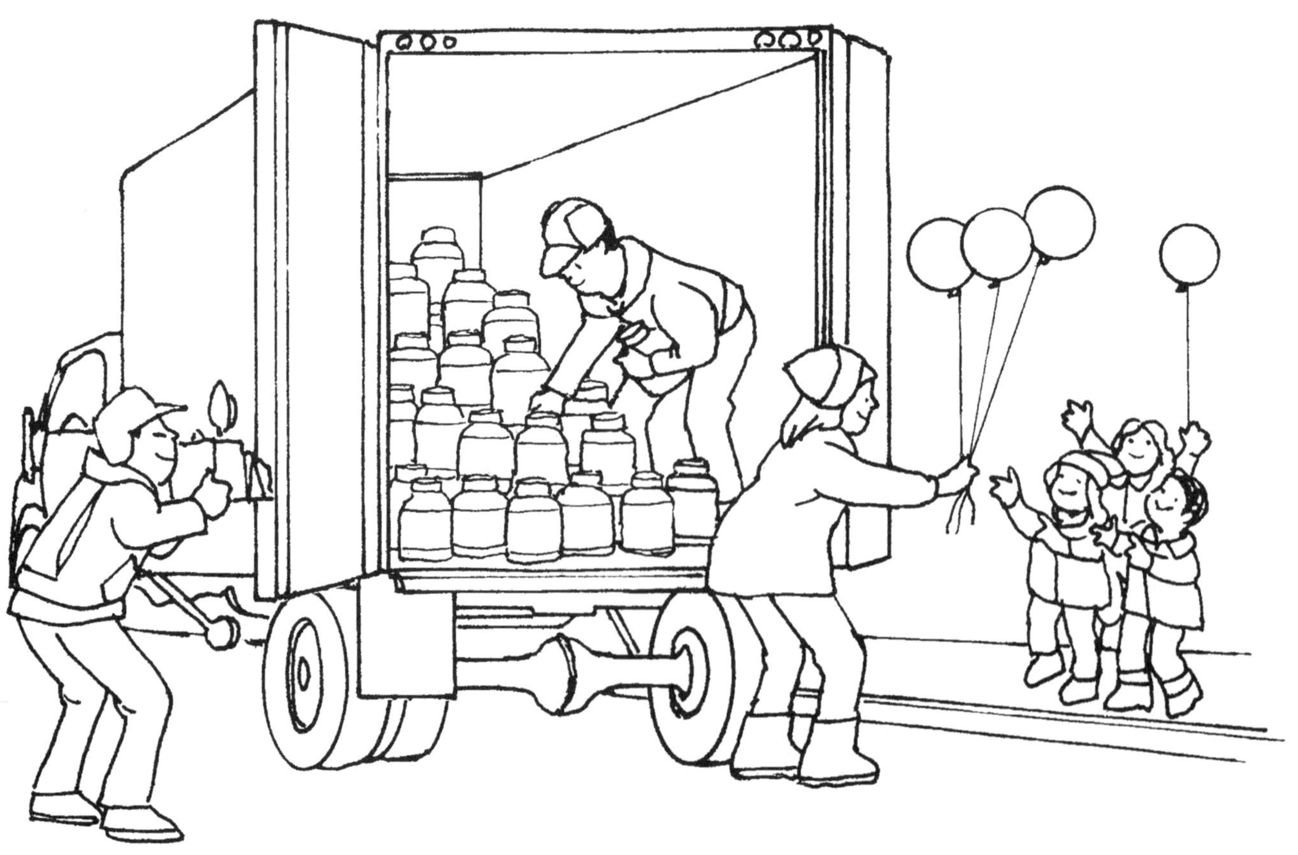

Follow-Up Questions

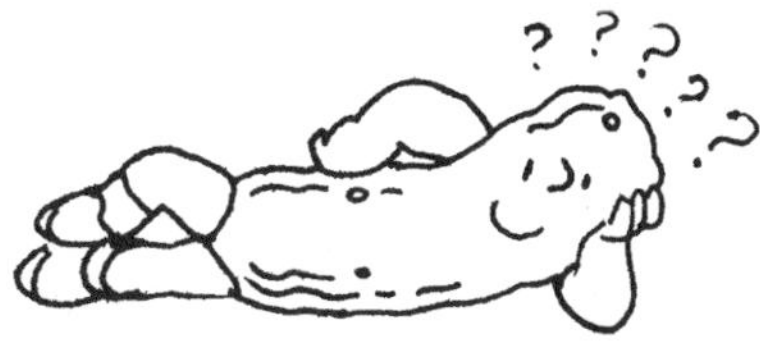

1. What fun, safe secrets did the children have? ____________
____
____

2. Was it all right for the teacher to keep her secret from the principal?
____

3. How did Mark show he cared for Carlos? ____________
____

4. Was it safe for Carlos to talk with the counselor? __________

5. Will Mrs. Jones tell all the students Carlos' secret? ________

6. What kinds of jobs might people do at the pickle factory? ____
____
____

7. How did the pickle company show adaptability? ____________
____

8. The teacher started the writing project on her own. Mark went to see the counselor without being told. What is the word for starting something yourself? ____________________

9. If the pickle company sent three cases of pickles and each case held 12 jars, how many jars of pickles went to Pickle Mountain School? ____________________

10. The deliveryman blew up five bags of balloons. Each bag held 100 balloons. How many balloons did he blow up? ________

    If 10 balloons popped, how many balloons were left? ______

Answers To Follow-Up Questions:

1. What fun, safe secrets did the children have? *(They knew where the most four-leaf clovers were, and they had an envelope with change that they were saving for a present for their teacher.)*
2. Was it all right for the teacher to keep her secret from the principal? *(Yes or no. Either answer could be justified.)*
3. How did Mark show he cared for Carlos? *(He told Mrs. Jones that there was something bothering Carlos.)*
4. Was it safe for Carlos to talk with the counselor? *(Yes.)*
5. Will Mrs. Jones tell all the students Carlos' secret? *(No.)*
6. What kinds of jobs might people do at the pickle factory? *(Make pickles, put pickles in jars, load pickles on trucks, etc.)*
7. How did the pickle company show adaptability? *(They rescheduled their visit because of the snow.)*
8. The teacher started the writing project on her own. Mark went to see the counselor without being told. What is the word for starting something yourself? *(Initiative.)*
9. If the pickle company sent three cases of pickles and each case held 12 jars, how many jars of pickles went to Pickle Mountain School? *(The pickle company sent 36 jars.)*
10. The deliveryman blew up five bags of balloons. Each bag held 100 balloons. How many balloons did he blow up? *(He blew up 500 balloons.)* If ten balloons popped, how many balloons were left? *(There were 490 balloons left.)*

THURSDAY,
THE THIRD DAY OF THIRD GRADE

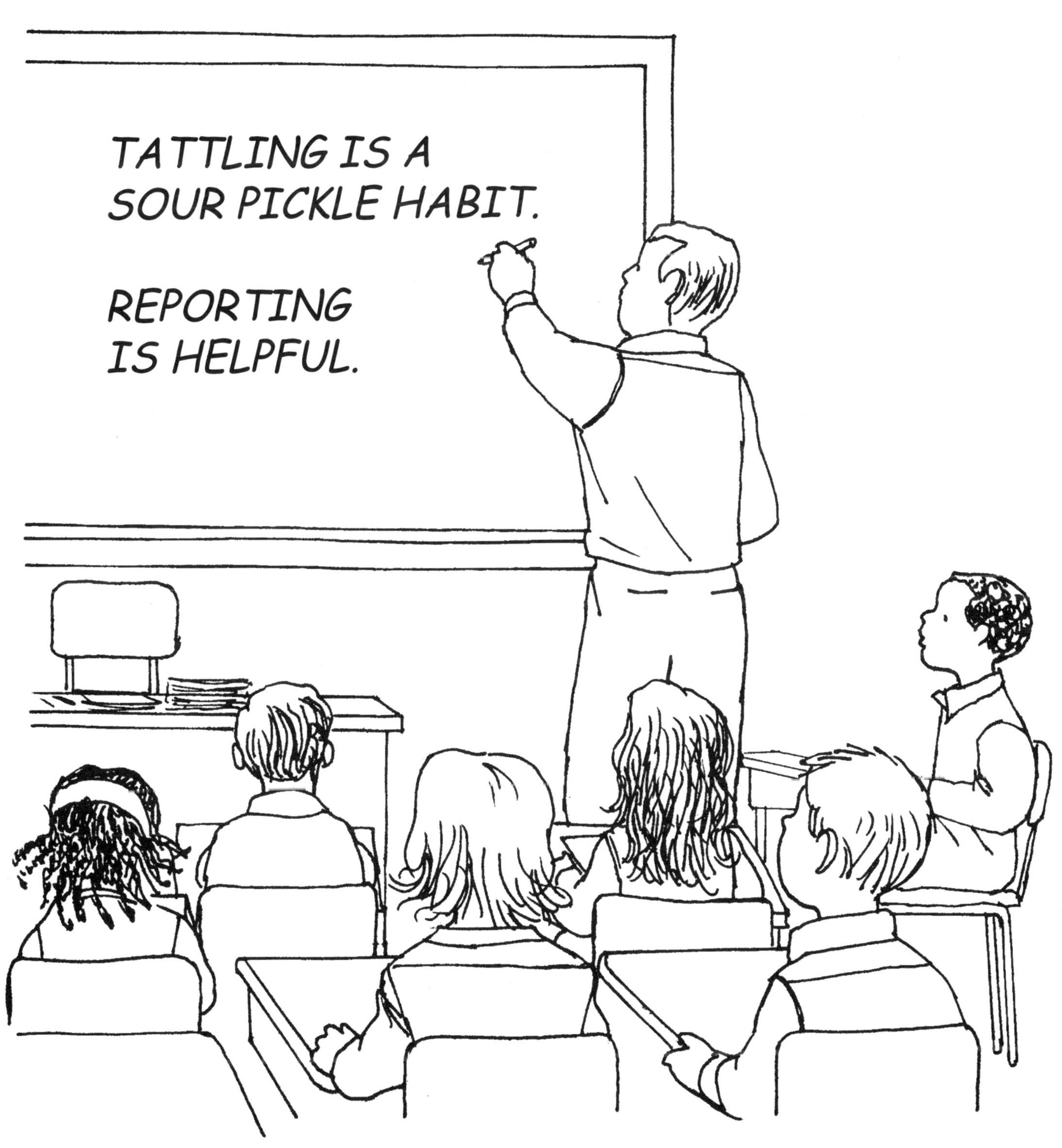

The third-grade students at Pickle Mountain School were getting used to a new room, a new teacher, and new work. All of the students already knew each other because they had been in classes together before or lived in the same neighborhood. By Thursday, the third day of the new school year, they were already starting to tattle on each other. Mr. Walker, the teacher, was already getting tired of it. He needed to put a stop to their behavior before another school day passed. So during recess, he placed a picture of a stoplight on each child's desk.

As the children came into the room after lunch, even before they took their seats, one girl told Mr. Walker: "Sandy crumbled her cookies into her milk." Mr. Walker just looked at the girl and said, "Sit down."

When all the children were seated, Mr. Walker wrote on the chalkboard in big letters: "TATTLING IS A SOUR PICKLE HABIT. REPORTING IS HELPFUL." Although he wanted the tattling to stop, Mr. Walker also wanted to make sure the students knew that sometimes there were things they needed to tell an adult.

Now the children were confused. First, there were these stoplights on their desks. And instead of starting the social studies lesson, Mr. Walker was writing on the chalkboard about tattling and pickles.

Mr. Walker turned to the class and began to speak: "There are things that happen that you should tell the teacher and things you should not. The times when you should tell the teacher are called *reporting*, and the times you should *not* are called *tattling*. Then he wrote the times you should tell on the board.

1. When someone could be hurt
2. When school property is being damaged
3. When the teacher has asked you to report a specific problem

Mr. Walker asked the students to point to the red on the stoplight and say this rhyme:

> *Red* means stop. Tattling is a flop.

Then he asked the students to point to the green on the stoplight and say this rhyme:

Green means go. An adult needs to know.

Then he said, "Green is for *report*. Red is for *tattle*."

Wanda was the student who *always* had a question, and this time was no exception. "If *red* means tattle and *green* means report," she asked, "what does *yellow* mean?"

Mr. Walker was ready with an answer, "*Yellow* means thinking time is short. Make up your mind if this is a tattle or a report."

Now the children understood. Mr. Walker then said, "I have a stoplight on my desk, just like yours. I'm keeping it there to remind you, when you come to my desk, to know whether you are tattling or reporting. But you also have a stoplight on your desk. Whenever you think of telling me something, look at your stoplight and decide whether you should."

The stoplight stayed on Mr. Walker's desk to remind the children when to tell. He even put a stoplight on his keychain and one on his whistle. Mr. Walker's tattling lesson goes everywhere.

Follow-Up Questions: 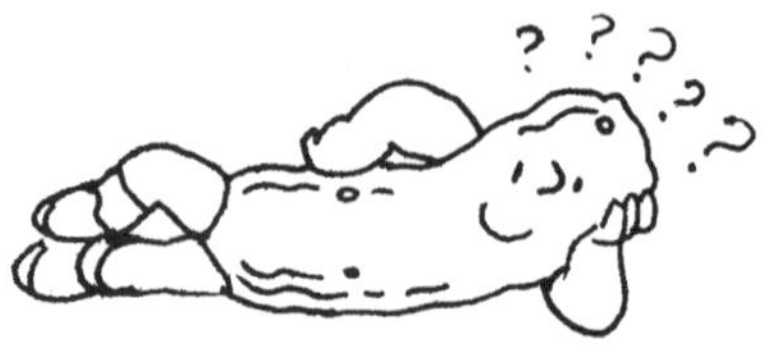

1. What problem did Mr. Walker have on the third day of school?

   ____

2. Are there times when a student should tell on another student?

   ____

   What are these times? ______________________________

   ____

3. When a bully is hurting or threatening to hurt someone, what should you do? ______________________________

   ____

4. How could you show compassion by reporting? __________

   ____

5. When could you show respect or responsibility by reporting?

   ____

   ____

6. What did *red* mean on Mr. Walker's stoplight? __________

   ____

7. What did *green* mean on Mr. Walker's stoplight? __________

   ____

8. What was the rhyme used for *yellow*? ________________

   ____

9. Would it be honest to tell on a student for something he did not do? ______________________________

10. What is a word that means you pause to carefully think about something? ______________________________

11. Mr. Walker had made a stoplight for each of the 23 children in his class. Only 19 children were at school that day. How many stoplights did he have left over? ________________

Answers To Follow-Up Questions:

1. What problem did Mr. Walker have on the third day of school? *(The children were tattling all the time.)*
2. Are there times when a student should tell on another student? *(Yes.)* What are these times? *(When someone could be hurt, school property is being damaged, or the teacher has asked you to report a specific problem.)*
3. When a bully is hurting or threatening to hurt someone, what should you do? *(You should report the situation because someone could get hurt.)*
4. How could you show compassion by reporting? *(If someone was in danger of being hurt, you could stop it from happening.)*
5. When could you show respect or responsibility by reporting? *(If school property is being damaged, you could show respect by reporting. If you were doing a specific task for a teacher, you would be responsible to report.)*
6. What did *red* mean on Mr. Walker's stoplight? *(Tattle—it is not necessary to tell.)*
7. What did *green* mean on Mr. Walker's stoplight? *(Report—it is good to tell.)*
8. What was the rhyme used for *yellow*? *(Yellow means thinking time is short. Make up your mind if this is a tattle or a report.)*
9. Would it be honest to tell on a student for something he did not do? *(No.)*
10. What is a word that means you pause to carefully think about something? *(Contemplation.)*
11. Mr. Walker had made a stoplight for each of the 23 children in his class. Only 19 children were at school that day. How many stoplights did he have left over? *(Mr. Walker had 4 stoplights left over.)*

CHOICES IN THE CITY

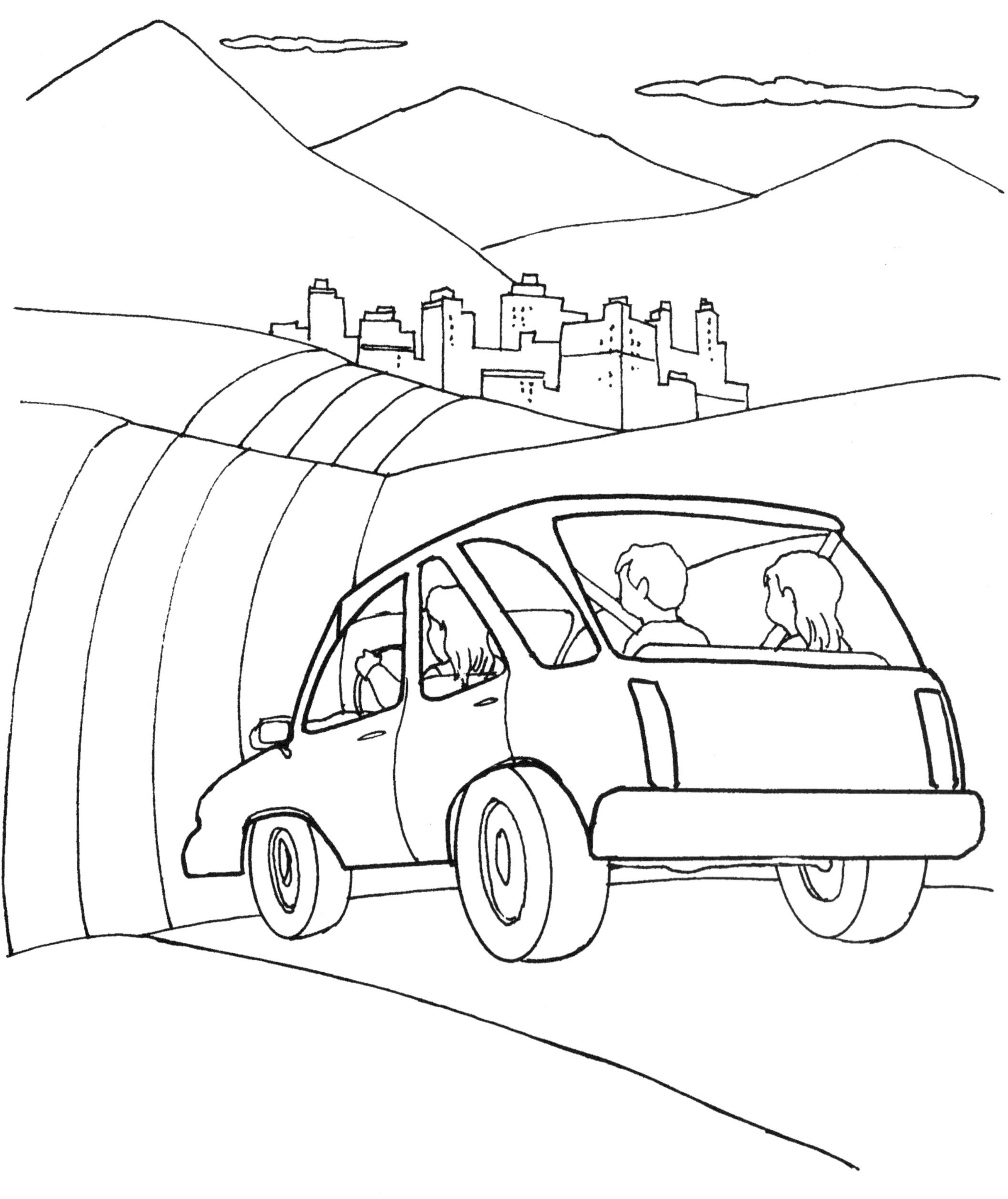

It took an hour and a half to drive to a city big enough to have a mall, a theater, and a big hospital. From Pickle Mountain the road began as narrow and curvy. But as they approached the city of Centerbrook, they were able to drive on a four-lane highway.

Franny and her brother Stan were absent from Pickle Mountain School. They had to go to Centerbrook. Franny had an appointment to see a special dentist about her teeth. After the appointment, Mom had other things to do before they could go to a movie. Mom, Franny, and Stan had lots of choices to make that day.

They had left home at 6:30 in the morning to get to the dentist by 8:30. Since they had not had breakfast, Mom said they could stop when they reached the big highway. There were two restaurants to choose from. At one restaurant, you sat at a table and a server brought you what you wanted. At the other restaurant, you gave your order at the counter. Mom only said to remember what time they had to be at the dentist. Stan really wanted the chocolate chip pancakes you could order from the server, but it would take half an hour to stop and eat there. So they ate at the restaurant where you ordered at the counter.

In the city, the dentist told them that Franny needed braces. There were choices of different kinds, which cost different amounts of money. This was a big decision that would have to be made at home.

They had two hours before the movie started. Aunt Elaine was in the hospital in Centerbrook. There was a mall and a big toy store. Both Franny and Stan had saved their allowances for three weeks to spend their money in the city. Mom also had to pick up a part for the lawnmower on their way out of town. The movie would be over at three o'clock, and the lawnmower store closed at four. They really had a lot of choices to make.

Even though Franny and Stan wanted to spend their money first, they agreed seeing Aunt Elaine was more important. Mom was happy about their decision, and she knew how happy Aunt Elaine would be to have company. When they arrived at the hospital, they saw many workers, some doing the same thing and others doing something completely different.

After seeing Aunt Elaine, they decided it really didn't matter whether they went to the mall or the toy store. Both were equally important. But they were hungry, so they chose the mall because they could eat lunch there. At the Food Court, Franny couldn't decide between tacos and chicken. She liked them both, so her choice was to go to the counter that had the shorter line.

Franny knew exactly what she wanted to buy with her allowance, but Stan wanted five different things. Of course, he didn't have enough money for all five things. He thought and thought, and he just couldn't decide what he wanted most. Mom and Franny told him to hurry and make up his mind, because the movie started in 20 minutes. Pressed for time, he chose a game he could play with his friends.

When they entered the movie theater, there were more choices to make. What did they want to drink with their popcorn? The movie was about to start, so they had to make a quick decision.

After the movie, they got to the lawnmower shop just before closing time. After Mom got the part she needed, there was time left over before they had to start home. Franny and Stan were lucky enough to play for an hour in the park.

It was past supper time when they came to the two restaurants on the big highway. Which one do you think they chose? Can you guess what Stan got for supper?

Follow-Up Questions: 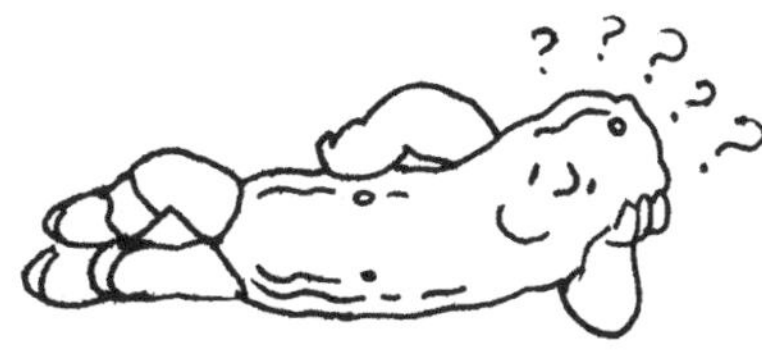

1. Do you think Franny's family went to the city every week? ____
2. Why did Stan not choose chocolate chip pancakes for breakfast?

   ____

3. What were the three most important things Franny, Mom, and Stan had to do in the city? ____________________

   ____

   ____

4. What things did they do for fun? ____________________

   ____

5. What choice was too important to be made quickly? ________

   ____

6. Which choices would not make a big difference a month after the trip? ____________________
7. How did Stan show adaptability at the store? ____________

   ____

   How did Franny show adaptability at lunch? ____________

   ____

8. How did Franny and Stan show both compassion and respect in the city? ____________________

   ____

9. Who were the workers they saw in the city? ____________

   ____

10. How can you predict what Stan wanted to eat for supper? ____

    ____

11. If Stan got $2.00 a week for his allowance, and he saved all of it, how much did he save in three weeks? ____________

Answers To Follow-Up Questions:

1. Do you think Franny's family went to the city every week? *(Yes or no. Either answer could be justified.)*
2. Why did Stan not choose chocolate chip pancakes for breakfast? *(Stan did not choose chocolate chip pancakes because they went to the restaurant where you ordered at the counter and were served quickly.)*
3. What were the three most important things Franny, Mom, and Stan had to do in the city? *(The three most important things to do were going to the dentist, visiting Aunt Elaine in the hospital, and going to the lawnmower shop.)*
4. What things did they do for fun? *(They went to the movie, mall, and park.)*
5. What choice was too important to be made quickly? *(The type of braces Franny should get.)*
6. Which choices would not make a big difference a month after the trip? *(Accept all appropriate answers.)*
7. How did Stan show adaptability at the store? *(He was able to decide on the game when he knew he didn't have a lot of time to make up his mind.)* How did Franny show adaptability at lunch? *(She picked the counter with the shorter line.)*
8. How did Franny and Stan show both compassion and respect in the city? *(They chose to visit Aunt Elaine in the hospital before doing the fun things they had planned.)*
9. Who were the workers they saw in the city? *(They saw workers in the dentist's office, restaurant, hospital, mall, movie theater, and lawnmower shop.)*
10. How can you predict what Stan wanted to eat for supper? *(He probably chose the chocolate chip pancakes he wasn't able to get for breakfast.)*
11. If Stan got $2.00 a week for his allowance, and he saved all of it, how much did he save in three weeks? *(He saved $6.00.)*

CHAPTER 4

ACTIVITIES FOR SPECIFIC TOPICS

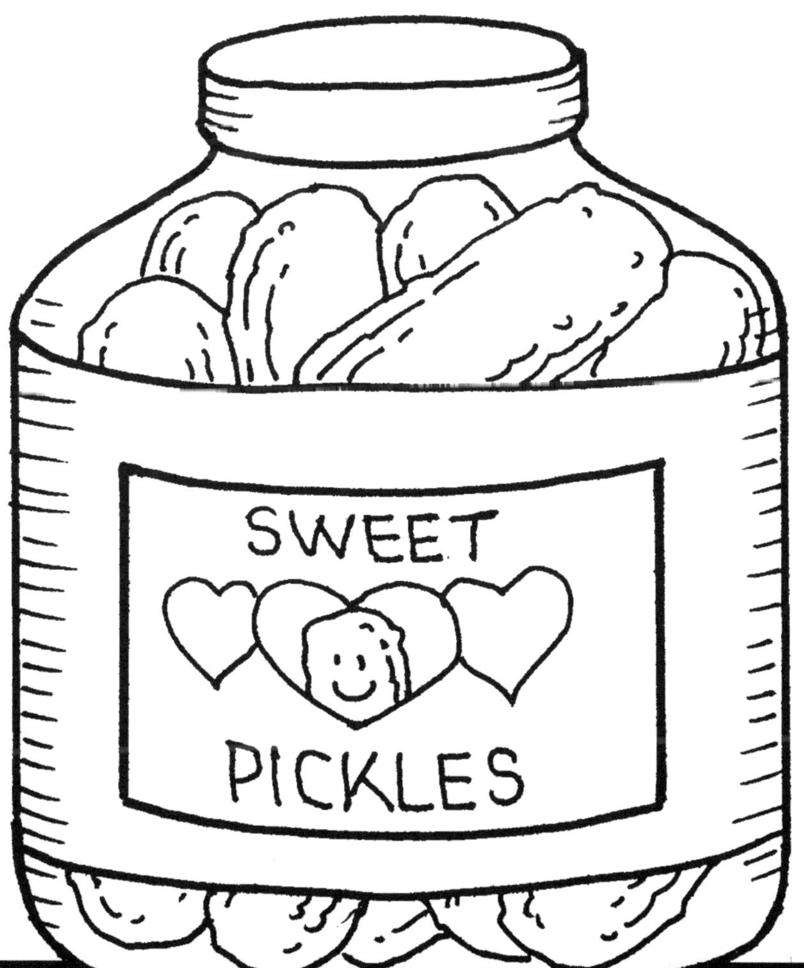

Name ______________________________

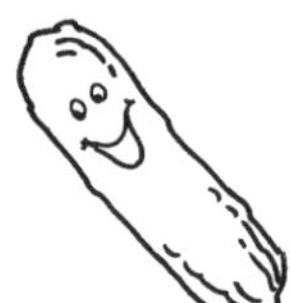

SWEET AND SOUR DREAMS

DREAMS ARE LIKE PICKLES.

Sometimes they are sweet. Sometimes they are sour.

Circle the words that you think fit the sentence.

1. When I wake up from a sweet dream, I feel ____________ .

   happy
   scared
   mad
   hopeful
   confused
   joyful
   excited
   worried

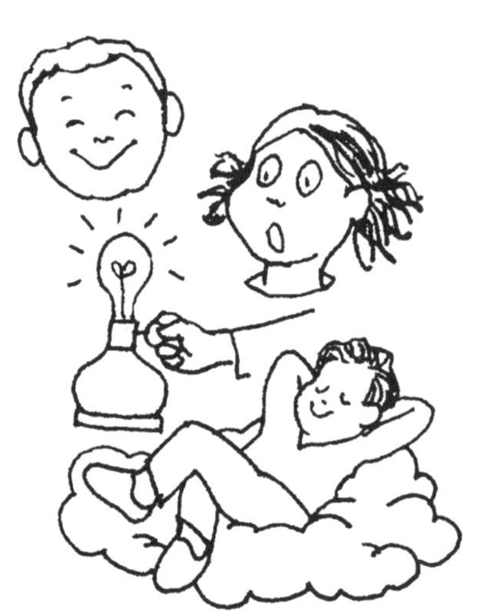

2. When I wake up from a sour dream, I feel ____________ .

   happy
   scared
   mad
   hopeful
   confused
   joyful
   excited
   worried

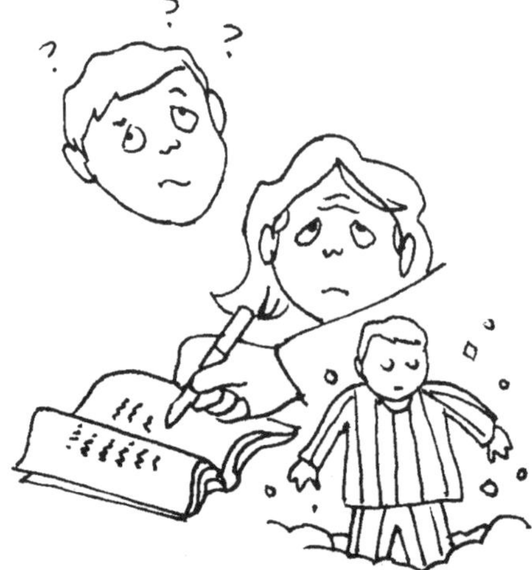

3. When I wake up from a sour dream, I could ____________ .

   talk with a grown-up
   plant flowers under my bed
   make up a new ending
   turn on the light
   hold a favorite toy
   go out and sleep on a cloud
   think about what parts of the dream could not be real
   pretend the dream is on TV and turn it off

4. When I wake up from a sweet dream, I could ____________ .

   talk with a grown-up
   watch my toys float around the room
   smile and enjoy it
   write it in a story
   go back to sleep
   go out and wash the car
   walk out in the snow in my pajamas

Name ______________________________

FALLING ASLEEP

Do you ever have trouble falling asleep? ______________________

Has it ever ended up being a sour pickle time?____________

Circle some things you might try when you have trouble falling asleep.

listening to soft music

singing a song to yourself

putting a favorite lotion on your hands

talking to a pet

holding a favorite toy

keeping something you like to smell nearby

reading a book

counting something imaginary, like sheep

thinking of good things that happened during the day

making up a story in your mind about going to a special place

Start with the letter "A" and think of something you like for every letter of the alphabet.

What is something you do when you can't fall asleep?

____

____

____

____

____

What is something different a classmate does to help himself or herself fall asleep?

____

____

____

____

USING "PICKLE CAT"

MATERIALS NEEDED:

For the Leader: Stuffed toy cat or full-bodied cat puppet, cat toy, stuffed toy dog or full-bodied dog puppet, Jack-in-the-Box (optional)
For the Students: Copy of *Pickle Cat* (page 157) and *Pickle Gets Mad* (page 158)

LESSON:

Begin the lesson by introducing the toy cat or cat puppet as *Pickle Cat.* Tell the students that Pickle Cat got his name because he, unlike other cats, *likes* to eat pickles. Distribute a copy of the *Pickle Cat* story to each student. Read *Pickle Cat* aloud with the students. Then ask the students to name some things they believe would make Pickle Cat mad. *(Pause for the students' responses.)* Tell Pickle Cat that to reward him for keeping the mice away, you want to give him a toy. *(Have Pickle Cat make soft meowing or purring sounds.)* Then have the dog grab the toy and run away. *(Make Pickle Cat shake and yowl loudly.)* Take the toy away from the dog and return it to Pickle Cat. *(Have Pickle Cat make soft meowing or purring sounds.)* Then ask the following questions:

1. Did Pickle Cat get mad over every little thing? *(No.)*
2. When did Pickle Cat get mad? *(Pickle Cat got mad when he had a good reason.)*
3. When Pickle Cat gets mad, does he hurt anyone? *(No.)*
   Does he destroy anything? *(No.)*
   Does he use any words that would get him in trouble with the principal, his teacher, or his parents? *(No.)*
4. Does Pickle Cat let you know when he is mad? *(Yes.)*
5. Does Pickle Cat stay mad a long time? *(No.)*

Next, tell the students that the class is going to sing the *Pickle Gets Mad* song. Distribute the lyric sheet to each student and review the directions at the top of the page. Sing the song with the students. If one is available, use a Jack-in-the-Box to show the students how to stay in one place when they pop up.

Conclude the lesson by reviewing the answers to the questions above and reminding the students that Pickle Cat's good anger-management habits are also good anger-management habits for them.

Encourage the students to take their papers home and share them with their parents.

VARIATIONS:

This activity may also be used to introduce a lesson on bullying. (see pages 271 and 284.)

PICKLE CAT

Pickle Cat is a strange name. Pickle Cat got his name because one day last summer, he ate a pickle. Can you believe he liked it? Yes, a cat liked a pickle! Now he waits for one any time the pickle jar comes out of the refrigerator.

Pickle Cat doesn't get mad very often, and that's a good thing. It's good because no one likes to be around a person or a cat who gets mad over every little thing that goes wrong.

I can say, "Your tail looks funny." What does Pickle Cat do? He just thinks, "That's silly and I'm not going to let you make me mad."

Or I can say, "Ha, ha, ha, I ate the last pickle." And what does Pickle Cat do? He doesn't get mad. Instead, he thinks, "I'm not going to starve without pickles."

And if I say, "I don't have any time to play with you today," he is disappointed. But he doesn't get mad.

He doesn't get mad without a very good reason. And even when he *does* get mad, he *doesn't*

- hurt anyone
- destroy things
- use words that will get him in trouble with the principal, his teacher, or his parents.

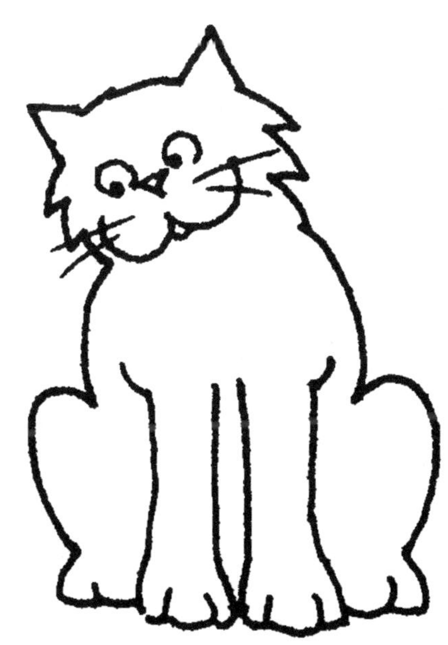

Pickle Cat lets you know he is mad. But he doesn't stay mad for a long time.

PICKLE GETS MAD

Sing this song to the tune of *Pop Goes The Weasel.* When you hear the word *when,* stand up and look mad. Sit down when you hear the word *us*.

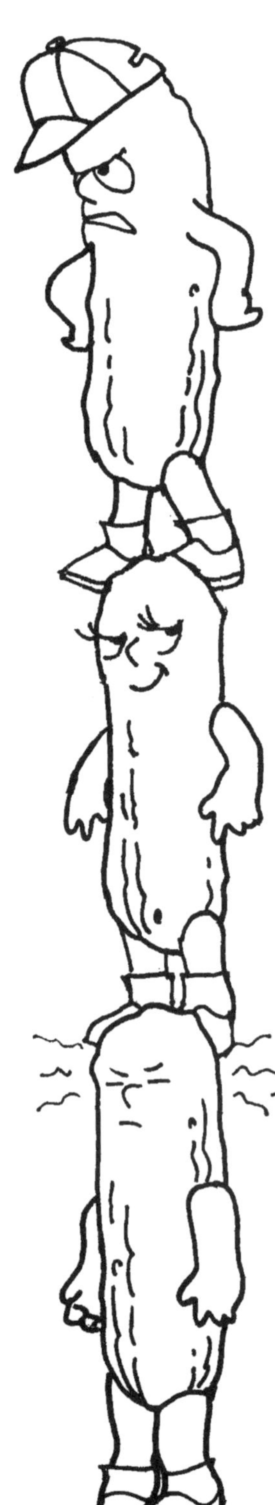

Pickle doesn't get mad very fast.
He thinks about it first.
Pickle does get mad sometimes.
When he does, he shows us.

Pickle doesn't hurt anyone.
He's careful what he does.
Pickle does get mad sometimes.
When he does, he shows us.

Pickle doesn't destroy anything.
He knows that it is wrong.
Pickle does get mad sometimes.
When he does, he shows us.

Pickle does not use any words
To cause trouble with adults.
Pickle does get mad sometimes.
When he does, he shows us.

Pickle doesn't stay mad very long.
He knows it doesn't help.
Pickle does get mad sometimes.
When he does, he shows us.

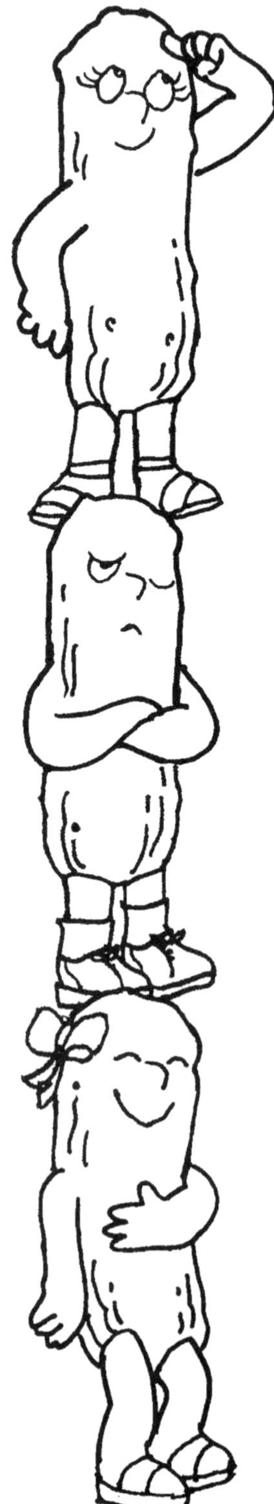

THE SWEET AND SOUR OF SEPARATION

Life is like a pickle. Sometimes it's sweet. Sometimes it's sour. This is true when parents separate, even though it may feel mostly sour.

We would not usually wish for parents to divorce. It can be a really, really sour time, but it won't stay that way forever. Sometimes something nice happens. Circle the things that have happened in your life.

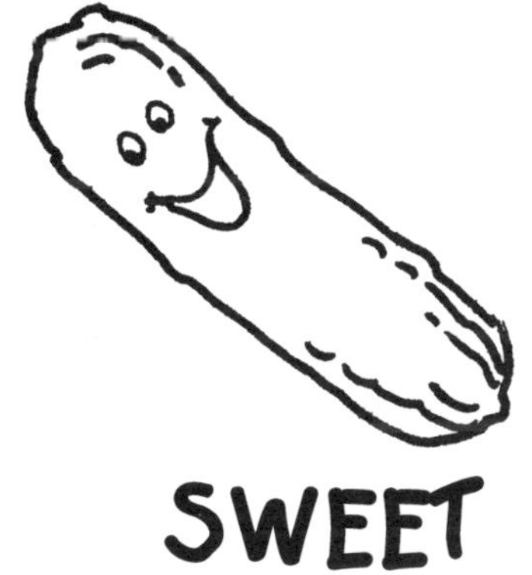

SWEET

I know the divorce is not my fault.

I know that grown-ups love me.

I know both my parents love me.

I'm not scared of fights any more.

I get to have birthdays at two houses.

I get to visit the parent I don't live with.

I have a stepparent I like.

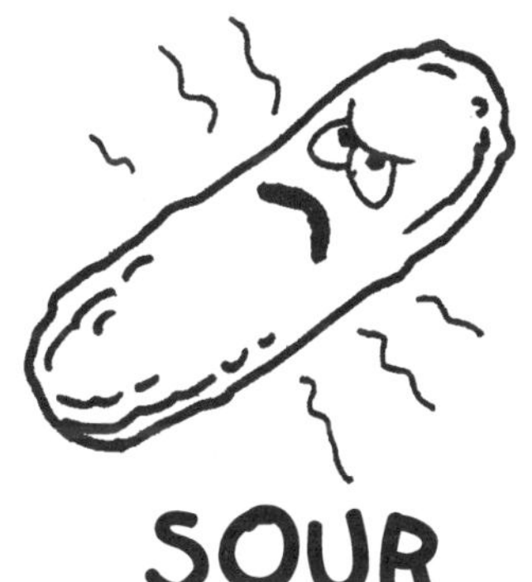

SOUR

Mom and Dad say bad things to each other.

I had to move, and I didn't like it.

I never hear from one of my parents.

We don't have as much money as we used to have.

Mom and Dad still fight.

I have to visit a parent when I don't want to.

I have a stepparent I don't like to be around.

Name ______________________________

DIFFERENT, BUT OKAY

At the grocery store, there are more than 20 different kinds of pickles. You might not like them all, but they are all safe to eat.

There are all different kinds of families. Being different is okay as long as the children are safe. What would you do if you knew a child who was not safe?

Look at the families on Bread and Butter Lane. Circle the one that is most like yours. In the large empty house, write the names of everyone who lives at your house. If you have a mom or dad who lives in another house, write that parent's name in the other empty house on Candied Dill Lane.

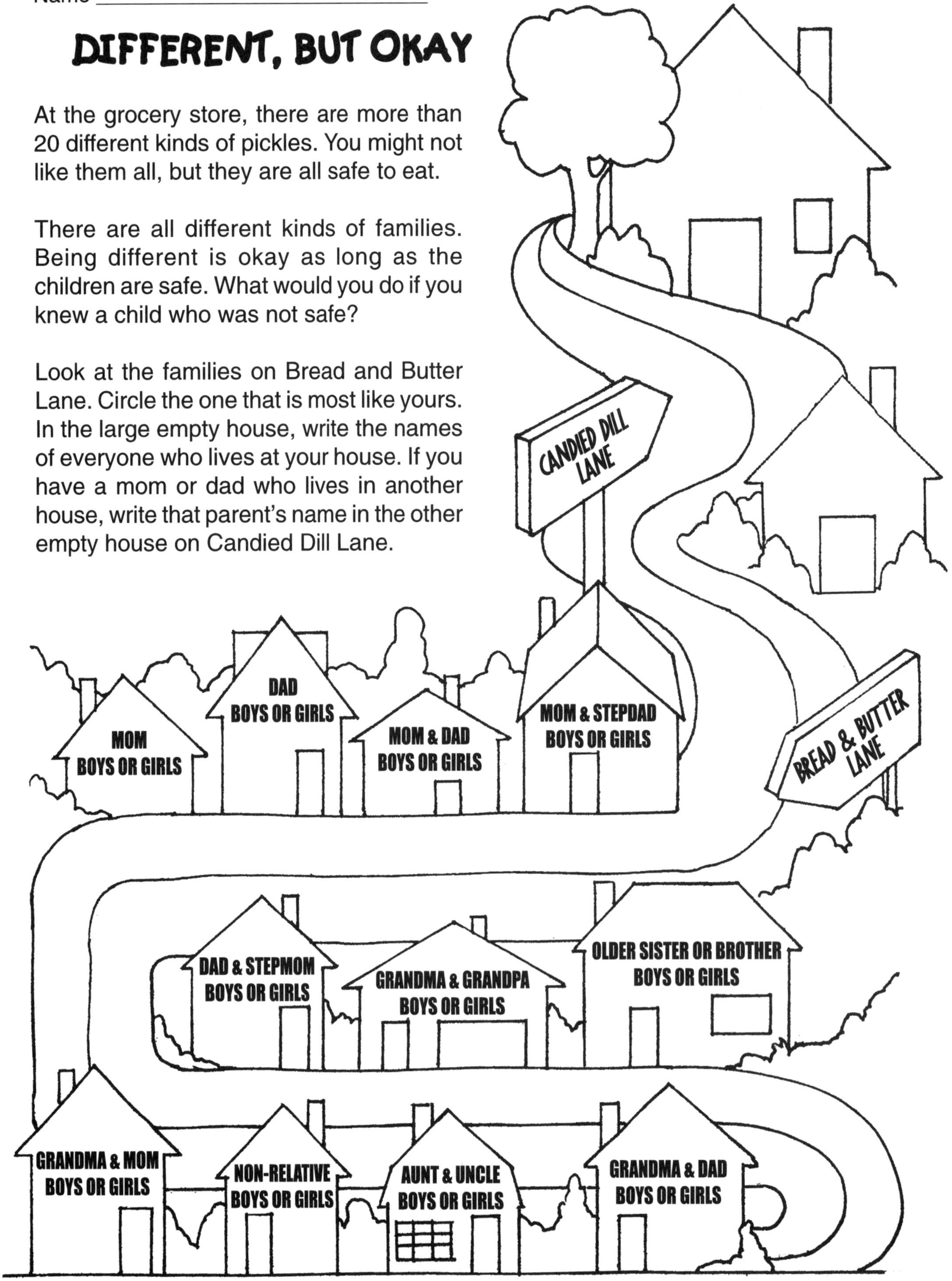

PICKLE PARADE

Listen.

You might hear something important.

Don't complain about where you are in line.

The whole line is going to the same place.

Look at the back of the person in front of you.

This prevents zig-zag lines.

Bulletin boards are for looking at, not touching.

Pictures get dirty and fall down.

Keep your hands and feet to yourself.

No pushing, hitting, or kicking allowed.

If you see a friend, wave instead of talking.

Teachers like quiet lines.

Hold the door for the person behind you.

Each person is polite to the person behind him or her.

NO SOUR PICKLES AT THE DOOR

MATERIALS NEEDED:

For the Leader: Some type of magic wand or conductor's baton

LESSON:

Introduce the lesson by saying:

> "If I am going into the bank and there are 10 people behind me, I will hold the door for the person behind me. Then that person holds the door for the next person. Sometimes we even pass along a smile. No one fights over who holds the door or who doesn't hold the door. Everyone takes a turn, and there are no sour pickles."

Teach the following song to the tune of *London Bridge:*

> Hold the door for the person behind you
> Person behind you, person behind you.
> Hold the door for the person behind you.
> Manners are magic.

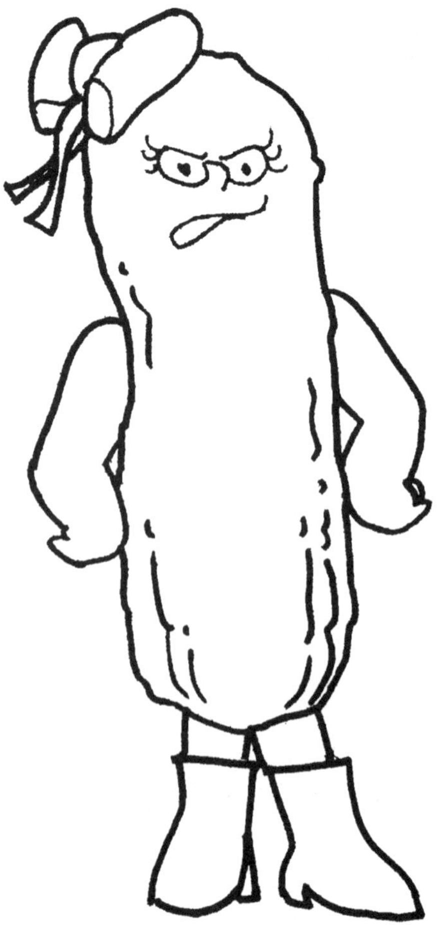

Have the children line up to go through the classroom door into the hall. Choose one student to be the leader. Give the leader the magic wand. Tell the leader to open the door and walk through it, holding it open for the next student in line. As that student comes through the door, the leader should pass the magic wand to him/her. The leader should then start a line in the hall. The student receiving the magic wand will then repeat the process, which will continue until all of the children have left the room and are in line in the hall.

Note: This is a good lesson to share with all of the teachers in your school.

Name ______________________________

SECRET CODE

(MANNERS)

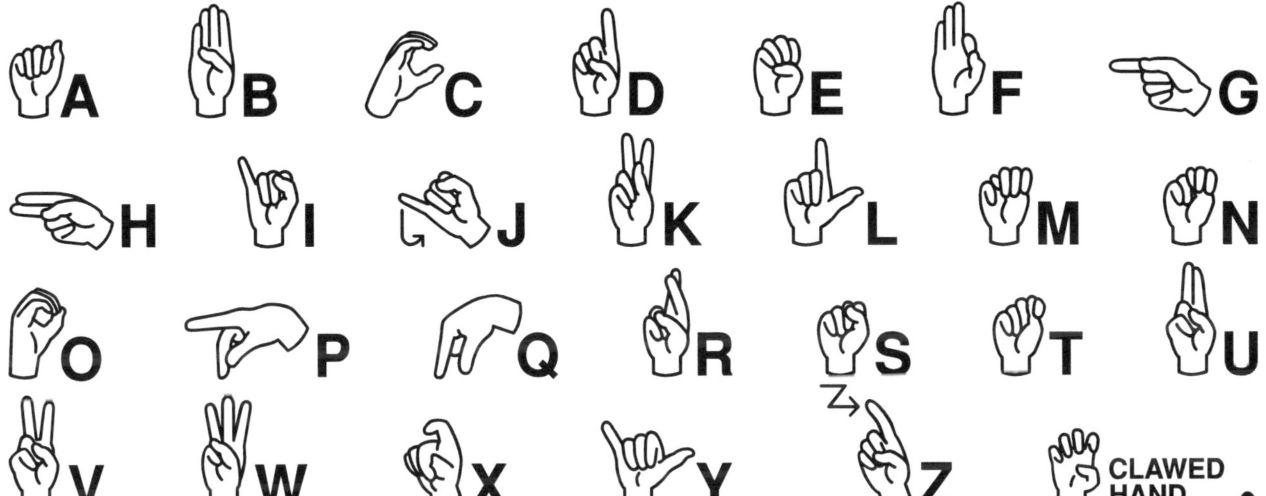

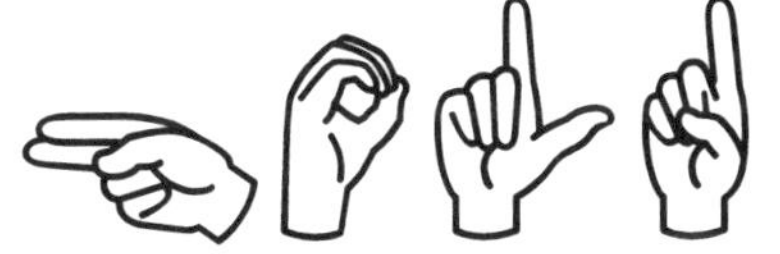

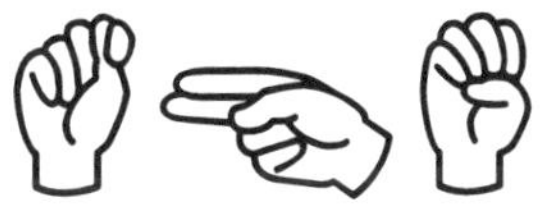

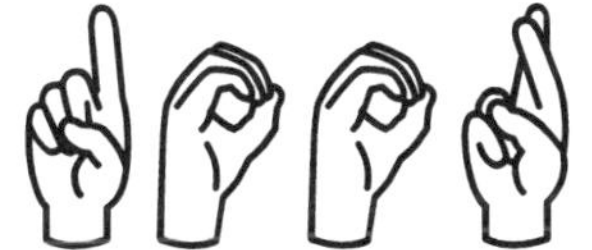

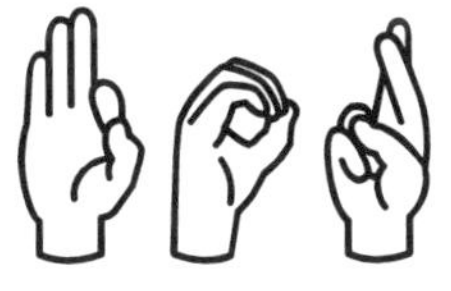

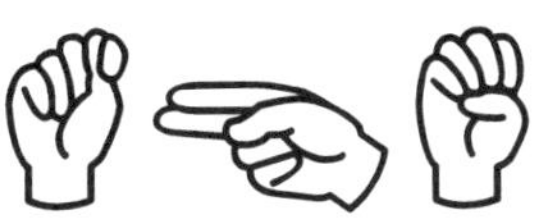

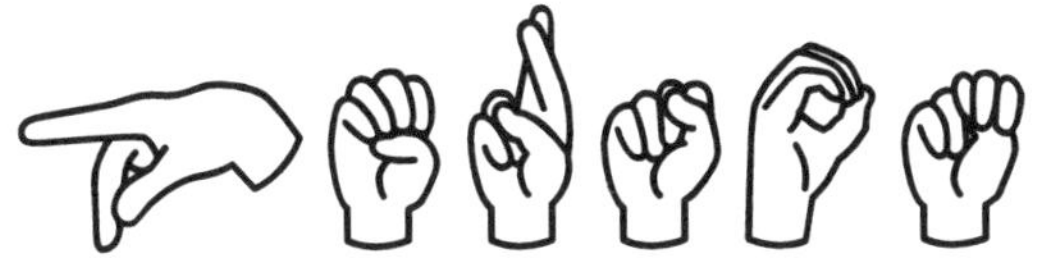

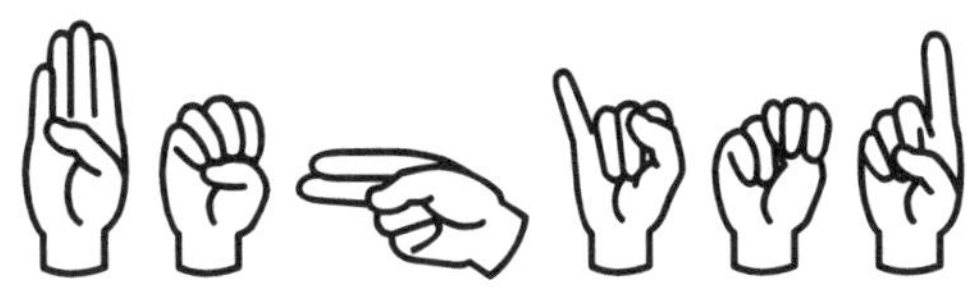

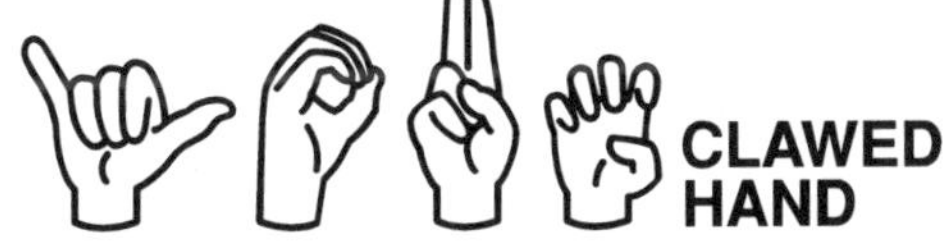

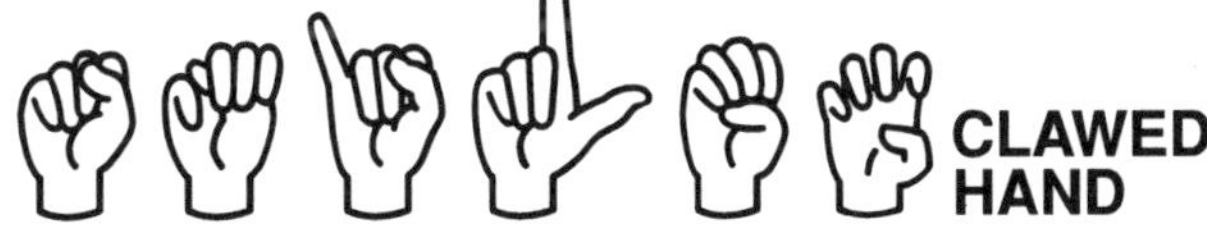

SWEET PICKLE TIPS FOR OPENING GIFTS

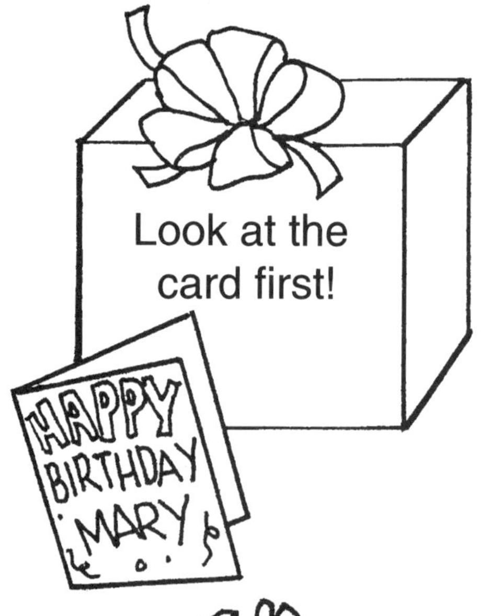

Look at the card first!

Make opening gifts a sweet pickle time for everyone.

WOW! This is great!

Say something nice about the gift (even if it's not exactly what you want).

Enjoy each present before rushing to open the next one.

Always say, "Thank you." When you have opened all your gifts, never ask, "Are there any more for me?"

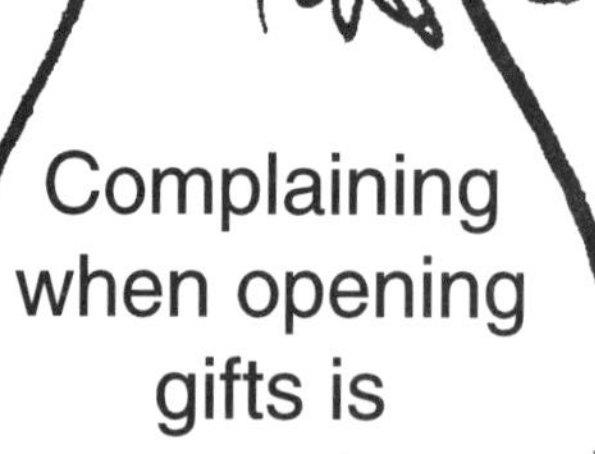

Complaining when opening gifts is never okay.

If you get two of something, talk to a parent about it when others aren't around. If **asked** if you already have one, answer honestly and politely.

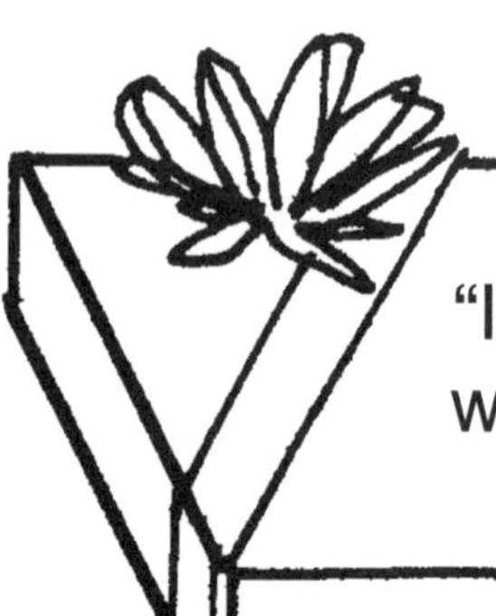

Never say, "I already have one of these," when opening a gift. Just say, "Thank you! This is nice."

HAPPY BIRTHDAY

PICKLE SWEEP ACTIVITY
(DRUG EDUCATION)

MATERIALS NEEDED:

For the Leader: Brooms, dustpans, paper strips labeled with actions that coordinate with your lesson

PRE-LESSON PREPARATION:

Write actions that coordinate with your lesson on paper strips. For example, if the lesson is aimed at drug education, your strips could say:

- eating bananas
- taking pills found on a bus
- drinking beer
- taking pills given by the nurse
- drinking milk
- smelling roses
- taking pills given by a teenager
- crossing at the crosswalk
- asking a parent before going someplace
- going away without asking your parents
- using cigarettes found on the playground
- taking illegal drugs
- chewing tobacco
- drinking alcoholic drinks
- inhaling second-hand smoke

LESSON:

Crinkle up the strips of paper and drop them on the floor. Have the students go around the room, read what is on the strip of paper, and pick it up if it says something they do not want to get rid of. Then distribute brooms and dustpans. Have the students sweep up the rest of the papers and put them in the trash. Explain that they are getting rid of things that are not good for them.

Name ______________________

KEEP OR SWEEP OUT

Directions: Read each sentence. Circle "keep" if the action it describes is OK. Circle "sweep out" if it would not be a good choice.

A friend gives you a bookmark she got on vacation.	Keep	Sweep Out
A friend gives you a purple pill he got on vacation	Keep	Sweep Out
A friend offers you a bottle of water from his refrigerator.	Keep	Sweep Out
A friend offers you a bottle of beer from her refrigerator.	Keep	Sweep Out
You take medicine from a bottle found on the playground.	Keep	Sweep Out
A friend opens a box of animal cookies and gives you some.	Keep	Sweep Out
Your mom gives you the right amount of medicine.	Keep	Sweep Out
A friend says to sniff the cleaning spray.	Keep	Sweep Out
A friend says to sniff a rose.	Keep	Sweep Out
A friend lights a cigarette and gives it to you.	Keep	Sweep Out
A friend gives you chewing gum.	Keep	Sweep Out
A friend gives you chewing tobacco.	Keep	Sweep Out

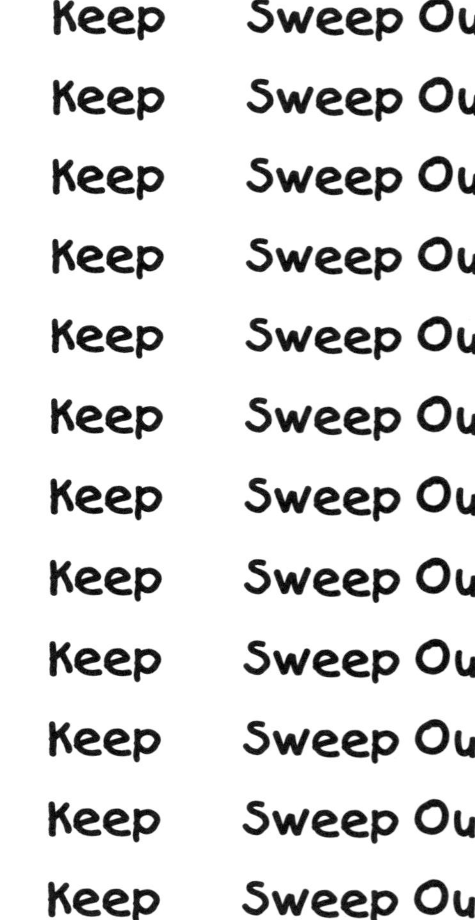

Name ______________________________

SWEEP OUT

Make an ✗ on the things you would sweep out to keep ***children*** safe.

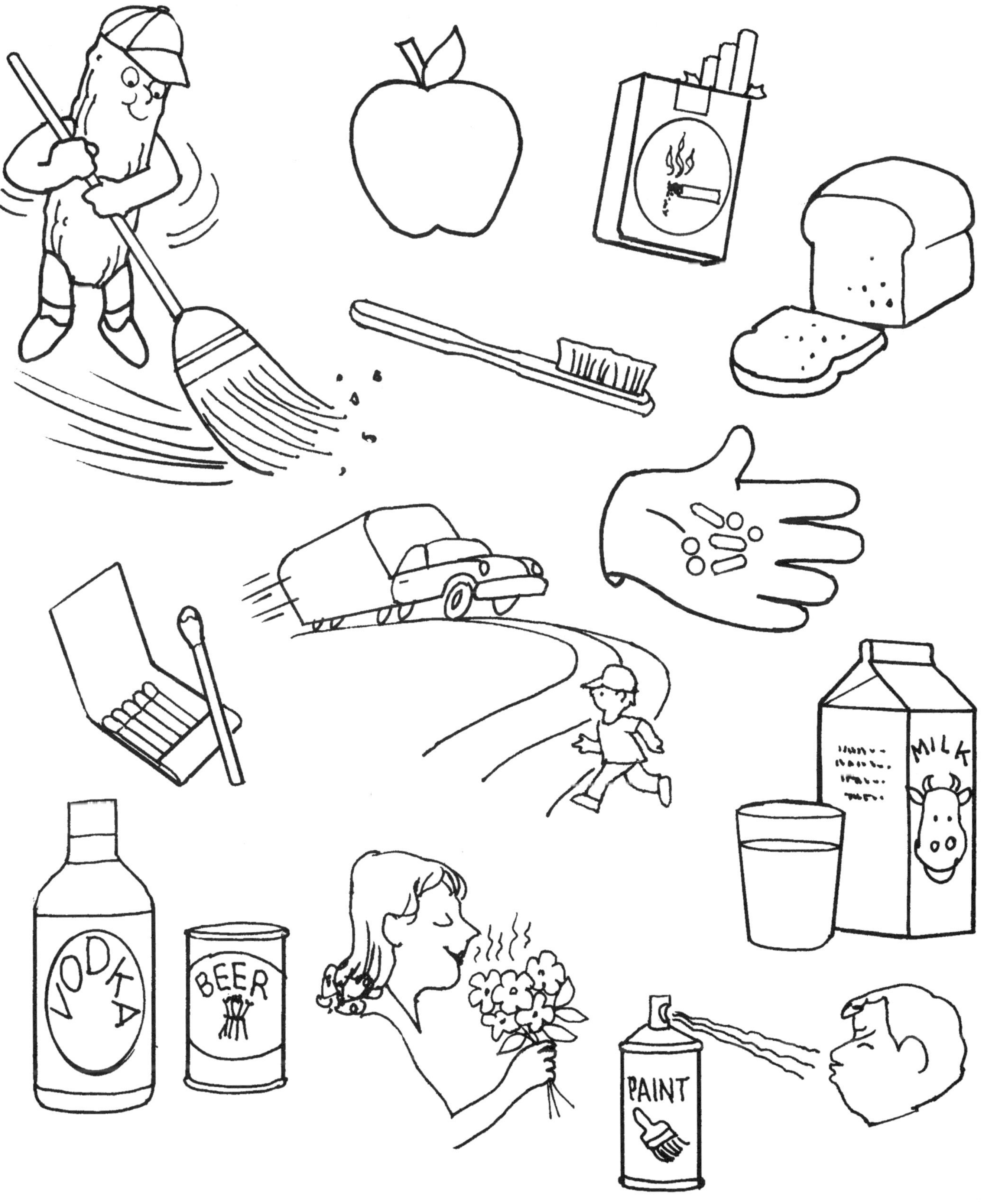

CARING WITH PENNIES

This is a great character-education project to do when emphasizing *compassion* or *thankfulness*. Bringing only *pennies* should be stressed to encourage the act of giving, not the amount of the gift. For each penny brought, the students think of one thing to be thankful for. It may be said silently to themselves, to an adult, or to an older student who could write it down. This can provide a means for integrating the guidance program with the reading and language curriculum. All school staff can participate in this project. Collection places can even be set up in the community to encourage parent and community involvement.

Choose a project suitable for children. We happened to choose Meals On Wheels and collected pennies in wagons. If you are collecting pennies to mail supplies to an organization, put the pennies in a mailbox. If you are going to purchase groceries, ask a local store to loan you a shopping cart. Put a container in the shopping cart to hold the pennies.

Begin by reading *Lunch For Susan's Grandmother* (pages 118-119). Then tell the students about the project. Explain whom they will be helping and how they will be helping by collecting pennies. Before the pennies leave the school, they can be used for math lessons. Make a list of possible assignments and let the teachers choose those suitable for the age group of the students they teach. Here is a list of some assignments that our teachers used:

- Figure out how old a penny is by subtracting the date on the penny from the current year.
- Determine how many pennies there are in a foot, yard, mile, pound, etc. (Older students have taken a bucket and guessed the number of pennies in it by using the number of pennies in a pound and weighing all the pennies collected to estimate the amount of money they had.)
- Make graphs showing the number of pennies from each decade that were collected.
- Count out the pennies required to buy a pretend ice cream cone, small toy, etc.
- Measure how tall a student is in pennies by marking the child's height with masking tape on the floor and covering the tape with pennies.

When you have finished using the pennies as a teaching tool, dump all of them in a pile and take pictures. Or call your local newspaper photographer to take pictures of the pennies and the students. The class may also take a field trip to a bank that has a coin-counting machine and watch the pennies being counted.

Beware! This project is contagious. Students' enthusiasm may surprise you.

PACKED LIKE PICKLES

This is a *caring* project designed to minimize both size and cost. To demonstrate this service project, use a jar of sweet gherkins to show how a lot of little things are packed close together. Continue by telling the children that a lot of little unbreakable items can fit into a small box.

This is a project that all students can participate in, even though they may live in households which cannot afford to buy something. Students can help by bringing small boxes for packaging, even if they don't have money to buy items. No matter who donates the items, it is crucial that all students participate in packaging them.

A variation of this project, if shipping is not a factor, is to pack lots of small items into a pair of socks. Examples could be: trial-size soaps and shampoo, combs, brushes, toothbrushes, and other inexpensive items. These items can get heavy in a hurry and might cost too much to ship, but they are good choices if someone is driving the donation to its destination. One task is for students to write a note listing the contents of the sock and attach it to the pair of socks when they are tied together. (*Note:* Sometimes you can find seasonal socks really cheap when the holiday or season is over.)

When doing caring projects, emphasize which items people really need. For example, a toothbrush and toothpaste are more important than a toy. It's all right to include a toy, but the essentials should come first.

Personal Reflection: I am reminded of a caring project that went sour when I took some of my students to help deliver packages. It was during the holiday, and gifts went to a large distribution center. My students wanted what they saw there—bicycles, videogame systems, fancy dolls, etc. Their packages of essentials and small toys didn't seem very important to them. In a society where children are bombarded by TV and print advertising, it is important to emphasize the act of giving. It is the *thought* that counts.

Name ______________________________

MANUAL ALPHABET

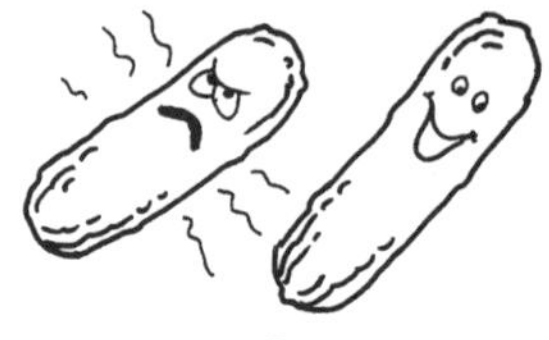

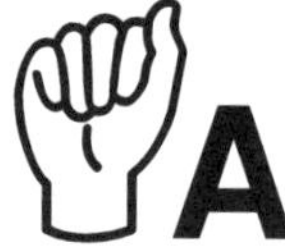 A 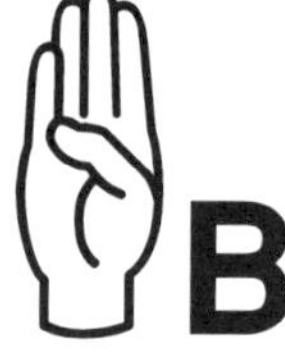 B 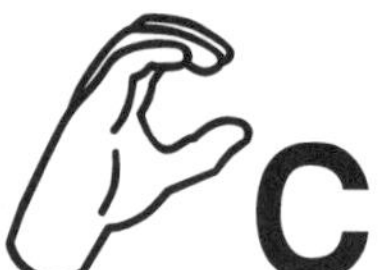 C 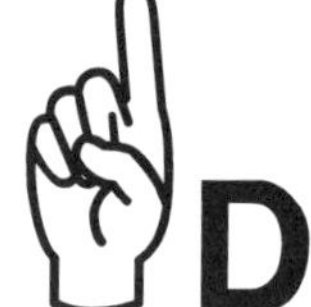 D

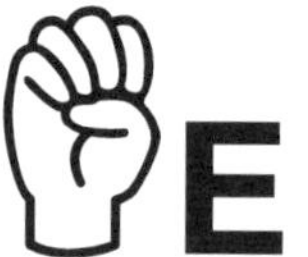 E 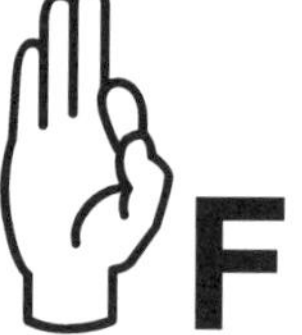 F 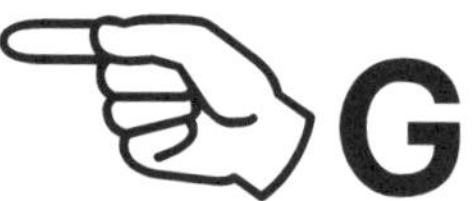 G 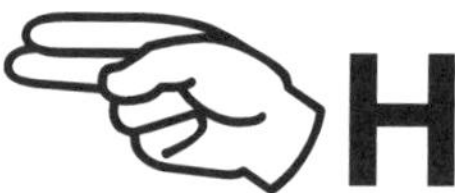 H

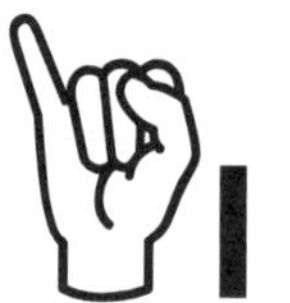 I 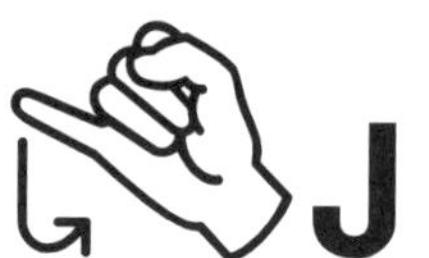 J 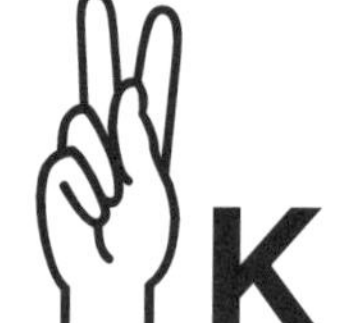 K 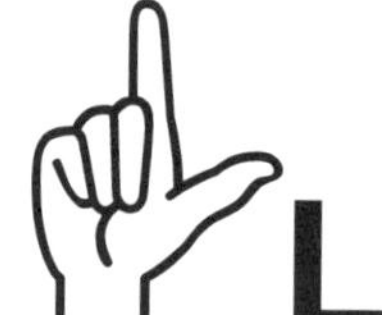 L

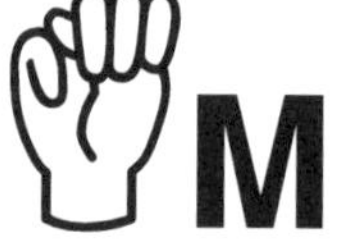 M 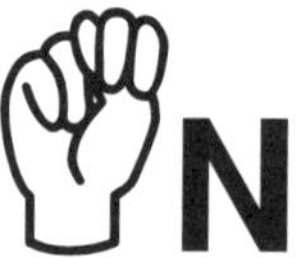 N 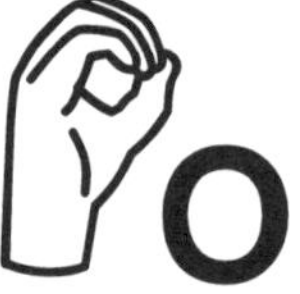 O 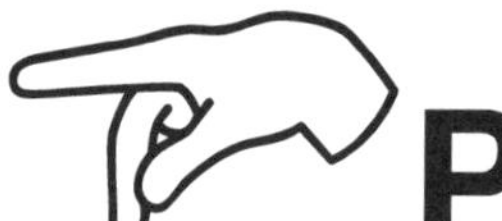 P

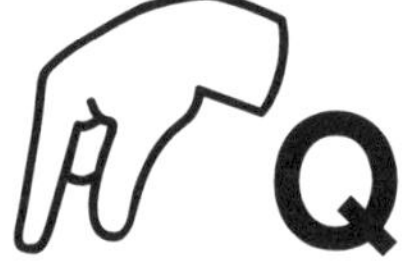 Q 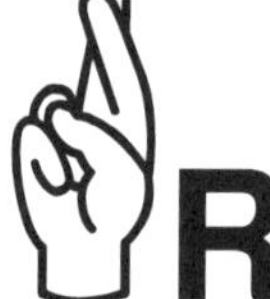 R 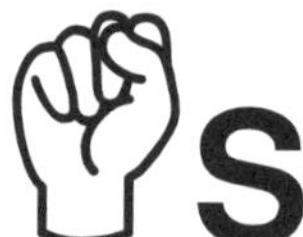 S 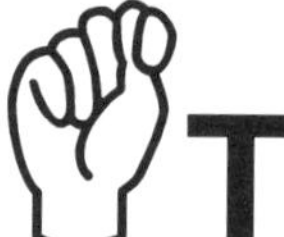 T

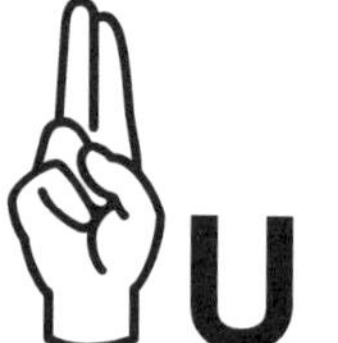 U 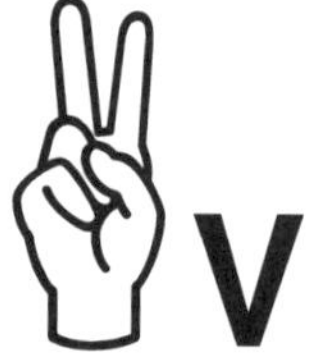 V 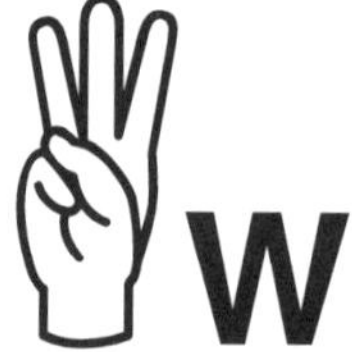 W 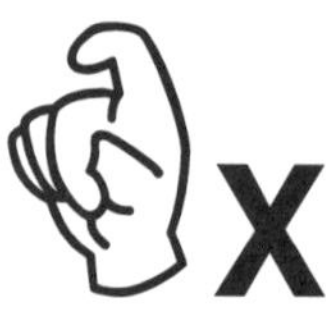 X

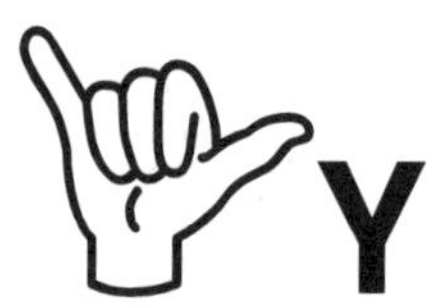 Y 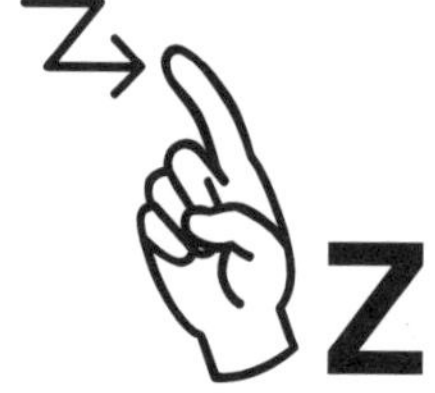

Z 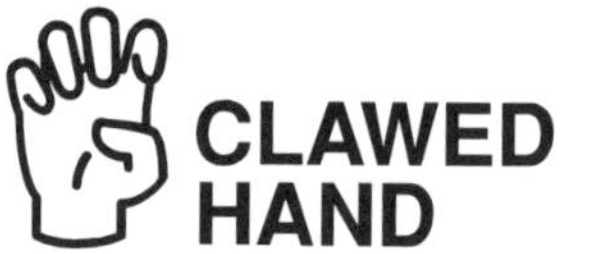 CLAWED HAND .

Name ______________________________

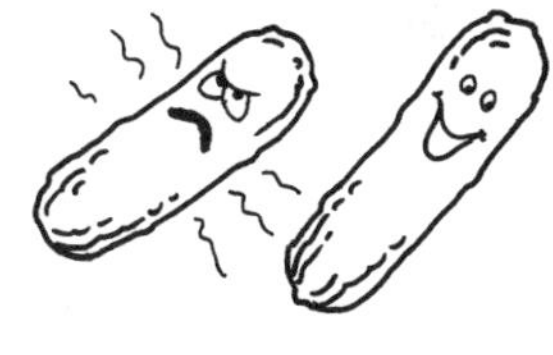

SAYING WORDS THREE WAYS

ENGLISH	SPANISH	SIGNING
1. girl	chica	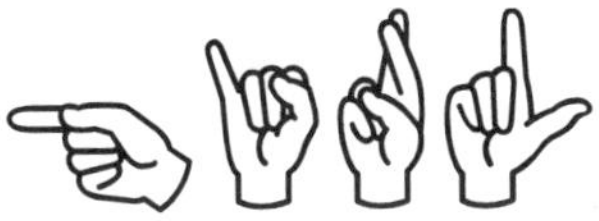
2. boy	chico	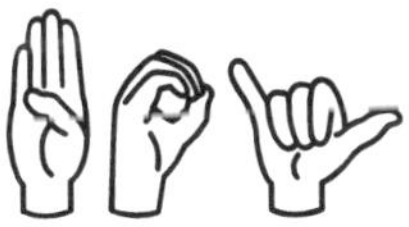
3. happy	feliz	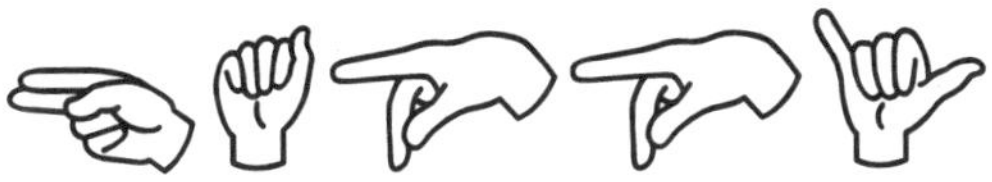
4. sad	triste	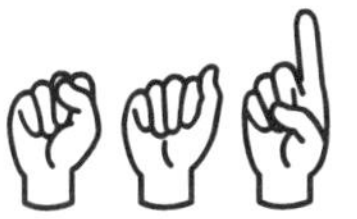
5. thanks	gracias	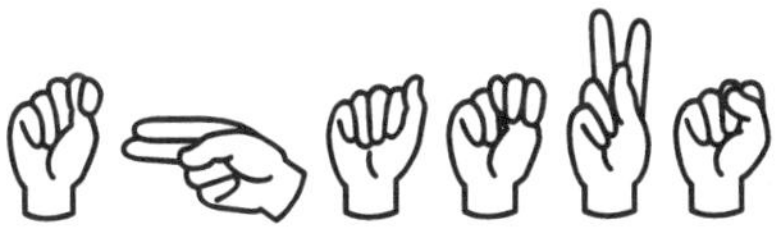
6. cat	gato	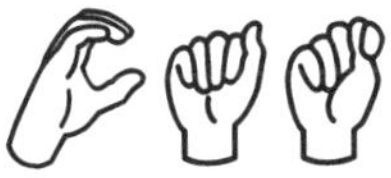
7. dog	perro	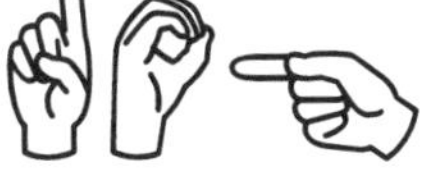
8. drink	beber	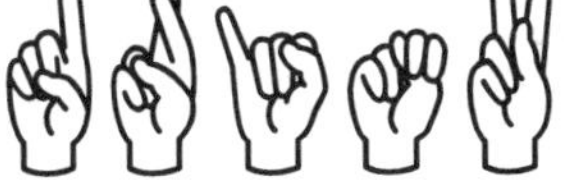

"WHEN" BRAND PICKLES

"WHEN" brand pickles come in five varieties, as you will see on the labels on this page. Copy the labels and glue them on the plastic jars. You may make a "Mixed" jar for review. On the following pages are questions to cut out in the shape of pickles to put in the jars. You may also want to make student copies of these pages to work as a review of the lesson. You may use the blank pickle outlines to write additional questions.

Using two plates or bowls, label one "Yes" and the other "No." Have a student pull a pickle from any jar. Discuss the question on the pickle pulled out of the jar and place it in the appropriate plate or bowl. Since all students may not agree, this is a good time to review *differences* and *respect*.

WHEN
BRAND PICKLES
When should you tell on another student?

WHEN
BRAND PICKLES
When should you tell a secret?

WHEN
BRAND PICKLES
When should you ask people to give you things?

WHEN
BRAND PICKLES
When is a choice important?

WHEN
BRAND PICKLES
When should you laugh?

WHEN
BRAND PICKLES
Mixed Questions

"WHEN" SHOULD YOU ASK? PICKLES

Directions: Cut out the "pickles" and place them in the appropriate jar. (See page 172.)

You have never lost your pencil before, but today it fell on the bus floor and rolled where you could not reach it. You know your counselor has extras. ***Should you ask for one?***

Your counselor has collected teddy bears for years and has more than 30. ***Should you ask for one?***

Children are carrying balloons at a store's grand opening. ***Should you ask the clerk for one?***

A vase of flowers is sitting by the cash register at the new store. ***Should you ask for it?***

A box of candy with a bow on it is sitting on the bank counter. ***Should you ask for it?***

A bowl of little wrapped candies is sitting on the bank counter. ***Should you ask for one?***

Mike has a special cupcake in his lunchbox for his birthday. ***Should you ask for it?***

You have a blister on your foot. Your teacher has bandages in her desk. ***Should you ask for one?***

Your little sister really likes ladybugs. Your friend has a big stuffed ladybug pillow. ***Should you ask for it?***

Your friend has a box of turtle stickers. Many of them are just alike. ***Should you ask for one?***

Name ______________________________

"WHEN" SHOULD YOU ASK? PICTURES

Directions: Make an **✗** the things it would ***not*** be okay to ask someone to give to you to keep.

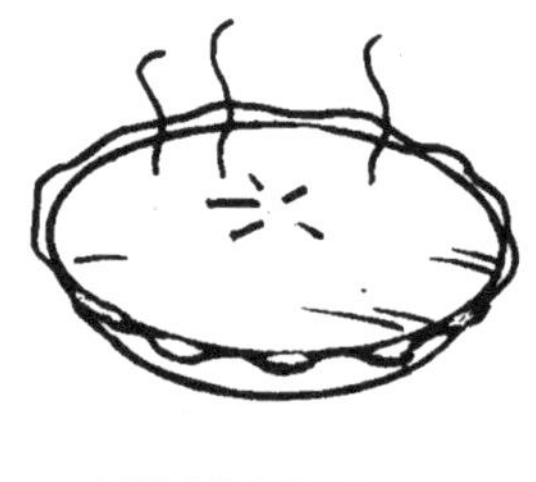

WHOLE PIE

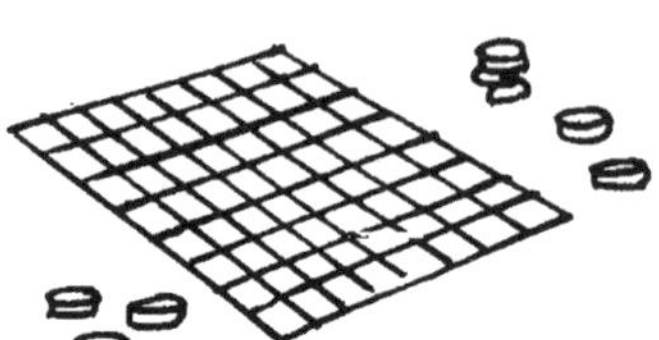

GAME

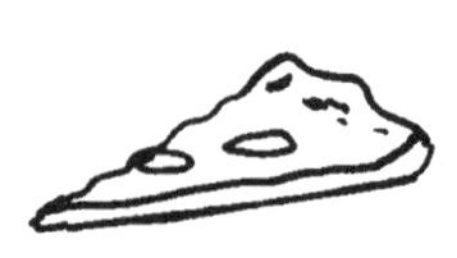

PIECE OF PIZZA

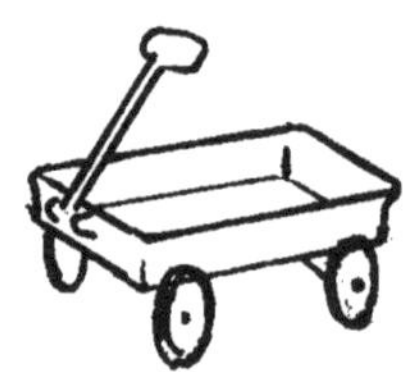

WAGON

STICKER

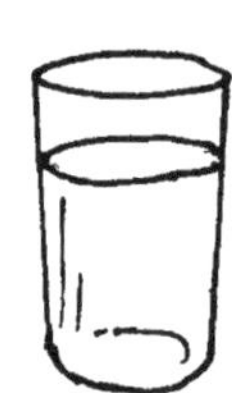

DRINK OF WATER

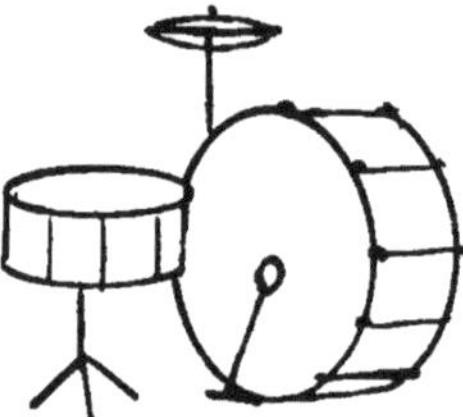

DRUM SET

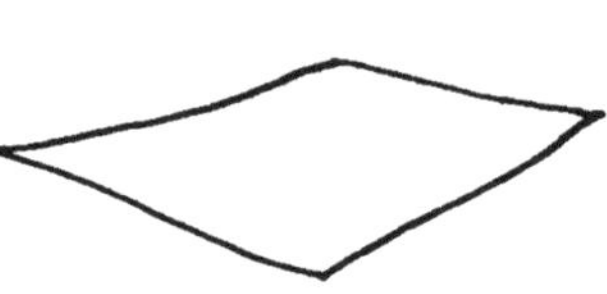

PIECE OF PAPER

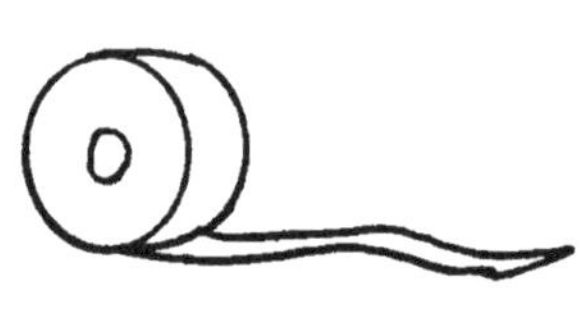

PIECE OF TAPE

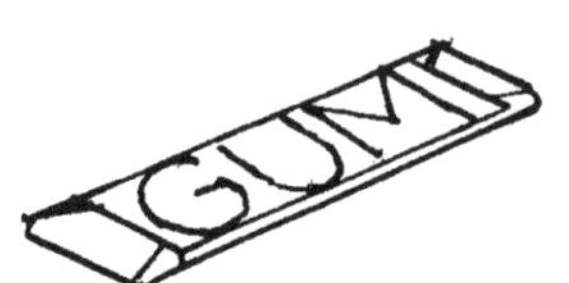

GUM

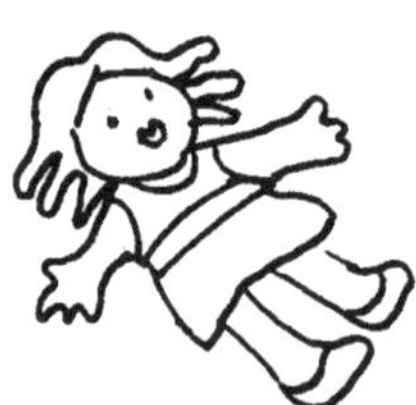

DOLL

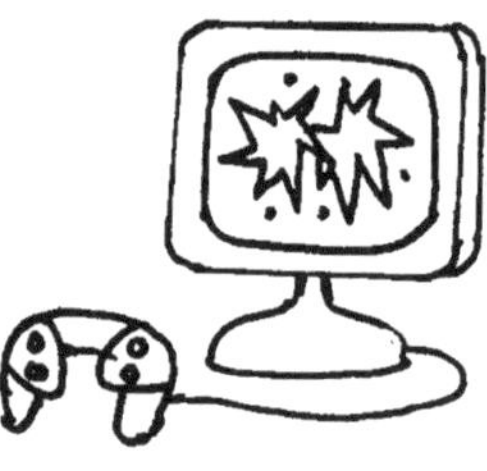

VIDEOGAME

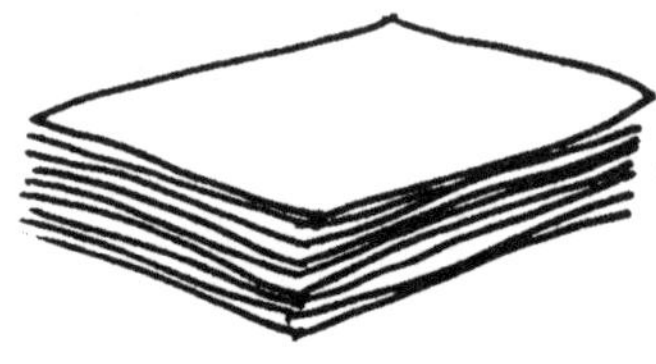

WHOLE PACKAGE OF PAPER

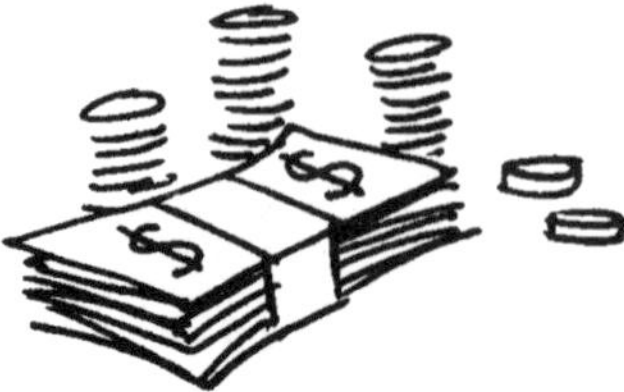

MONEY

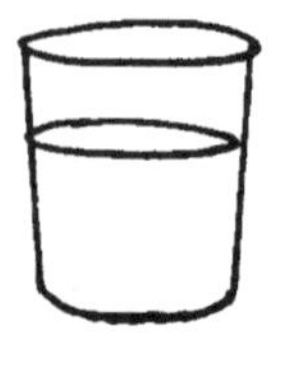

GLASS OF MILK

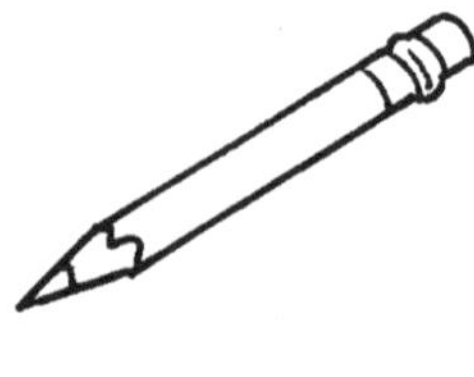

PENCIL

"WHEN" SHOULD YOU LAUGH? PICKLES

Directions: Cut out the "pickles" and place them in the appropriate jar. (See page 172.)

Fran tripped and fell into a patch of clover. She grinned and said, "Help me find a four-leaf clover."
Should you laugh?

Fran tripped and fell into a patch of clover. She ripped the sleeve of her blouse and began to cry.
Should you laugh?

Zach was reading aloud. He read the word wrong and was upset with himself.
Should you laugh?

Zach was reading aloud. He read the word *gazed* wrong and laughed at the silly sentence he made. He read, "The cow grazed up in the sky."
Should you laugh?

Victor's homework flew out of his hand and landed in a mud puddle. He kept saying how much trouble he would be in.
Should you laugh?

Victor's homework flew out of his hand and landed in a mud puddle. He laughed and hoped his teacher would like a mud pie.
Should you laugh?

Maria was painting a rainbow when the wind blew her paper right across her shirt. She said her mom would laugh and say she was the pot of gold at the end of the rainbow.
Should you laugh?

Maria was painting a rainbow when the wind blew her paper right across her shirt. She was upset because the teacher might think she was being careless.
Should you laugh?

A bully put on Sam's glasses and started laughing.
Should you laugh?

A bully pulled on the jumprope which made Sarah fall.
Should you laugh?

Name ______________________________

SECRET CODE

(LAUGHING)

A B C D E F G

H I J K L M N

O P Q R S T U

V W X Y Z CLAWED HAND . BENT HAND ,

BENT HAND

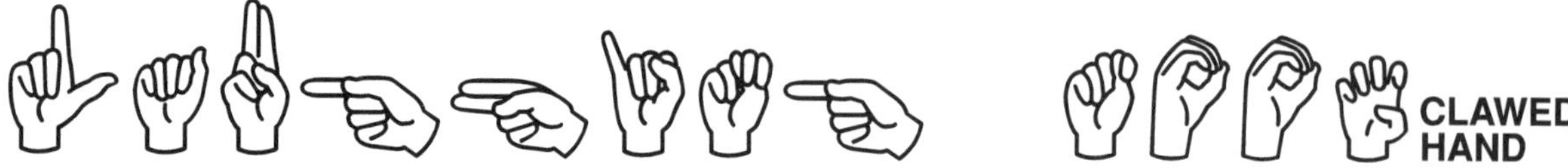

"WHEN" SHOULD YOU TELL? PICKLES

Directions: Cut out the "pickles" and place them in the appropriate jar. (See page 172.)

Bill is writing on his own lunch box.
Should you tell?

Bill is writing on the classroom wall.
Should you tell?

Jamal is running in circles on the playground.
Should you tell?

You saw the kid who likes to bully other kids hit Jamal with a rock.
Should you tell?

Pam is trying to trip students going to the pencil sharpener.
Should you tell?

Pam is making silly faces at students going to the pencil sharpener.
Should you tell?

Carmen's glue is dripping on the computer keyboard.
Should you tell?

Carmen put a crayon in her glue.
Should you tell?

Mike threw a rock at the window.
Should you tell?

Mike threw a paper airplane at the window.
Should you tell?

"WHEN" SHOULD YOU TELL? PICKLES

Directions: Cut out the "pickles" and place them in the appropriate jar. (See page 172.)

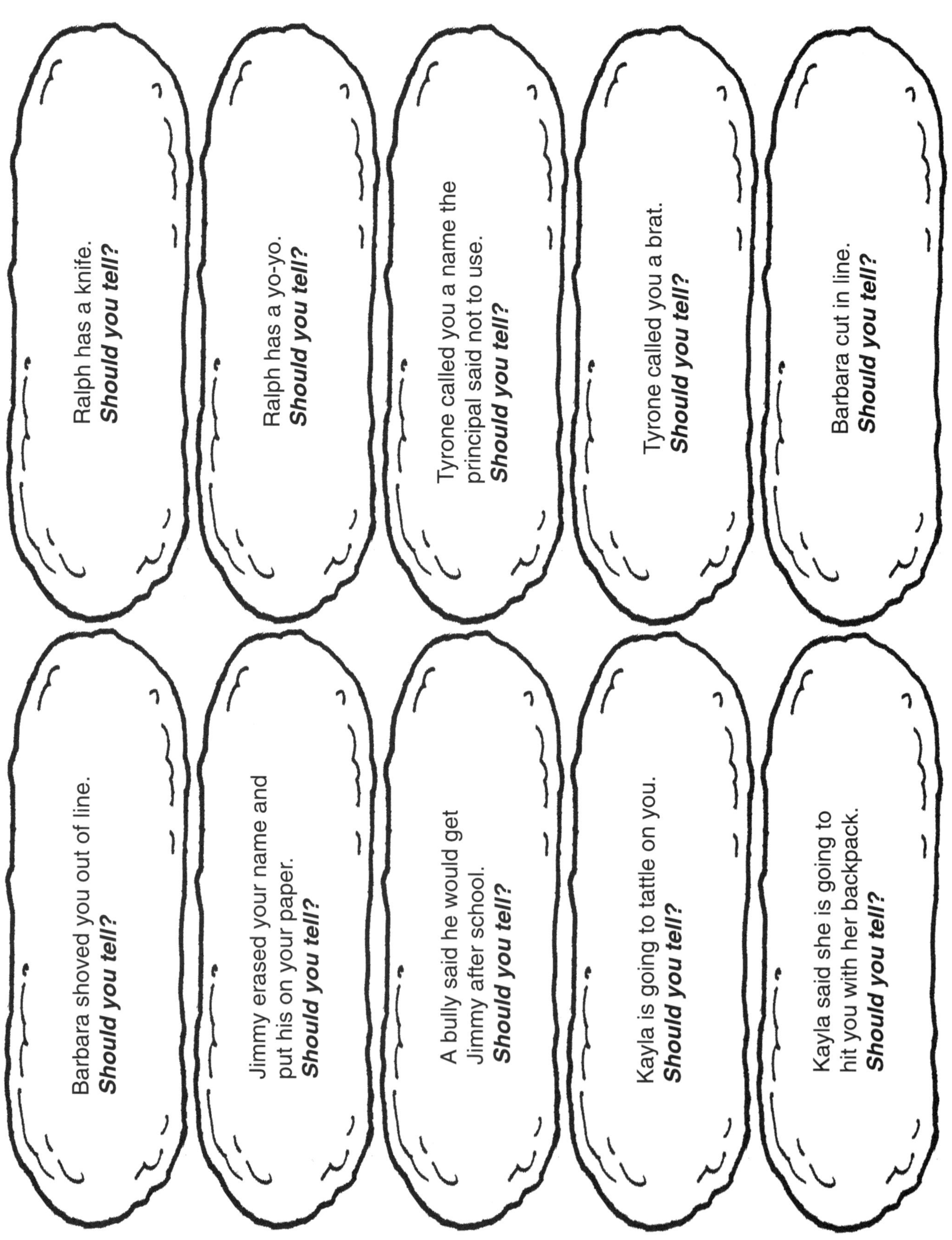

Name ______________________________

PLAYGROUND REPORTING

Directions: Circle the pictures that show something that should be reported to an adult.

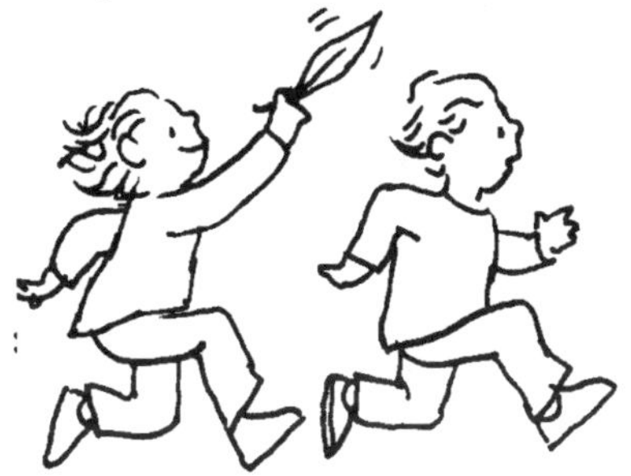

Chasing someone with a feather

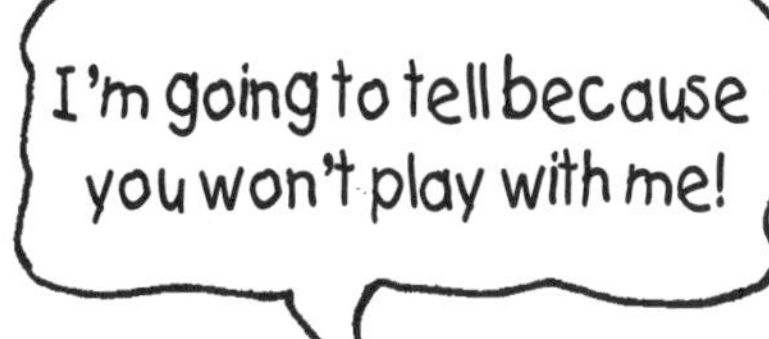

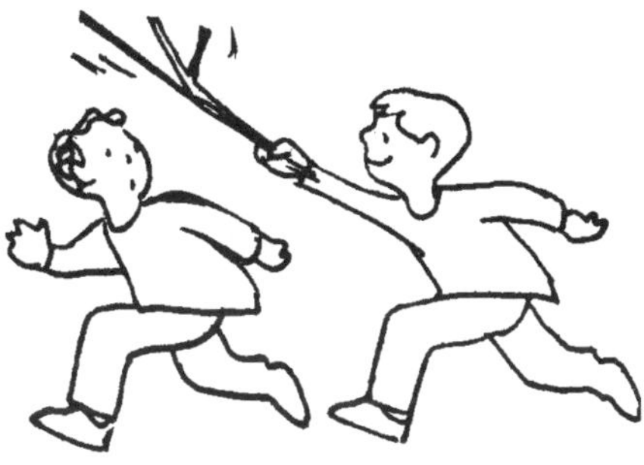

Chasing someone with a stick

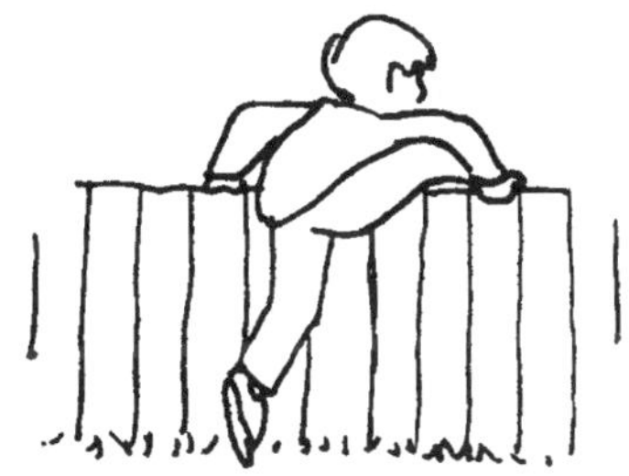

Climbing over a fence

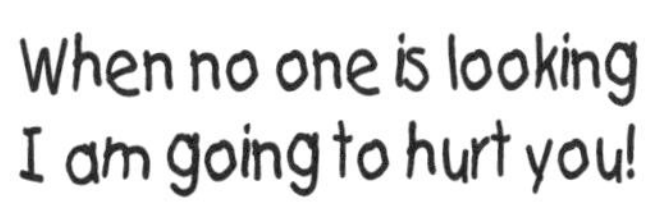

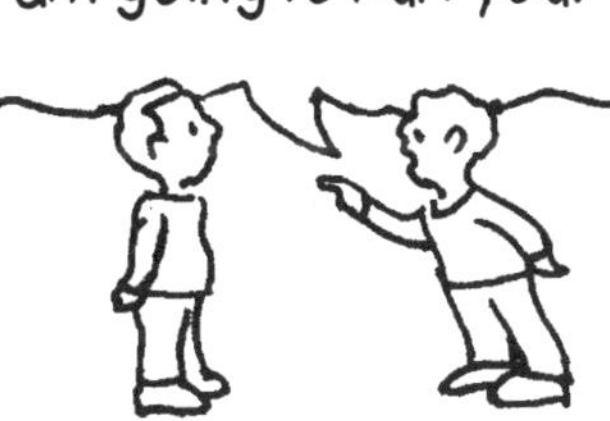

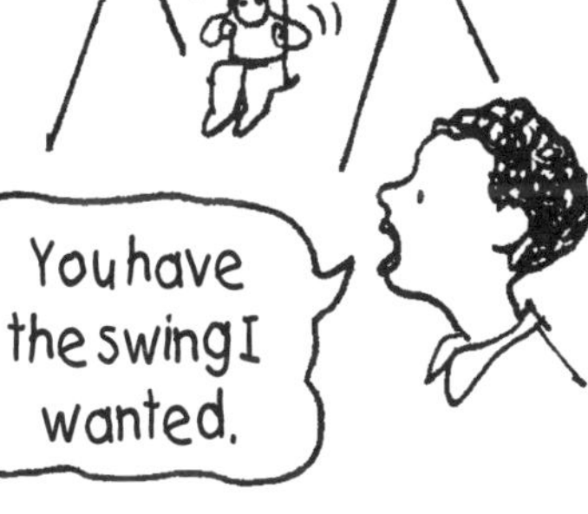

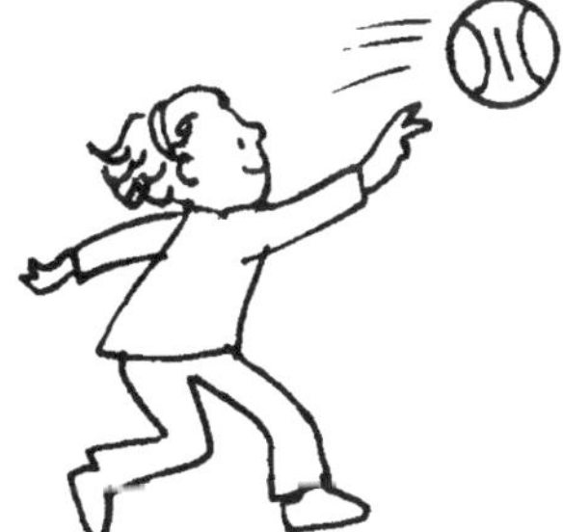

Throwing a ball

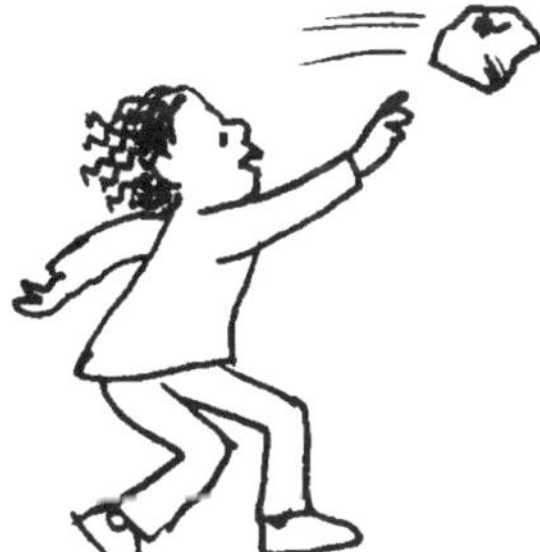

Throwing a rock

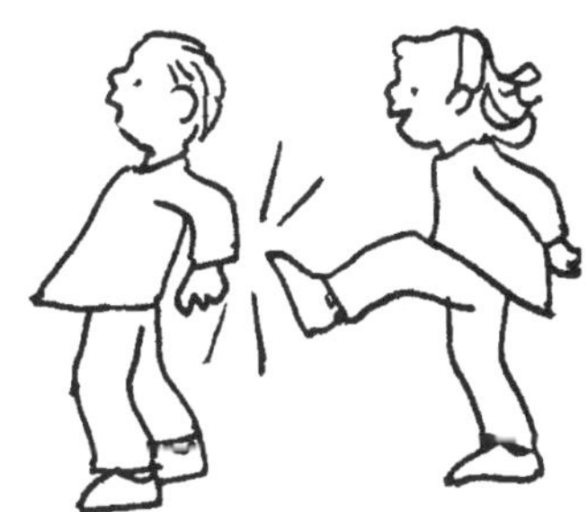

Kicking

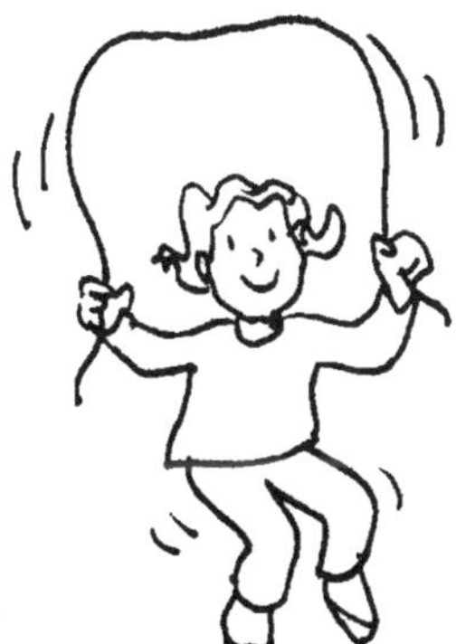

Jumping rope

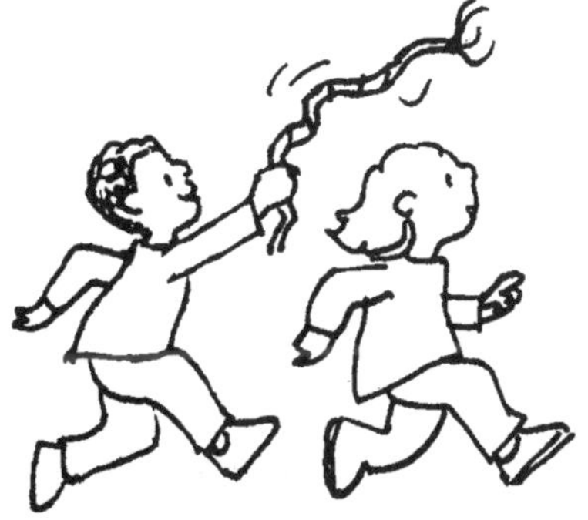

Chasing someone with a rope

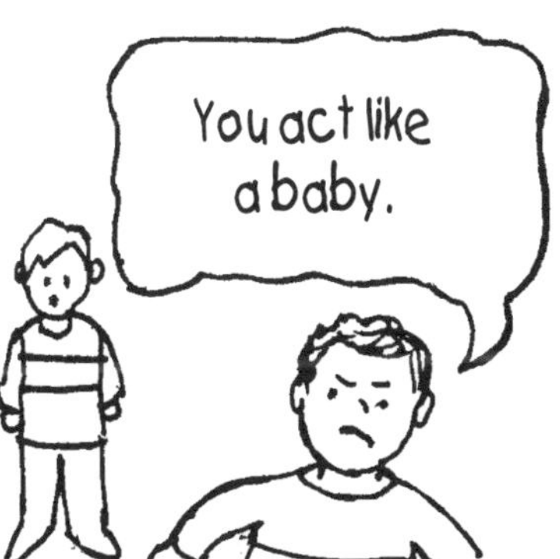

TATTLING/REPORTING GUIDELINES

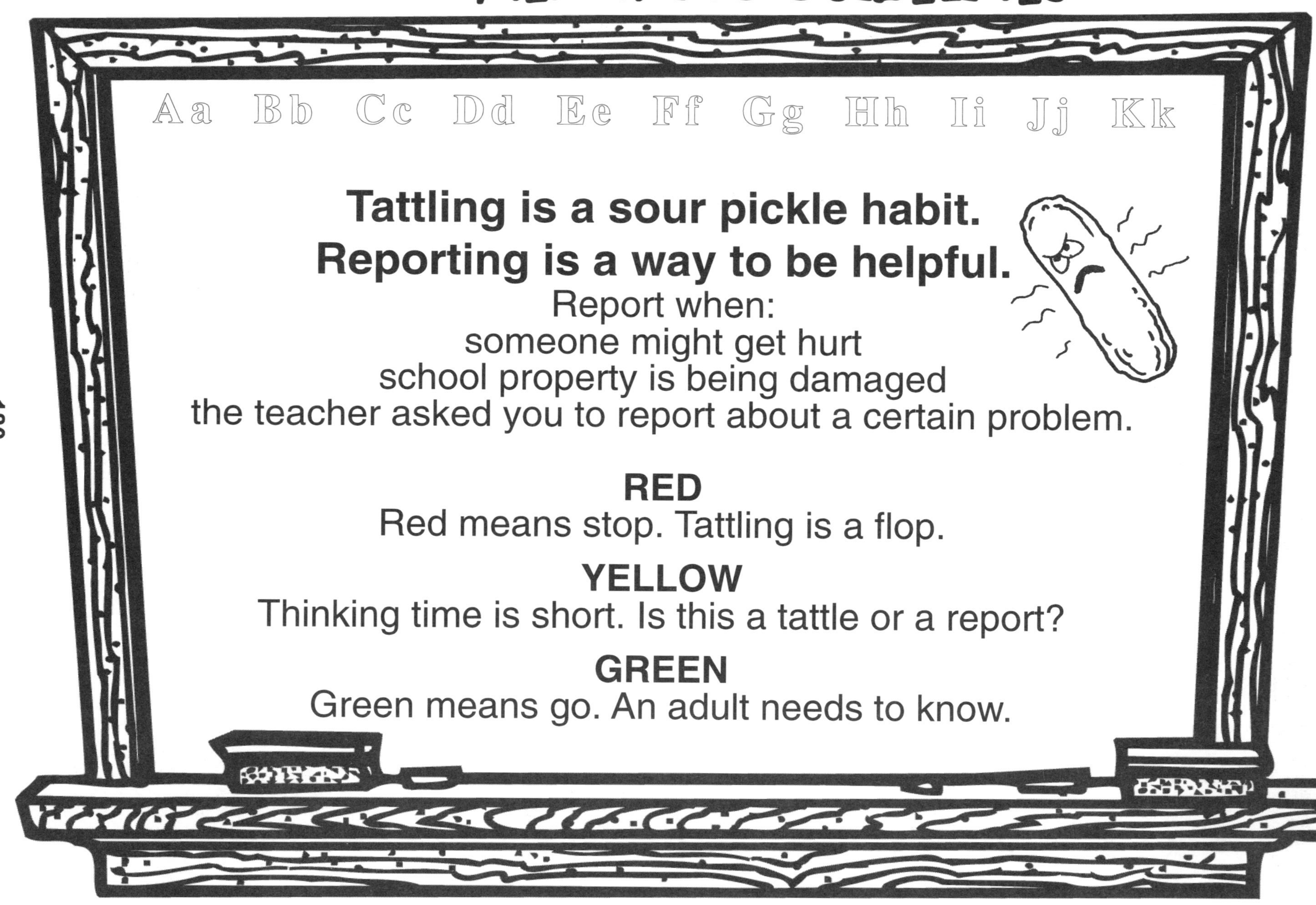

Tattling is a sour pickle habit.
Reporting is a way to be helpful.

Report when:
someone might get hurt
school property is being damaged
the teacher asked you to report about a certain problem.

RED

Red means stop. Tattling is a flop.

YELLOW

Thinking time is short. Is this a tattle or a report?

GREEN

Green means go. An adult needs to know.

STOPLIGHT FOR TATTLES AND REPORTS

RED MEANS STOP.

TATTLING IS A FLOP.

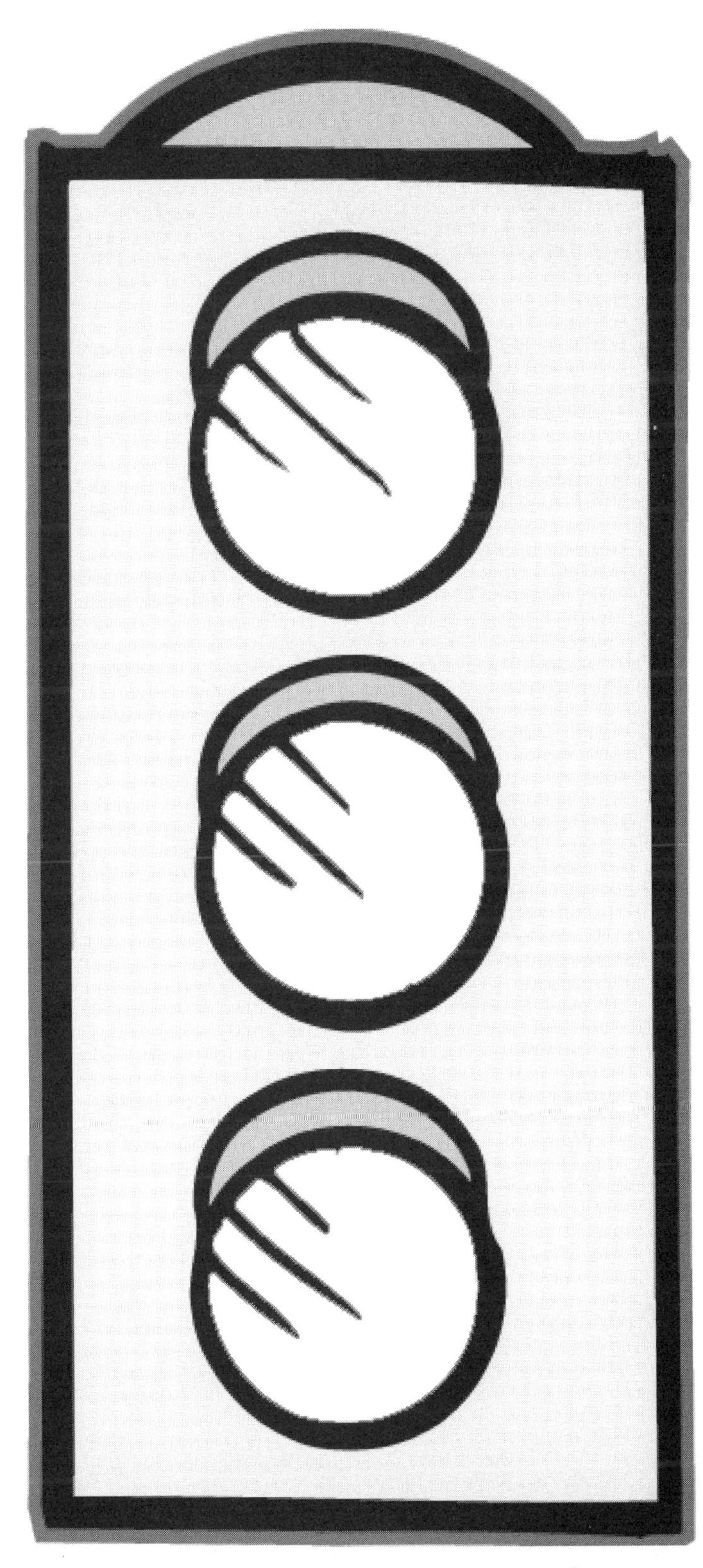

YELLOW MEANS THINKING TIME IS SHORT.

IS THIS A TATTLE OR A REPORT?

GREEN MEANS GO.

AN ADULT NEEDS TO KNOW.

Name ______________________________

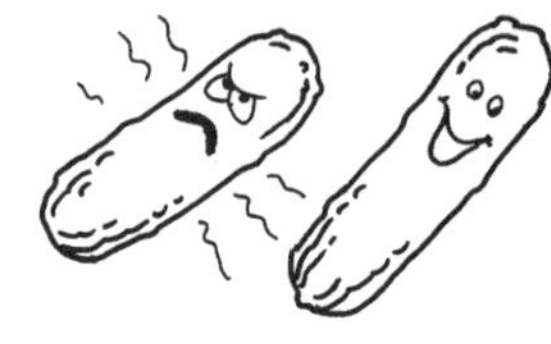

SECRET CODE
(TATTLING)

A B C D E F G

H I J K L M N

O P Q R S T U

V W X Y Z CLAWED HAND . BENT HAND ,

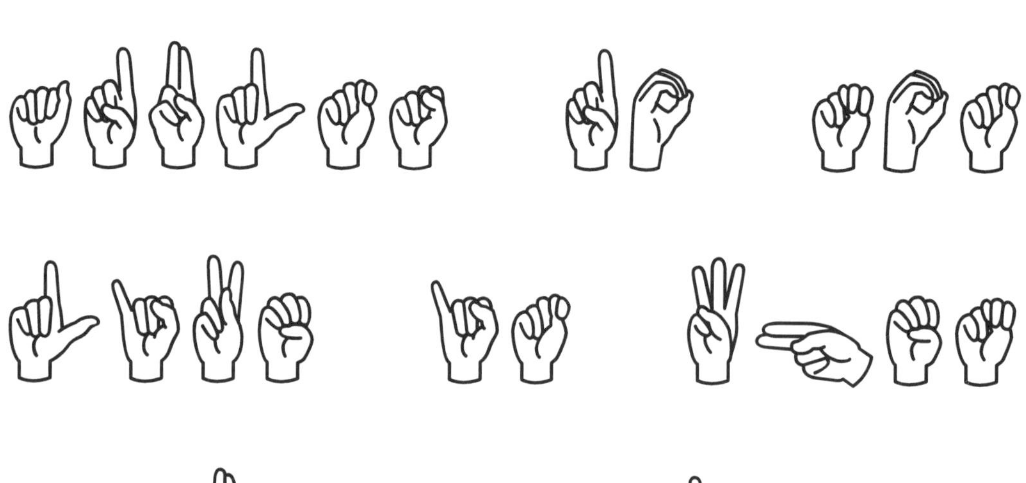

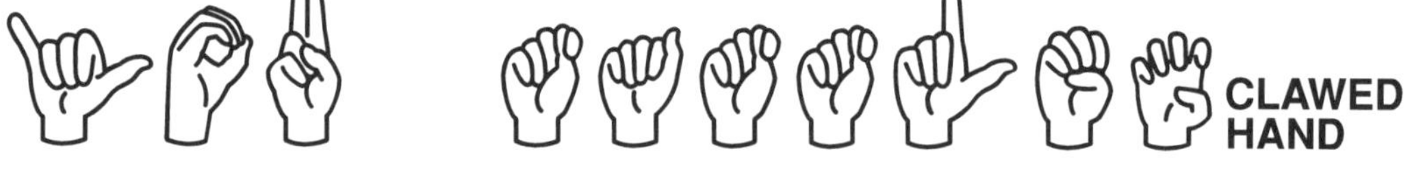

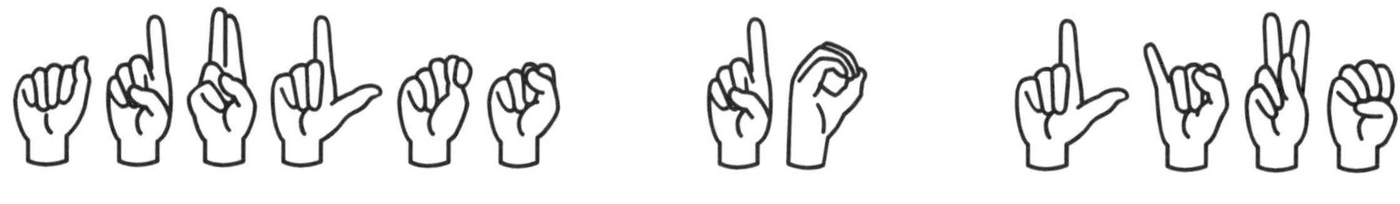

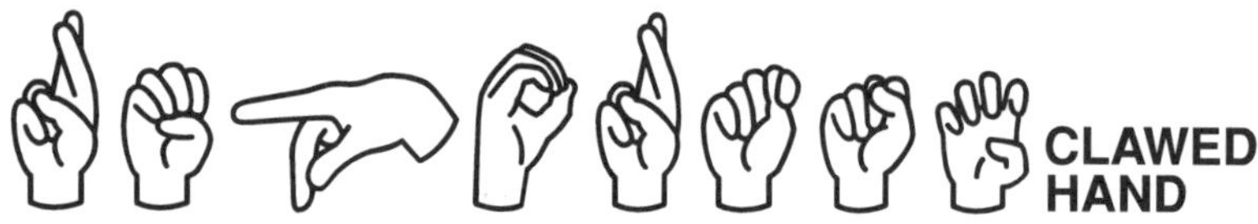

"WHEN" SHOULD YOU TELL A SECRET? PICKLES

Directions: Cut out the "pickles" and place them in the appropriate jar. (See page 172.)

Mary's father told her he stopped at the florist to order her mother some flowers. He said it was a secret. ***Should she tell?***

Mom told Ian's brother that Ian was getting a puppy. It was a secret. ***Should he tell?***

A teenager showed Chip some secret pills that were supposed to make him very happy. ***Should he tell?***

Jane heard two big kids talking about hurting another kid. They said nobody better find out. ***Should she tell?***

Lance showed his best friend four big bruises he got when someone in his house drank too much. ***Should his friend tell a grown-up the secret?***

Bianca told you she likes Carlos, but it's a secret. ***Should you tell?***

Bruce stole Sam's homework. Mike saw him do it. ***Should he tell?***

A man tried to get Sissy to take candy and get into his car. He said it was a secret. ***Should she tell?***

Louis told you he was saving part of his allowance to buy a present. ***Should you tell?***

Whitney told you she was making a surprise card for her dad. ***Should you tell?***

"WHEN" SHOULD YOU TELL A SECRET? PICKLES

Directions: Cut out the "pickles" and place them in the appropriate jar. (See page 172.)

Kevin is being bullied by a group of boys on his way to school. They threaten to beat Kevin up if he tells. ***Should he tell?***

Shanna didn't want her dad to know a big boy took her umbrella. ***Should she tell?***

The strangers at the store took a picture of Kano and said not to tell. ***Should he tell?***

Chris is baking her grandmother a surprise birthday cake. ***Should she tell?***

Yvonne broke her grandmother's vase and went home without telling. ***Should she tell?***

A student felt uncomfortable when touched by a man at the fair. ***Should the student tell?***

Robin felt nervous around a man who sometimes visited her house. ***Should she tell?***

Linda saw the teacher's husband leave a flower on her desk. He said it was a secret and not to say how it got there. ***Should she tell?***

Name ______________________________

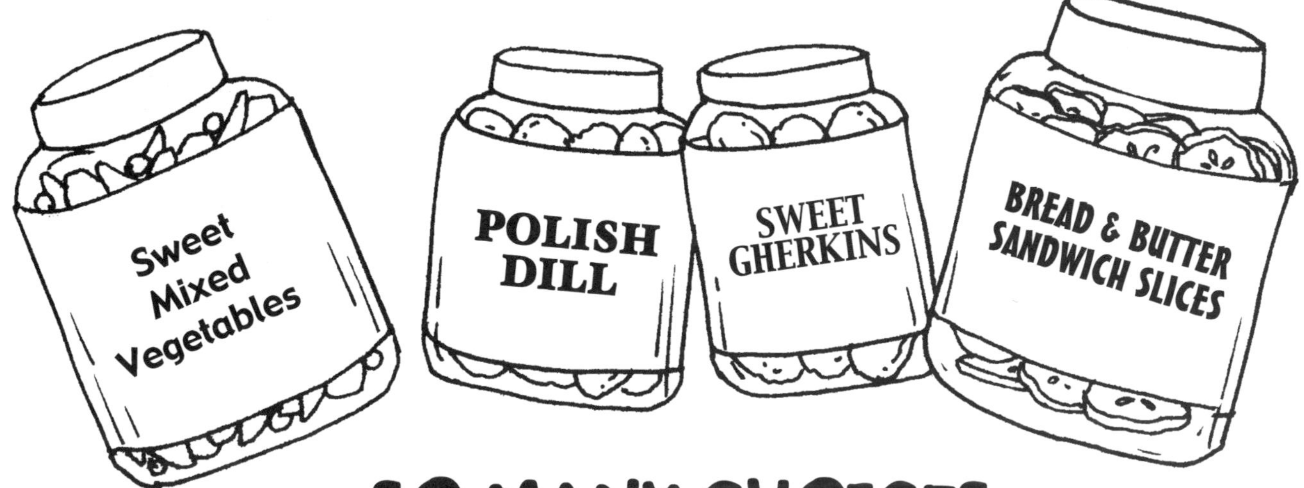

SO MANY CHOICES

There are so many choices to make! Sometimes we worry too much and too long over choices that don't really matter.

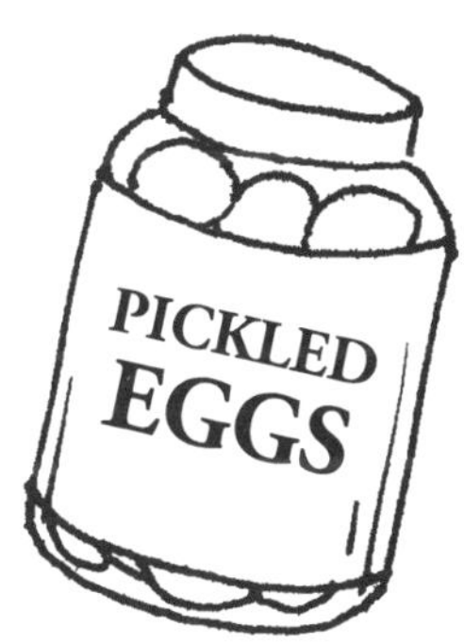

Look at the jars of pickles. We could take lots of time studying them at the store. A year from now, will it matter which one we choose? A month from now, will it matter which one we choose? Probably not.

Some choices are very important. You must think before making some choices, because they will matter to other people, or to yourself, long after the choice is made.

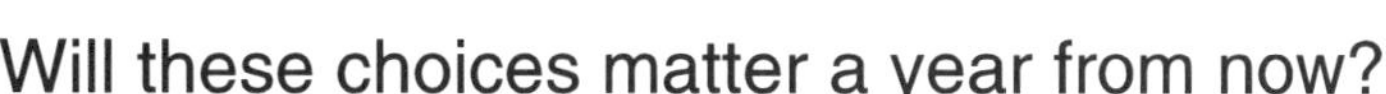

Will these choices matter a year from now?

what you eat for dinner	**YES**	**NO**
which shirt you wear today	**YES**	**NO**
which coat you buy	**YES**	**NO**
which fast-food restaurant you go to	**YES**	**NO**
whether you enroll in baseball or soccer	**YES**	**NO**

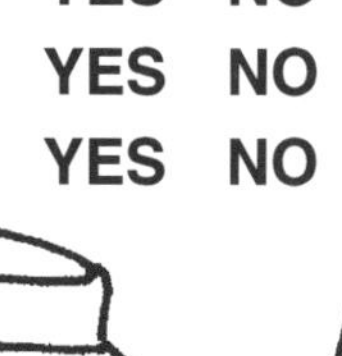

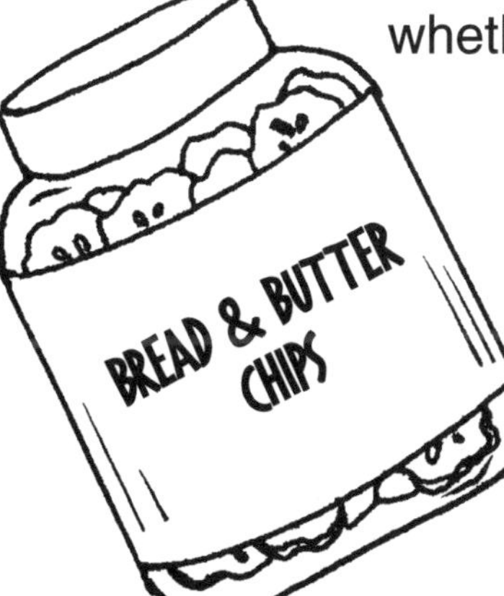

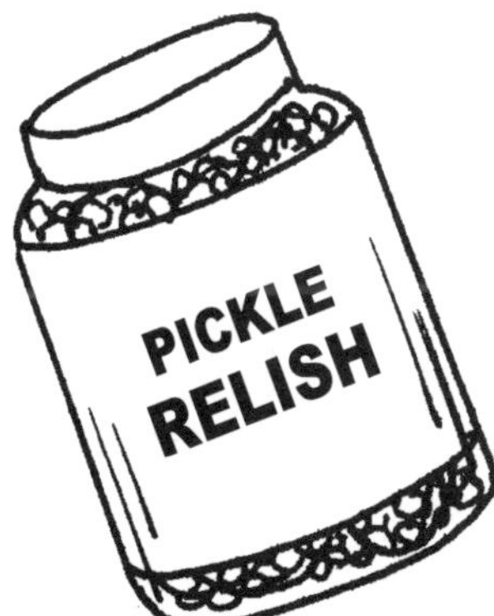

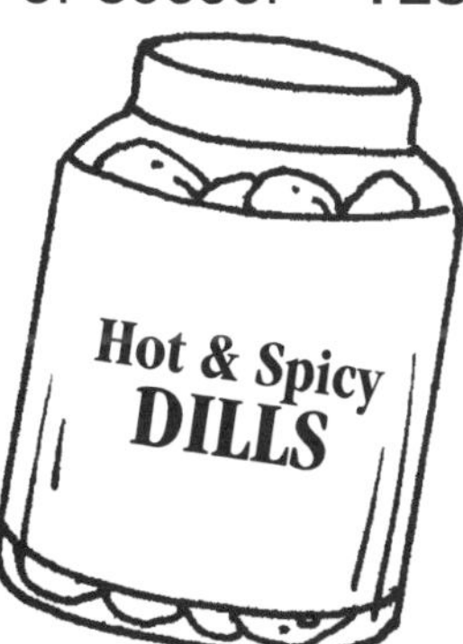

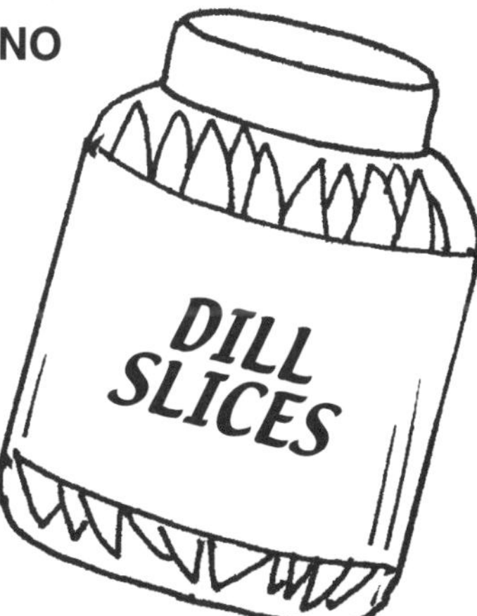

"WHEN" IS A CHOICE IMPORTANT? PICKLES

Directions: Cut out the "pickles" and place them in the appropriate jar. (See page 172.)

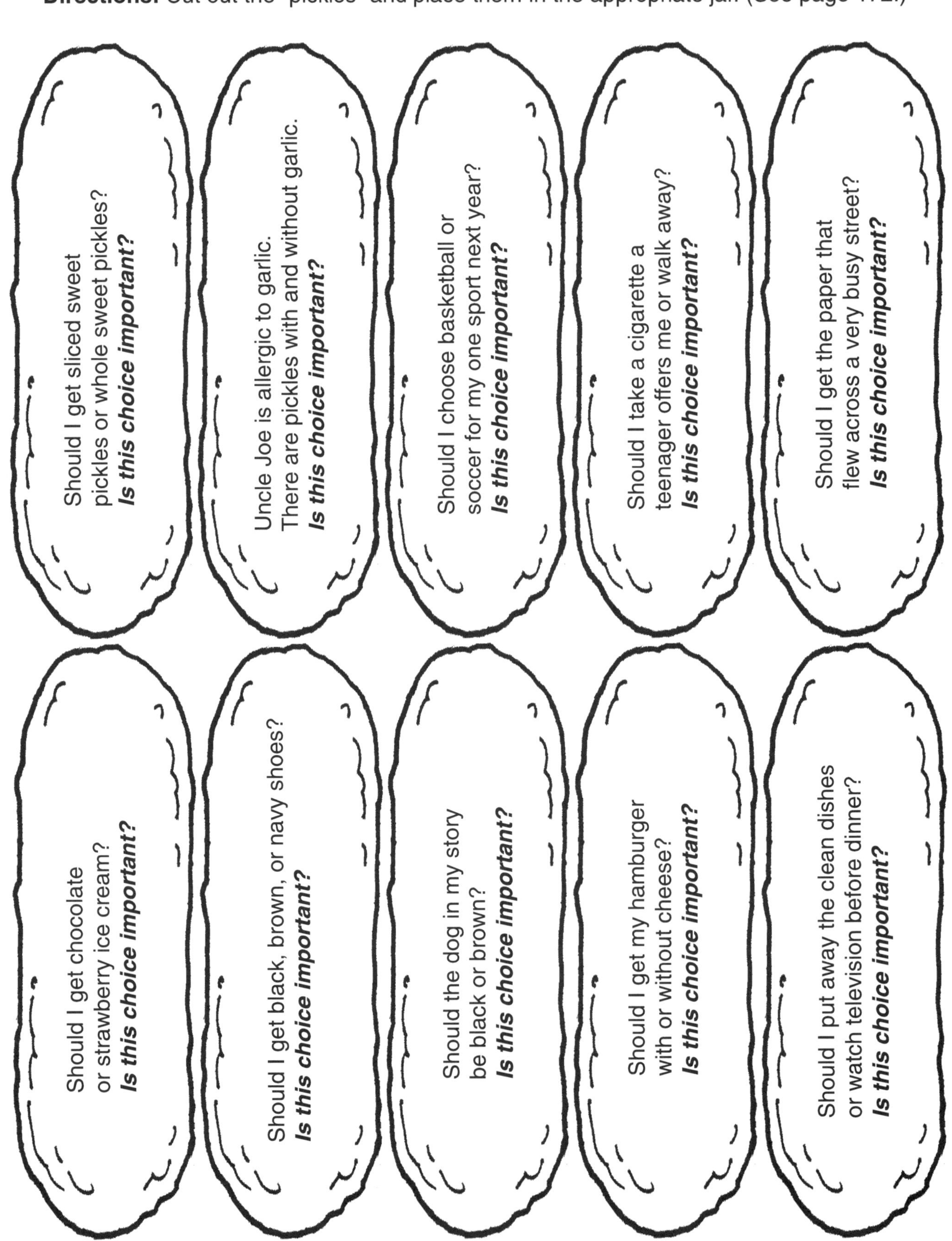

"WHEN" IS A CHOICE IMPORTANT? PICKLES

Directions: Cut out the "pickles" and place them in the appropriate jar. (See page 172.)

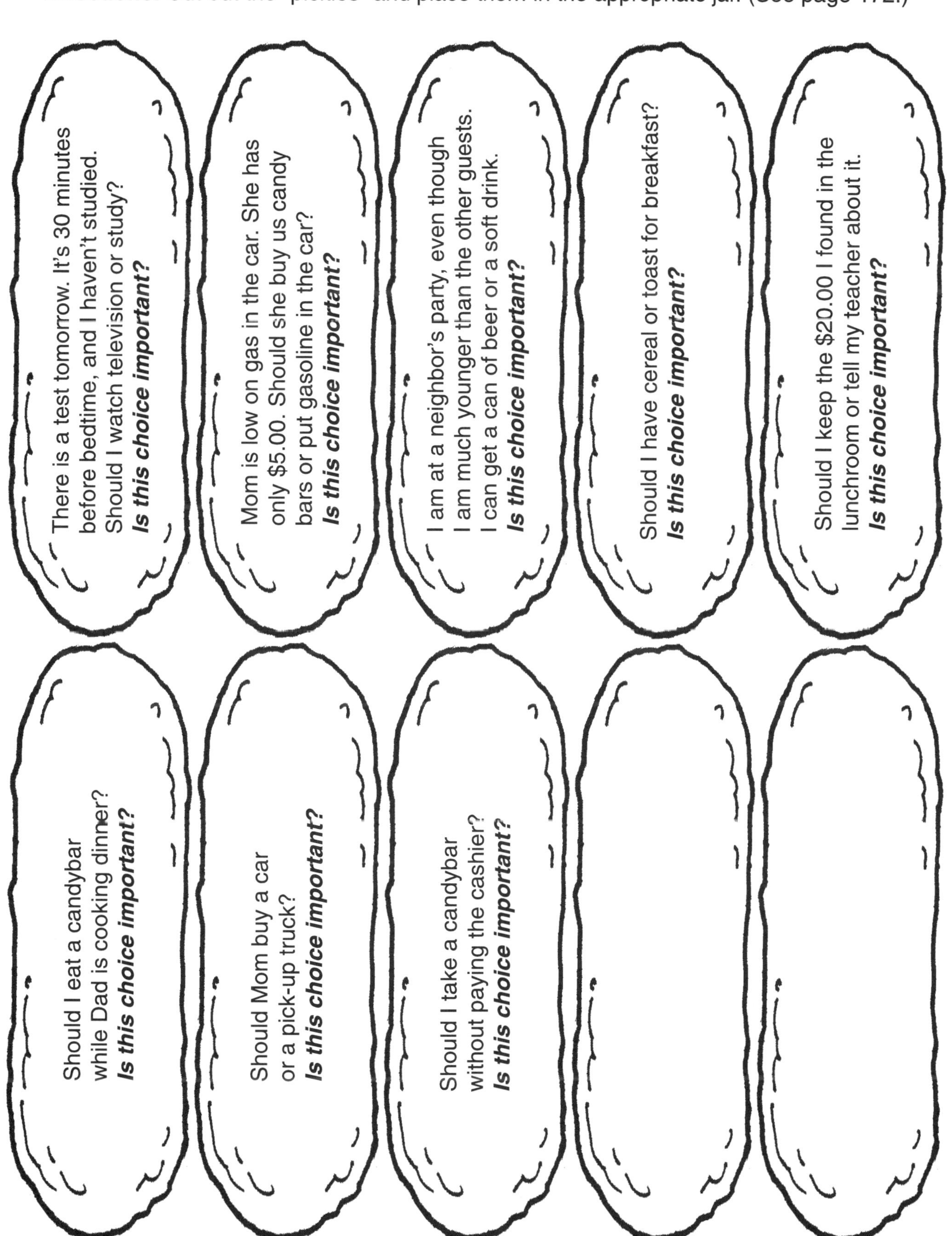

Name ______________________________

WE CARE ABOUT EACH OTHER PHRASES

Directions: Circle the phrases that show that we care about each other.

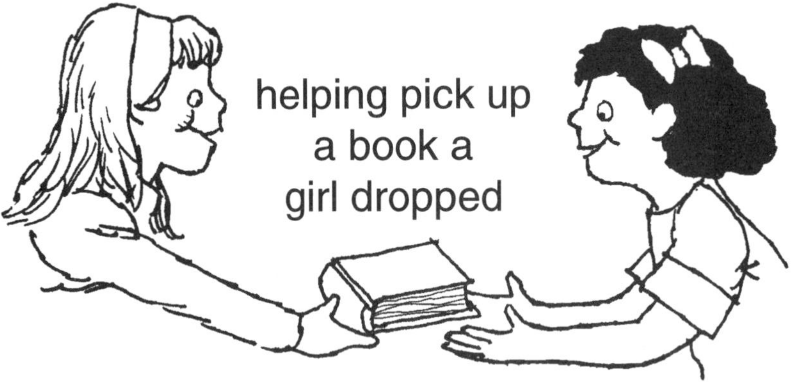

helping pick up a book a girl dropped

taking three of the four cookies on a plate

helping a boy chase a paper in the wind

flushing the toilet

saying something nice about someone

telling a boy his "show and tell" is dumb

taking the new student to the playground

covering your mouth when you sneeze

making fun of a hurt student

being quiet while the teacher is reading

helping raise money for a family whose house burned down

laughing at the girl who dropped her tray

pushing in line

sending a thank-you note

Name ______________________________

WE CARE ABOUT EACH OTHER PICTURES

Directions: Circle the pictures that show that we care about each other.

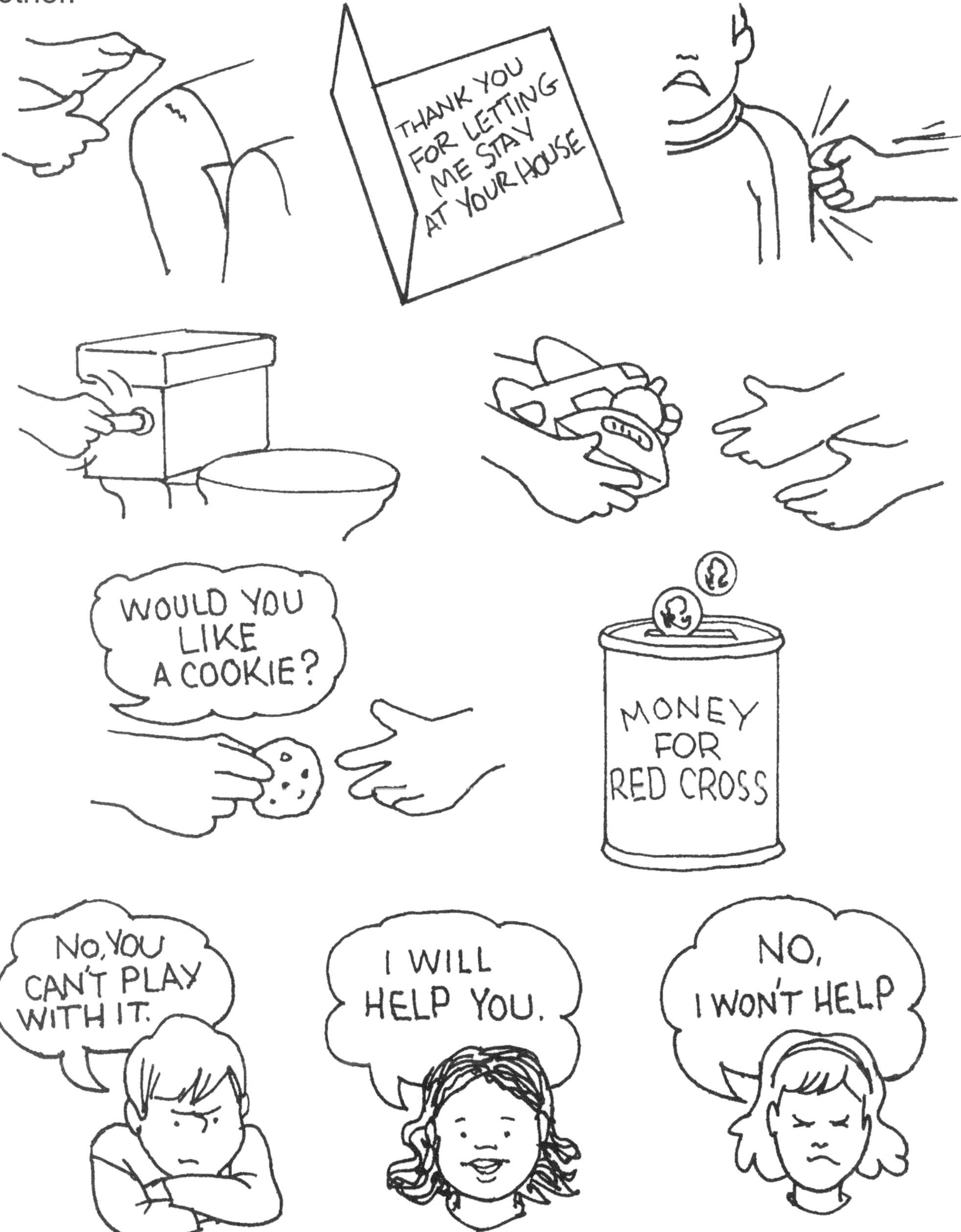

Name ______________________________

WE CARE ABOUT OURSELVES PHRASES

Directions: Circle the phrases that show that you care about yourself.

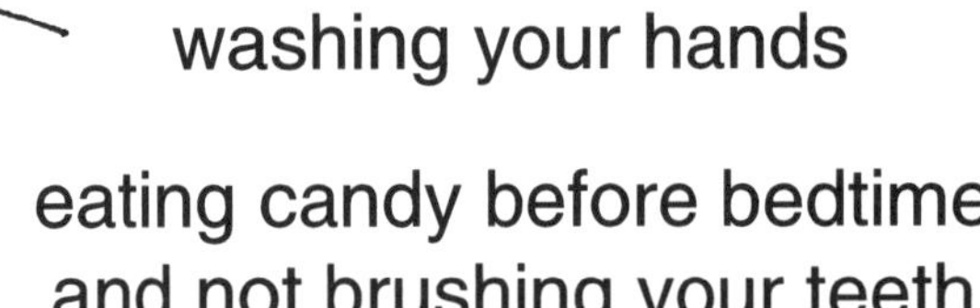

washing your hands

eating candy before bedtime
and not brushing your teeth

watching television for three hours right after school

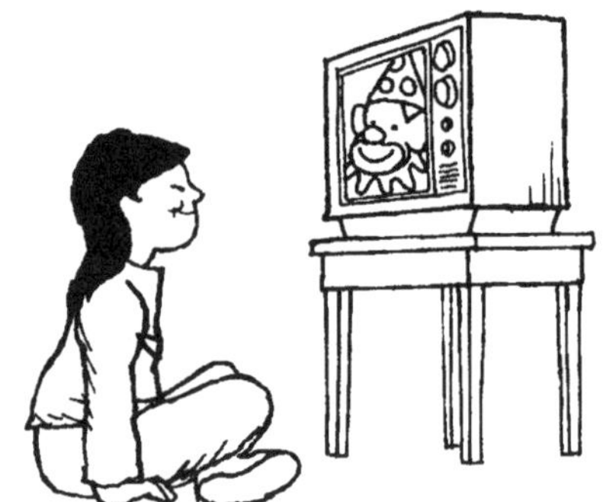

wearing sunscreen

learning to read

doing your homework

wearing a seatbelt

taking medicine without an adult's permission

turning in your schoolwork

smoking a cigarette

eating fruit

keeping a scary secret

playing with matches

telling a scary secret

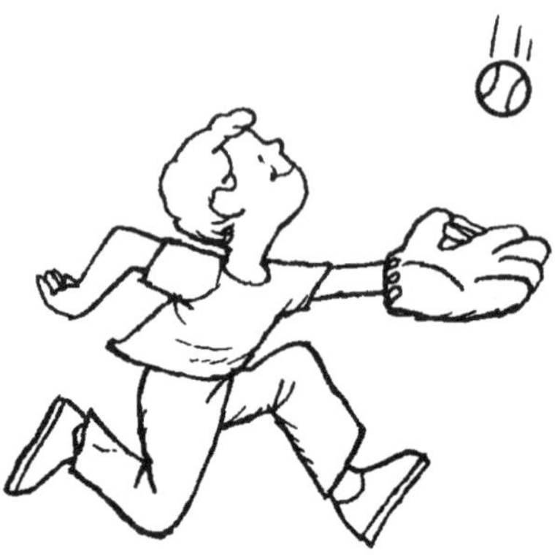

brushing your teeth

getting exercise

getting enough sleep

Name ___________________________

WE CARE ABOUT OURSELVES PICTURES

Directions: Circle the pictures that show that you care about yourself.

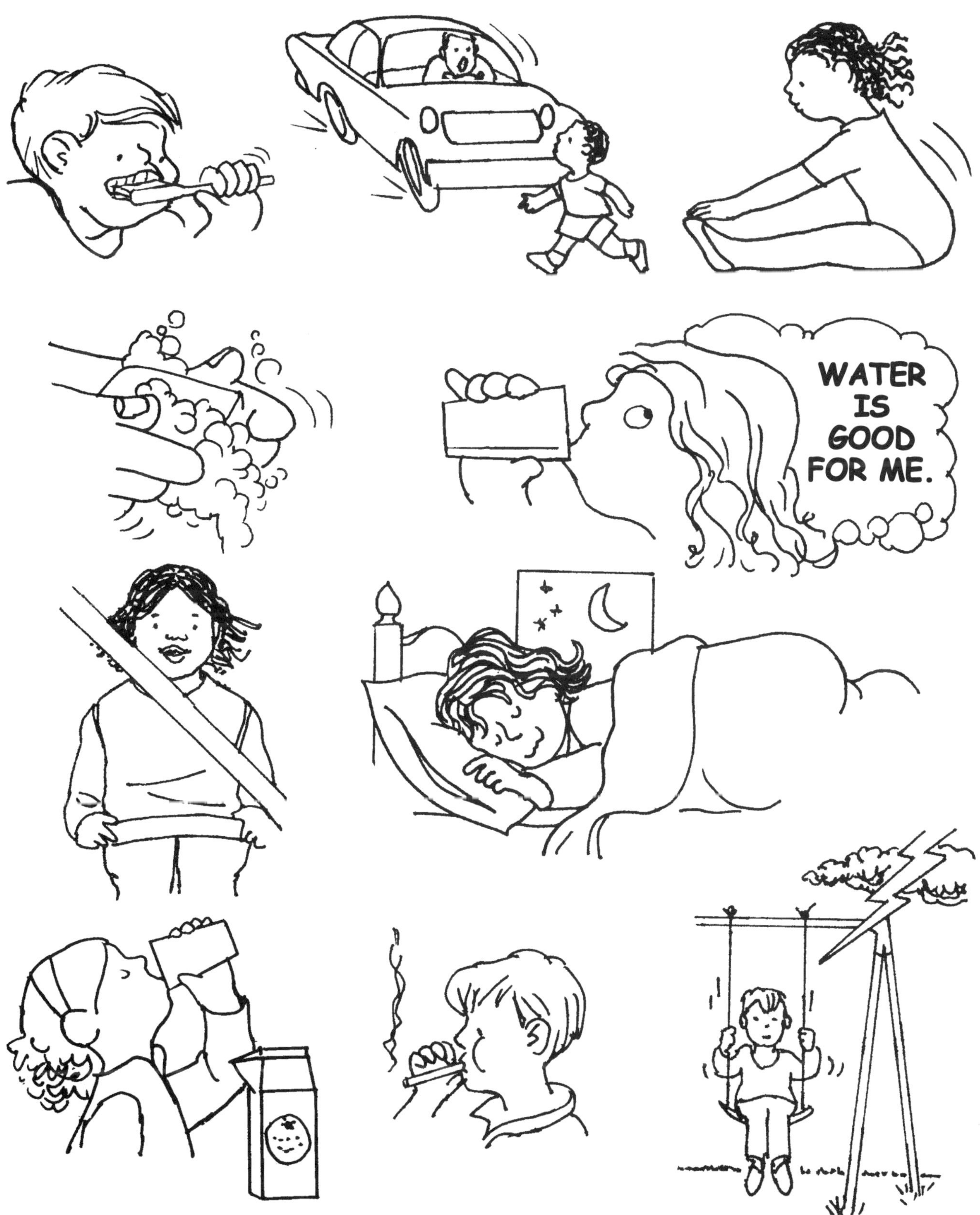

Name ______________________________

WE CARE ABOUT THE EARTH PHRASES

Directions: Circle the phrases that show that you care about the earth.

 planting flowers 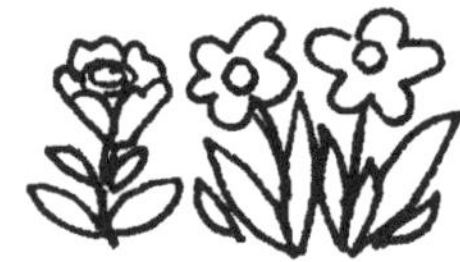

dropping gum on the sidewalk

putting gum in the trashcan

leaving spilled glue on the floor

telling a grown-up about broken glass

recycling cans and newspapers

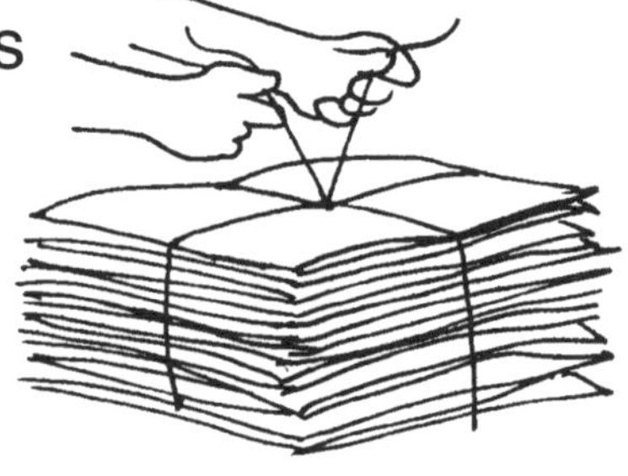

feeding the birds

tossing a can into the creek

throwing a paper cup out the car window

giving items you don't need to a helping organization

throwing unwanted items by the side of the road

picking up trash

leaving water running

turning off unneeded lights

buying products made from recycled materials

Name ______________________________

WE CARE ABOUT THE EARTH PICTURES

Directions: Circle the pictures that show that you care about the earth.

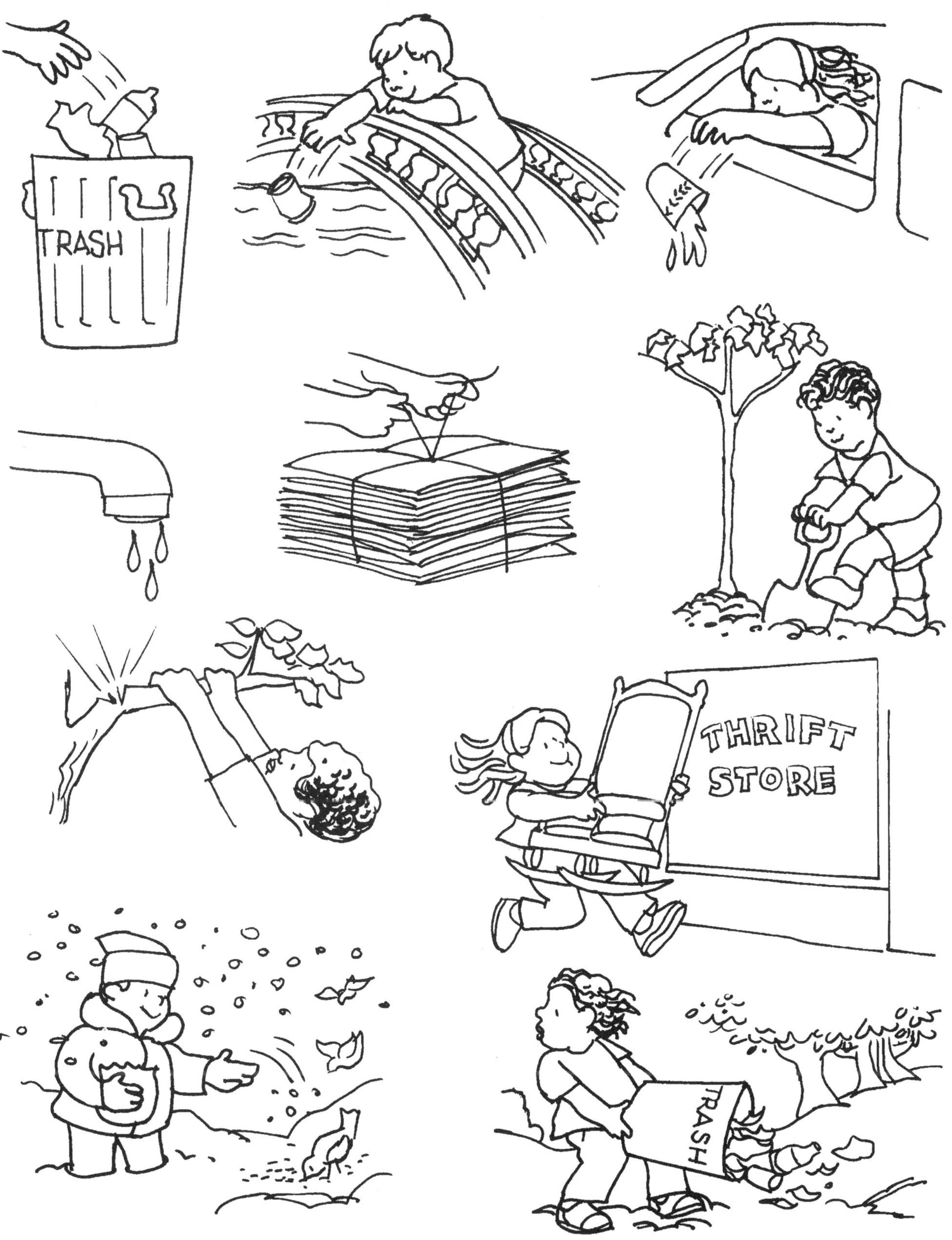

CHAPTER 5

CAREER EDUCATION

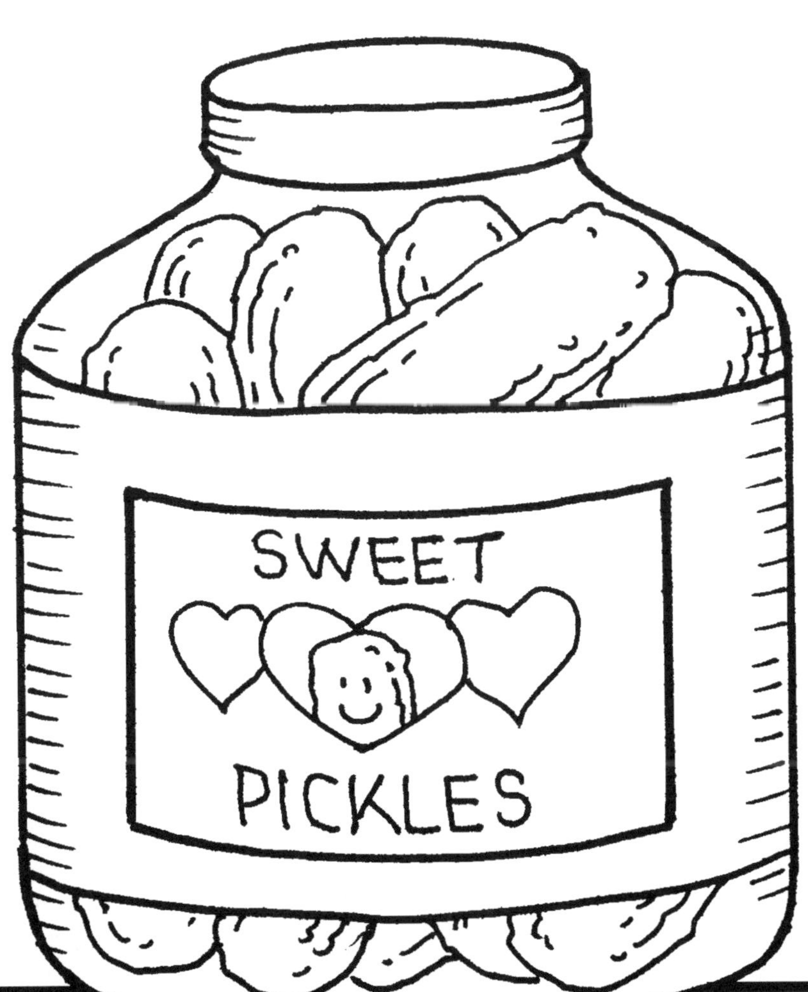

Name ______________________________

ALL JOBS ARE IMPORTANT

Any job that helps others and earns money for a family is important. Some jobs help other workers do their jobs. Read each sentence below and circle the jobs that are needed.

Before you can eat at a restaurant, which jobs **need** to be done?

food bought

dishes washed

food cooked

car washed

Before you fly in an airplane, which jobs **need** to be done?

plane checked by mechanics

shoes polished

cabin prepared by flight attendants

orders given by air traffic controller

Before you come to school each day, which jobs **need** to be done?

restrooms cleaned

teachers' plans made

haircut for principal

bus drivers ready to drive buses

Before you have a broken arm set, which jobs **need** to be done?

homework graded

supplies ordered

hospital cleaned

check-in forms completed

Before you can live in a house, which jobs **need** to be done?

house electricity turned on

plumbing in working order

pictures hung on wall

furniture moved in

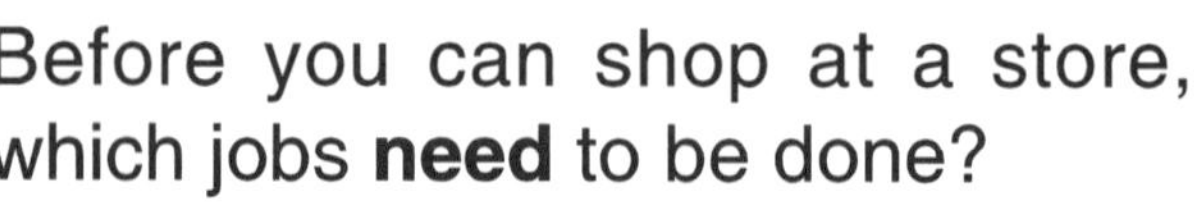

Before you can shop at a store, which jobs **need** to be done?

items shipped to the store

store clerks hired

items priced

music played

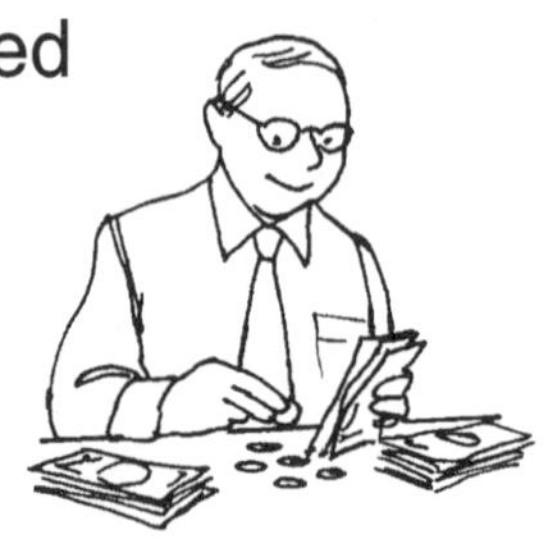

OCCUPATIONS LIST

1. **Accountants/Bookkeepers**
complete financial records
(Accountants have more specialized education.)

2. **Air Traffic Controllers**
Direct flights by giving information from a control tower to a pilot

3. **Airline Agents**
work with travelers checking in at the airport before a flight

4. **Architects**
draw plans and specifications, called blueprints, for buildings

5. **Bricklayers**
build with bricks or concrete blocks

6. **Carpenters**
build things from wood

7. **Cashiers**
in charge of paying and receiving money

8. **Commercial Drivers**
drive vehicles that deliver products or transport people

9. **Computer Operators**
use programs to accomplish tasks on a computer

10. **Cooks/Chefs**
prepare food (Chefs have more specialized training.)

11. **Counselors**
listen to people and help them look at their choices

12. **Custodians/Janitors**
keep buildings clean and in good working order

13. **Dieticians**
plan meals meeting various health requirements

14. **Electricians**
repair or install electrical wires and electrical devices

15. **Executives**
make decisions about and run an organization or business

16. **Flight Attendants**
take care of passengers on airplanes

17. **Glaziers**
install glass

18. **Groundskeepers**
maintain the property outside a building

19. **Housekeepers**
keep rooms clean for patients or guests

20. **Inspectors**
check products to verify quality

21. **Insulation Workers**
install materials that make buildings energy-efficient

22. **Judges**
preside over courts of law and sentence criminals

23. **Laundry Workers**
wash and prepare clothes
or linens to be used again

24. **Librarians**
organize and check out a collection of
books and other information materials

25. **Line Workers**
perform specific jobs
on an assembly line

26. **Mechanics**
repair and keep vehicles
(cars, buses, airplanes, etc.)
in good running condition

27. **Medical Technicians**
perform specific tests or
therapies on patients

28. **Nurses**
provide help that assists a doctor or
that does not require a doctor

29. **Nurse's Aides**
take care of patient needs that
do not require a nurse or doctor

30. **Painters**
paint inside and outside of buildings,
paint roads, bridges, etc.

31. **Personnel Managers**
hire employees and keep up
with their effectiveness

32. **Pharmacists**
dispense medicine
prescribed by doctors

33. **Physical Therapists**
help patients regain strength and
flexibility following illness or injury

34. **Physicians**
diagnose and treat illnesses
(Many physicians specialize in a field
of medicine, such as pediatrics.)

35. **Pilots**
operate the controls of an
aircraft in flight or a ship at sea

36. **Plumbers**
install and repair water pipes
and related fixtures

37. **Porters/Skycaps**
carry baggage and do
errands for travelers

38. **Principals**
make decisions and oversee
activities of teachers and students

39. **Receptionists**
greet people who enter offices

40. **Secretaries**
do a variety of necessary office tasks

41. **Security Guards**
provide security for buildings
and employees

42. **Social Workers**
help people with family-related
problems find needed services

43. **Surveyors**
measure and draw maps
to determine boundaries

44. **Teachers**
provide instruction and
help students learn

SUPPLEMENTARY OCCUPATIONS LIST

1. **Bailiffs**
   maintain order in the courtroom
2. **Commercial Artists**
   provide drawings needed for projects like ads, pamphlets, etc.
3. **Cosmetologists**
   take care of hair, nails, or skin for customers
4. **Court Reporters**
   record all words spoken at a trial except what the judge asks to be omitted
5. **Editors**
   check articles before publication and decide what will be printed
6. **Engineers**
   use math and science laws to develop products, public projects (roads, bridges, airports), machines, etc.
7. **Food Servers**
   take food to tables, hand out food at counters, or dish out food in cafeteria lines
8. **Investigators**
   search for facts to determine what happened
9. **Lawyers (also called attorneys)**
   give advice about matters of law and represent clients in court
10. **Meteorologists**
    study and forecast the weather
11. **Millwrights**
    install or take care of machinery in a factory
12. **Newspaper Carriers**
    deliver newspapers to newsstands and individual customers
13. **Photographers**
    use cameras to take pictures for newspapers, magazines, individuals, etc.
14. **Police Officers**
    keep order and arrest people who do not obey the law
15. **Printing Press Operators**
    run machines that print papers with words and pictures
16. **Reporters**
    gather news to be presented to the public
17. **Roofers**
    install and repair roofs on buildings
18. **Sales Representative**
    find customers to buy products
19. **Sanitation Workers**
    collect trash and recycling materials from homes, businesses, and public places
20. **Telephone Operators**
    answer phones and direct calls to appropriate people
21. **Typesetters/Compositors**
    put words on a page to be printed
22. **Welders**
    use heat to join or shape pieces of metal

Name ___________________________

JOBS AT A PICKLE FACTORY

Directions: Circle the workers who might work at a large pickle factory every day. That means they don't come in just once in a while.

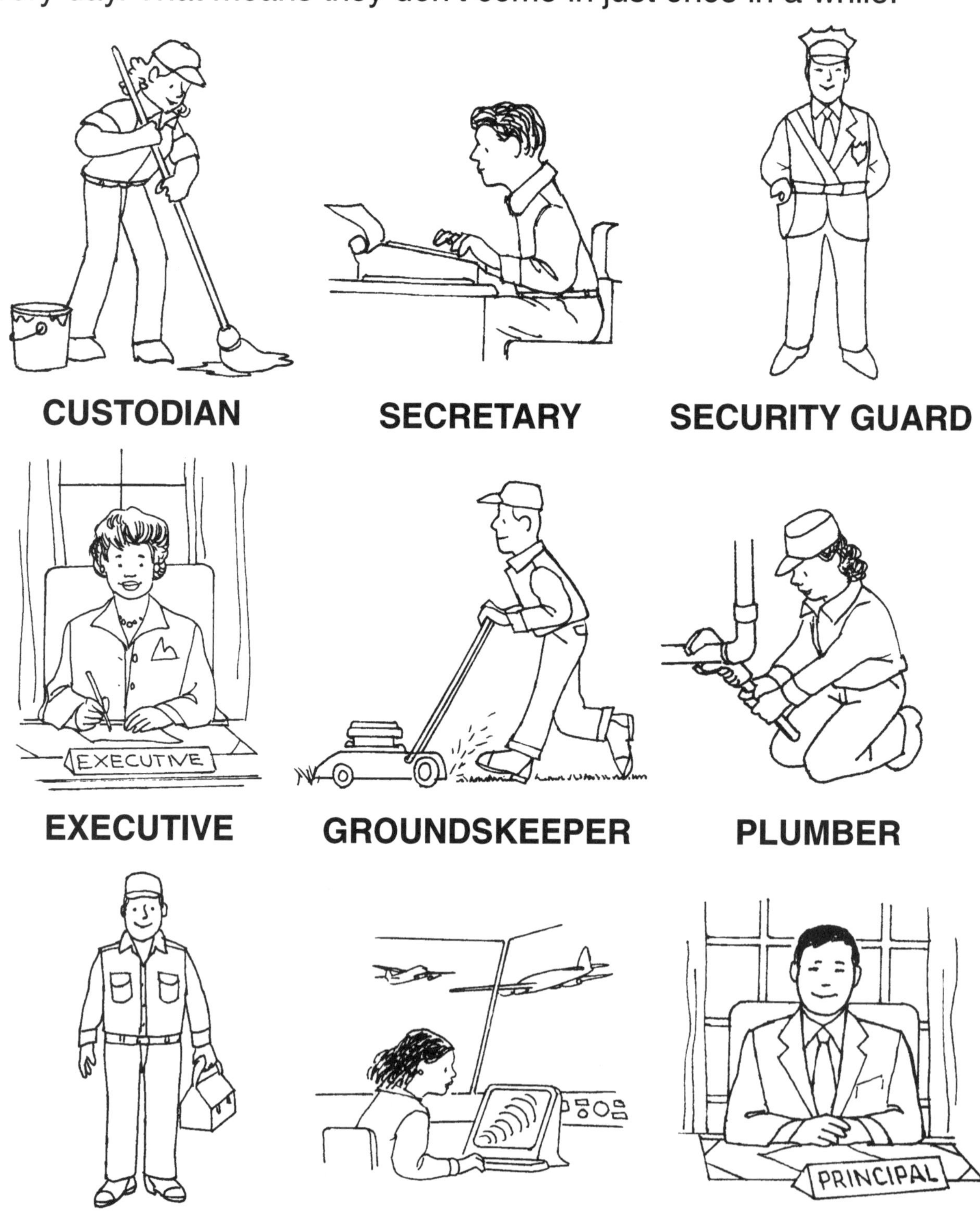

Name ______________________________

OCCUPATIONS AT A PICKLE FACTORY

Directions: Circle the workers who might work at a pickle factory every work day. That means they are not called in just once in a while to do a job.

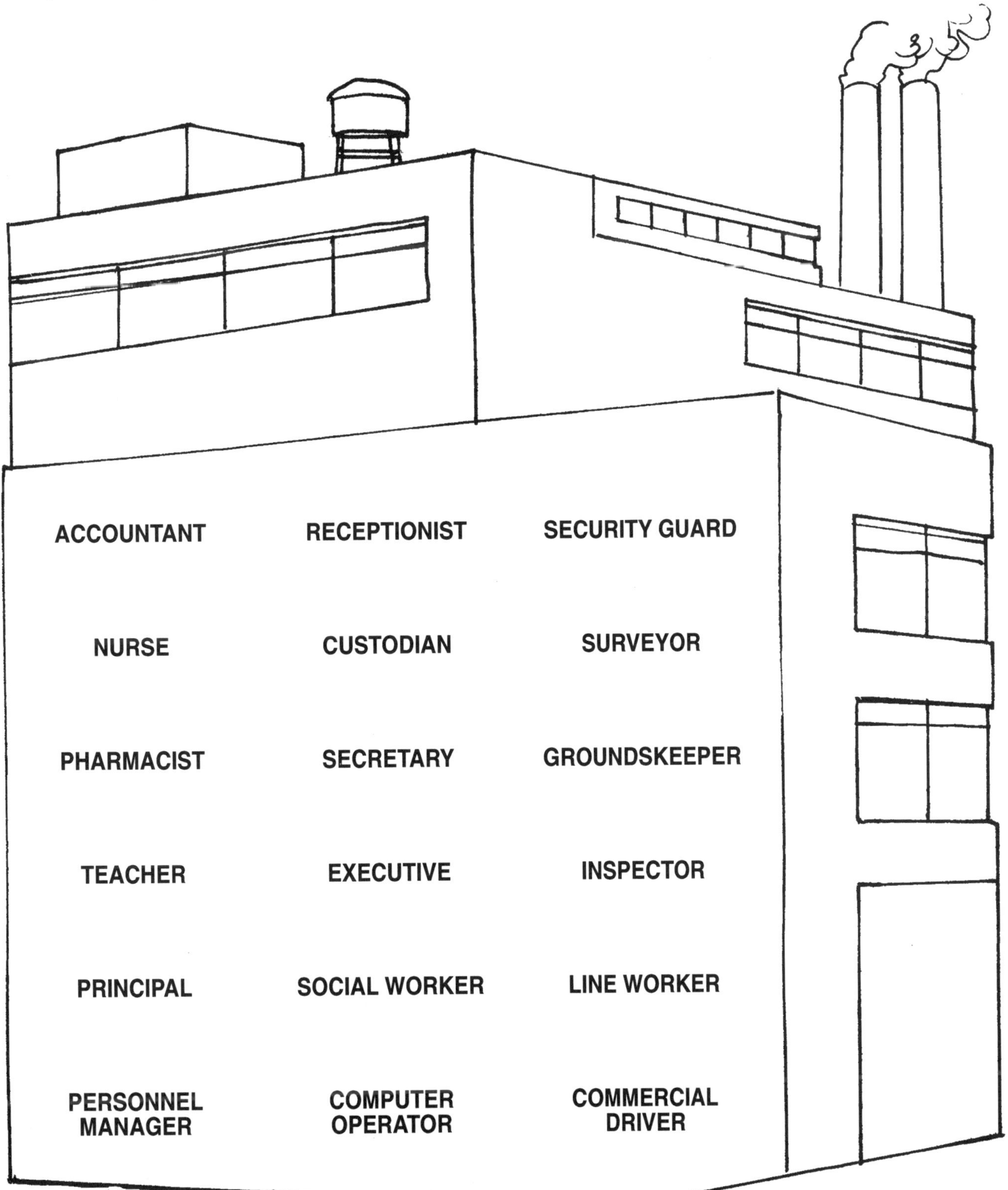

Name ______________________________

JOBS AT A HOSPITAL

Directions: Circle the workers who might work at a very large hospital every work day. That means they don't come in just once in a while.

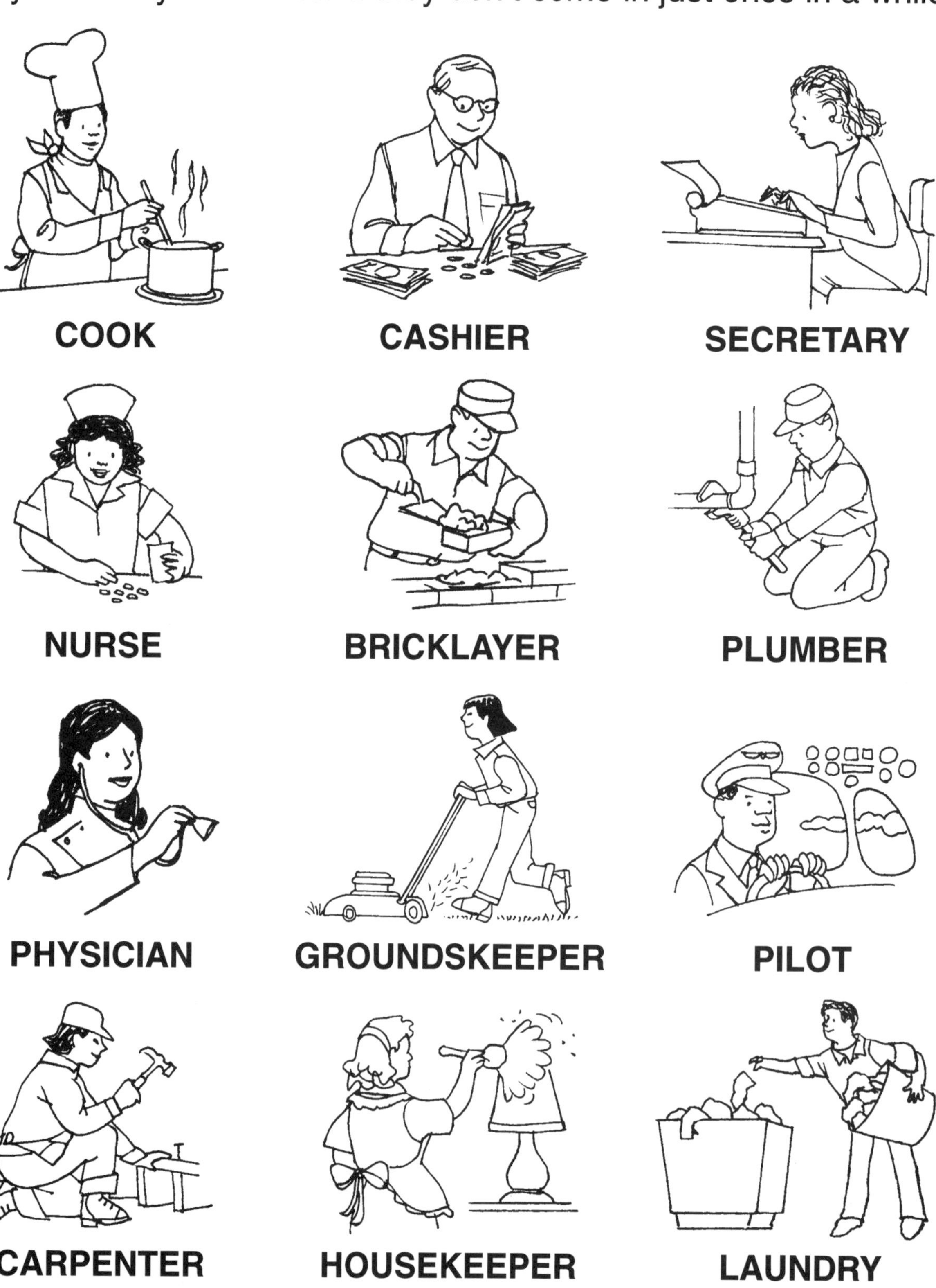

Name ______________________________

OCCUPATIONS AT A HOSPITAL

Directions: Circle the workers who might work at a very large hospital every work day. That means they are not called in just once in a while to do a job.

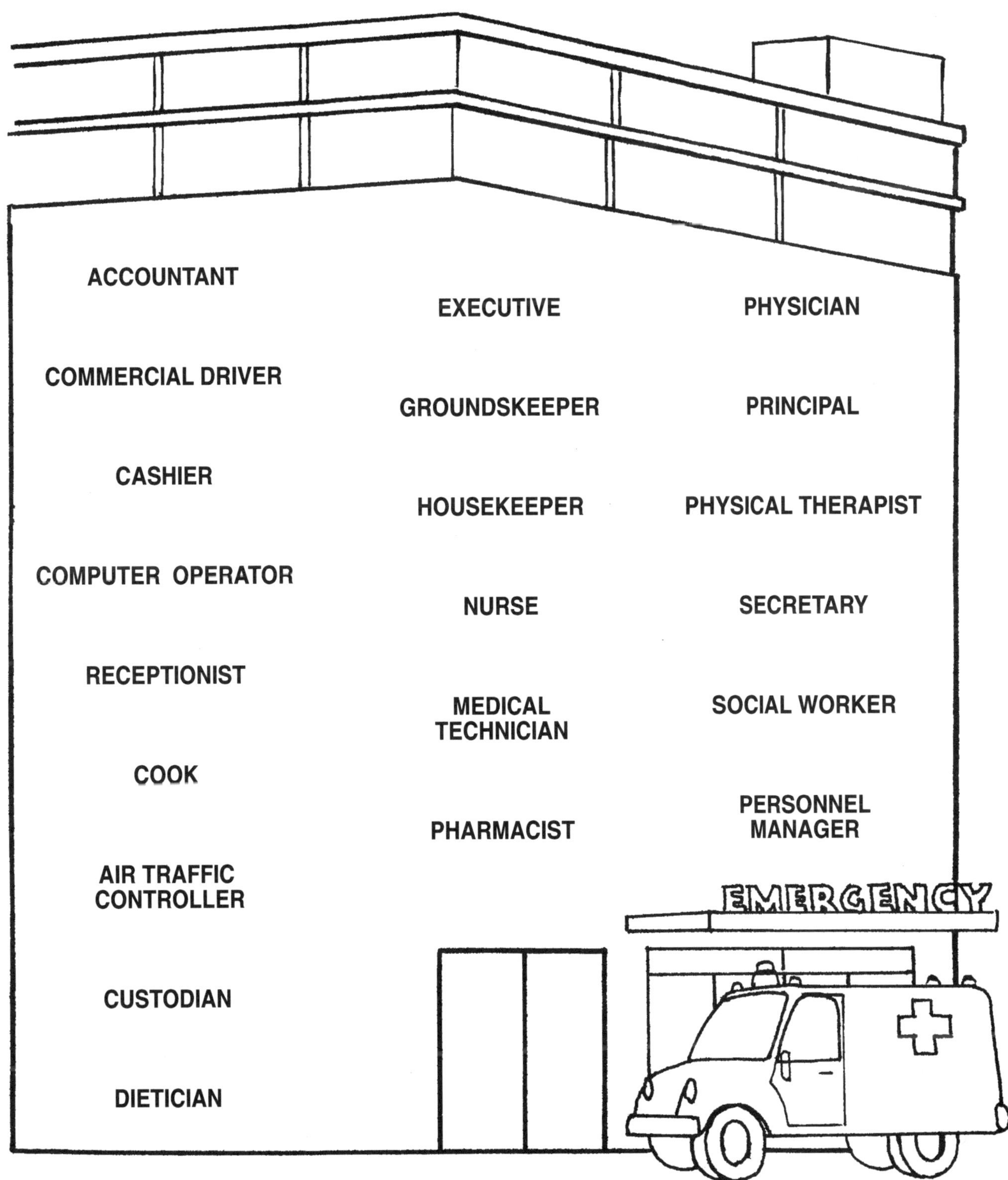

Name ______________________________

JOBS AT AN AIRPORT

Directions: Circle the workers who might work at a large airport every work day. That means they don't come in just once in a while.

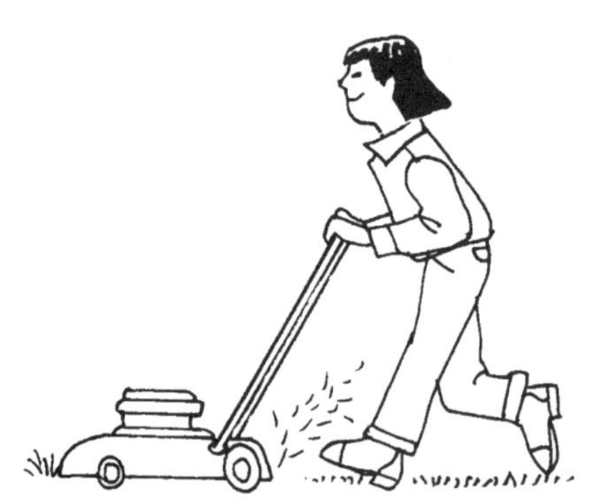
GROUNDSKEEPER

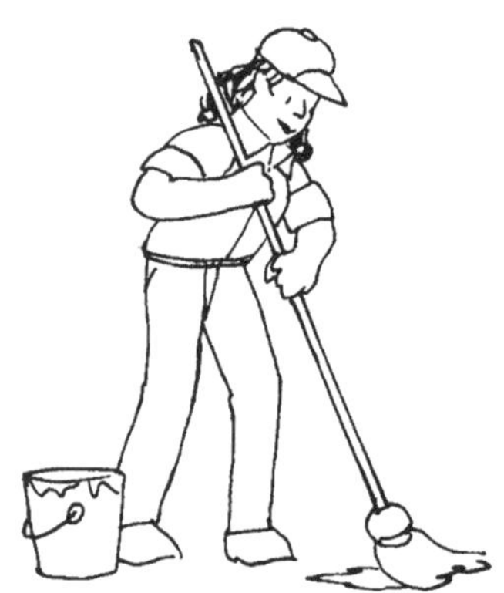
CUSTODIAN

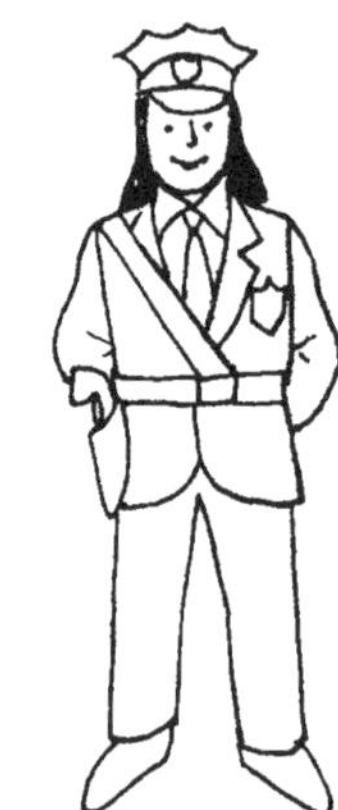
SECURITY GUARD

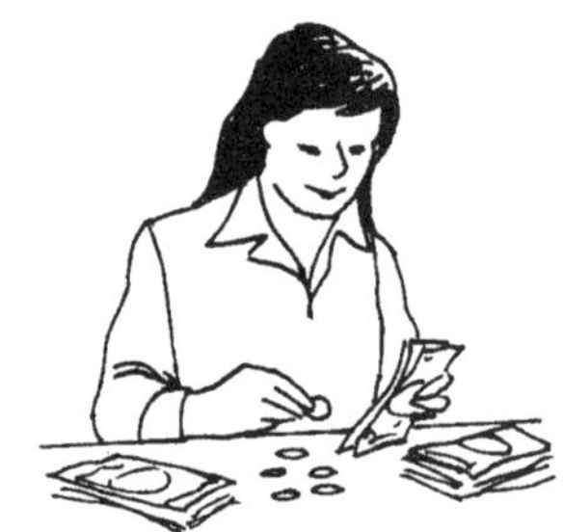
CASHIER

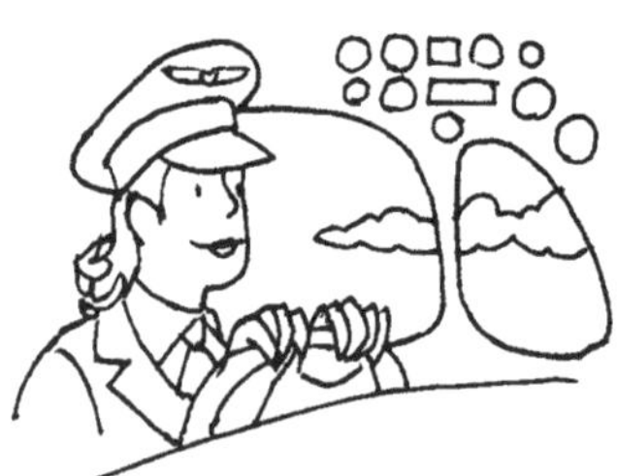
PILOT

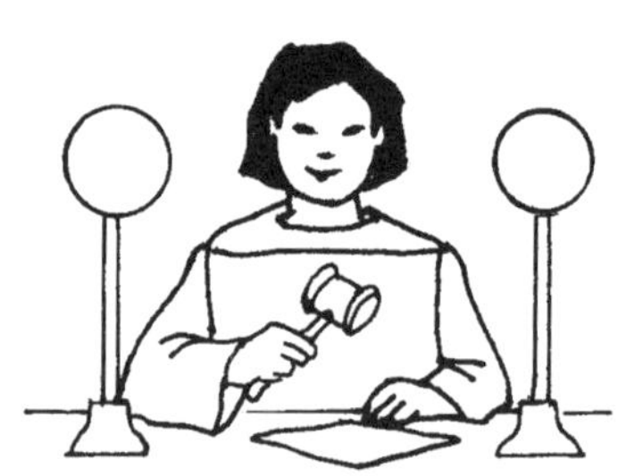
JUDGE

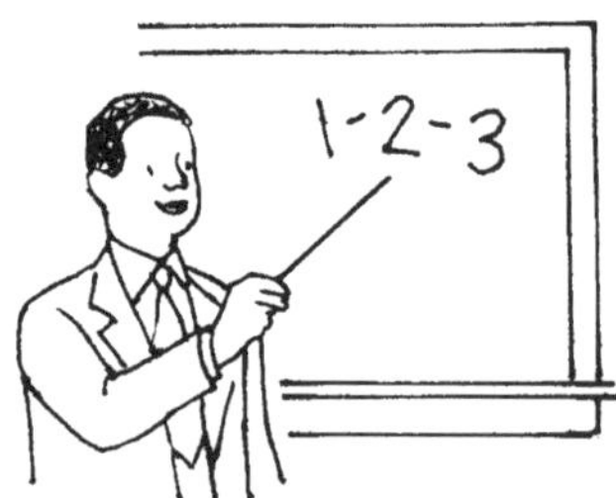

TEACHER

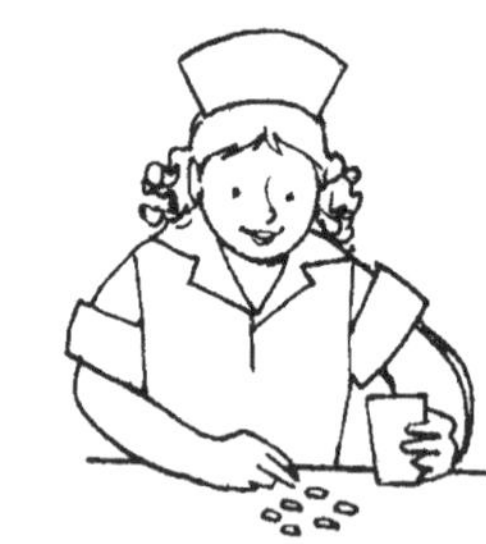
NURSE

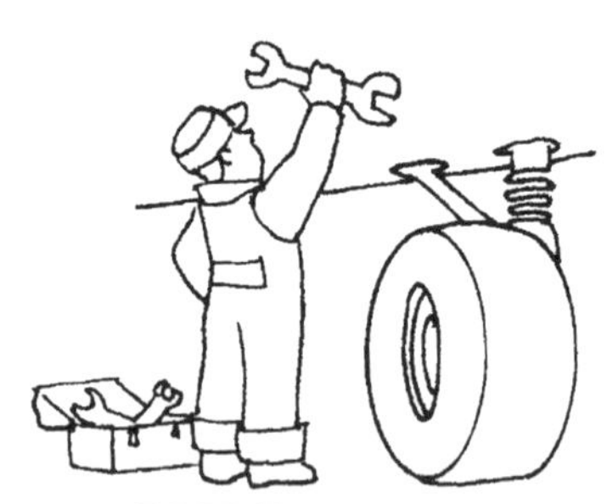
MECHANIC

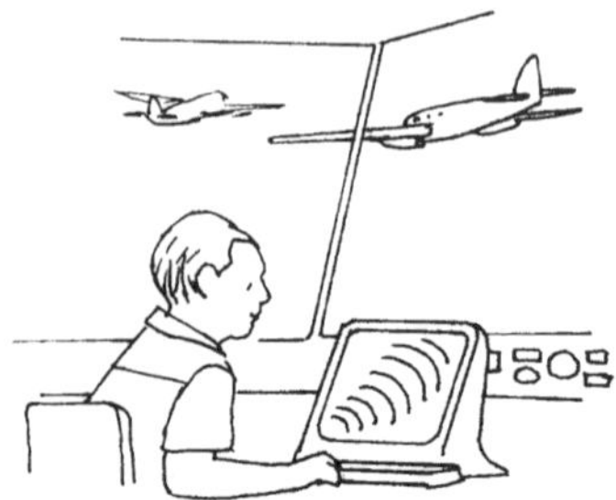
AIR TRAFFIC CONTROLLER

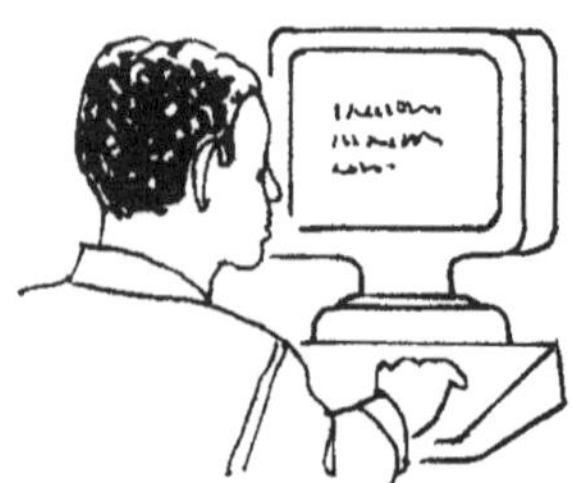
COMPUTER OPERATOR

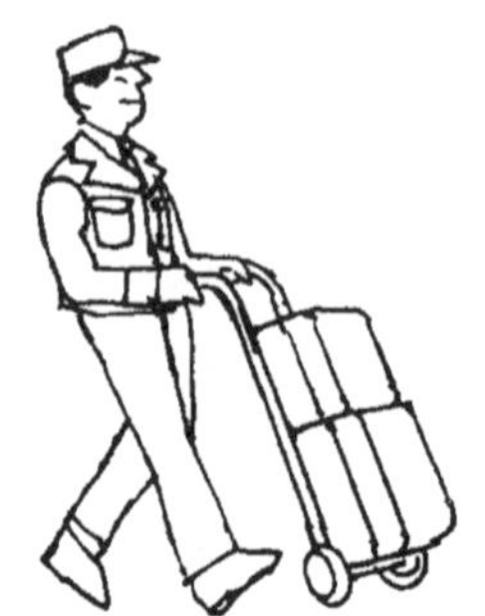
PORTER/SKYCAP

Name ______________________________

OCCUPATIONS AT AN AIRPORT

Directions: Circle the workers who might work at a large airport every work day. That means they are not called in just once in a while to do a job.

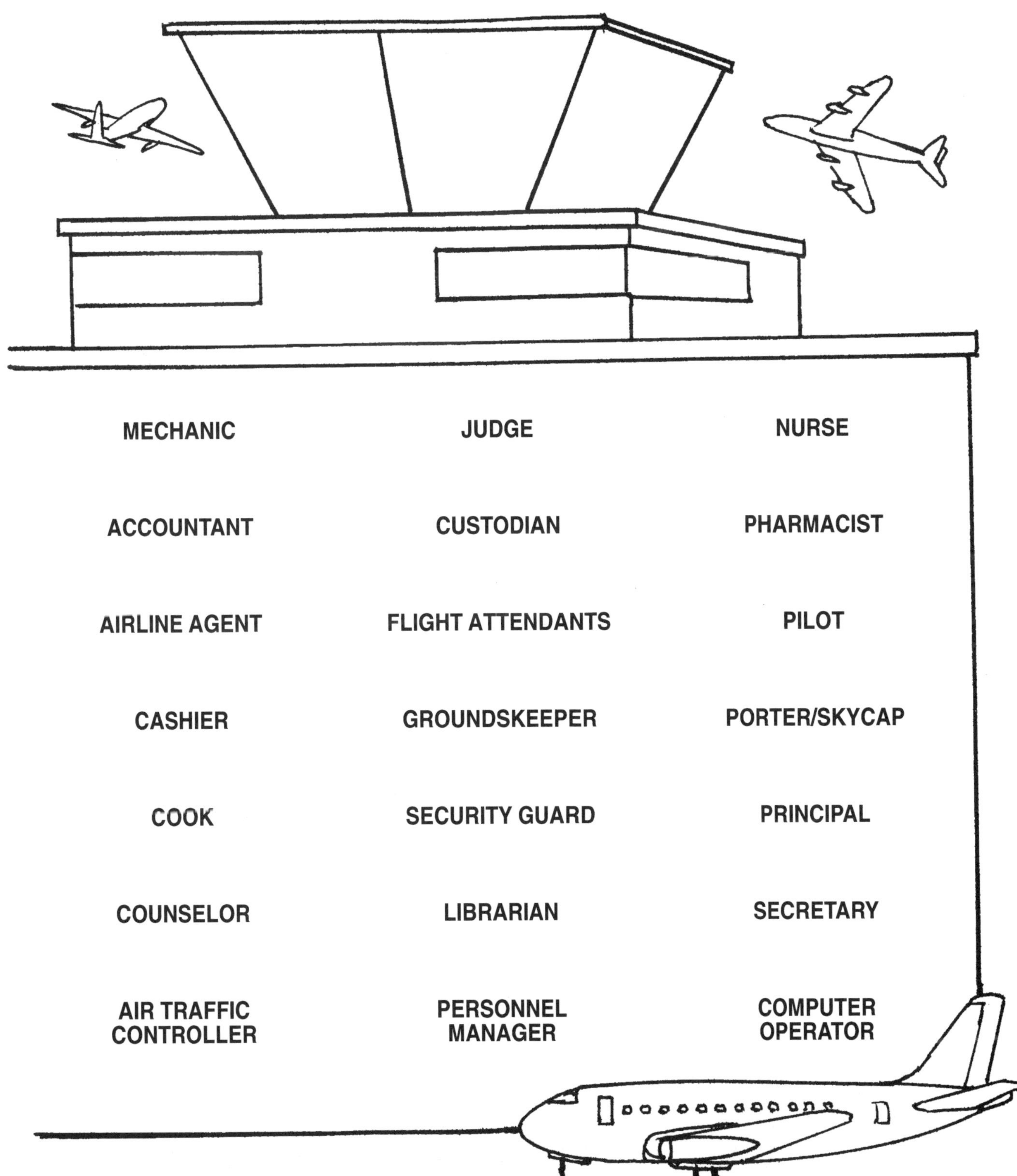

MECHANIC	JUDGE	NURSE
ACCOUNTANT	CUSTODIAN	PHARMACIST
AIRLINE AGENT	FLIGHT ATTENDANTS	PILOT
CASHIER	GROUNDSKEEPER	PORTER/SKYCAP
COOK	SECURITY GUARD	PRINCIPAL
COUNSELOR	LIBRARIAN	SECRETARY
AIR TRAFFIC CONTROLLER	PERSONNEL MANAGER	COMPUTER OPERATOR

Name ______________________________

JOBS AT SCHOOL

Directions: Circle the workers who might work at a school every work day. That means they don't come in just once in a while.

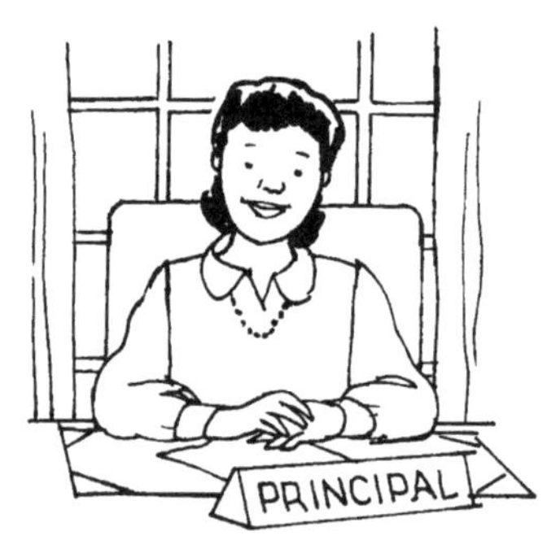

PRINCIPAL

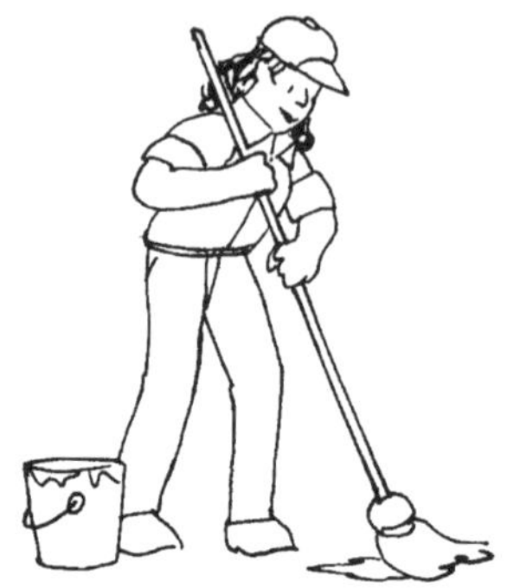

CUSTODIAN

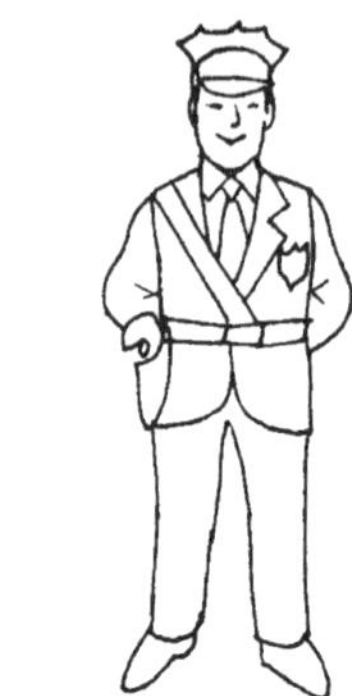

SECURITY GUARD

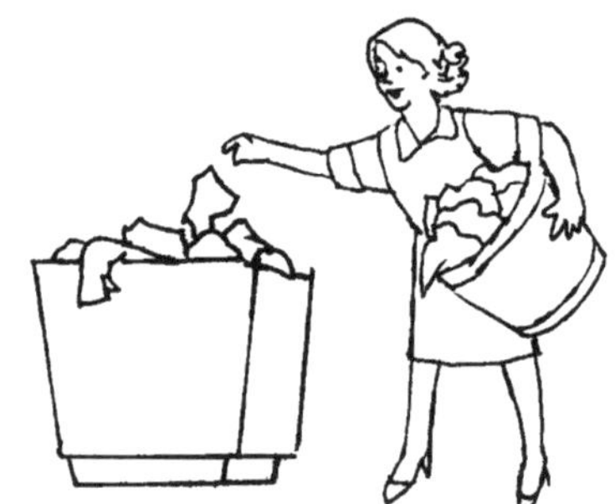

LAUNDRY WORKER

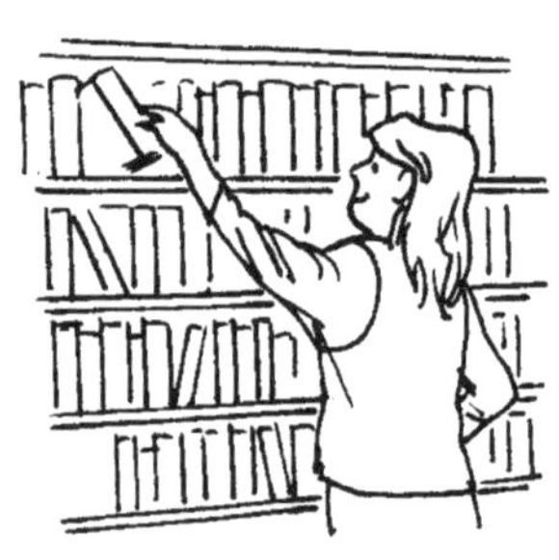

LIBRARIAN

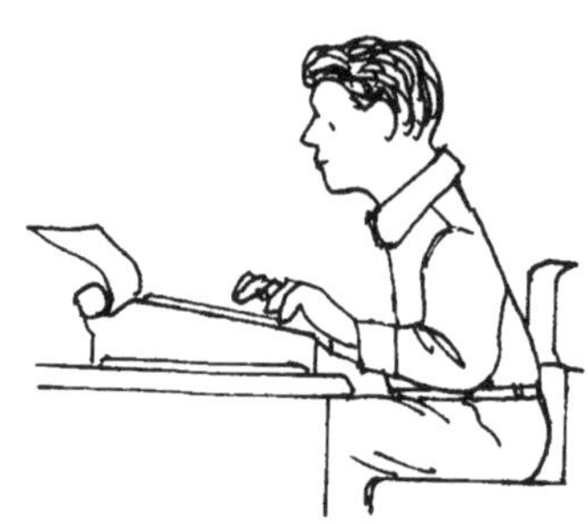

SECRETARY

COOK

NURSE

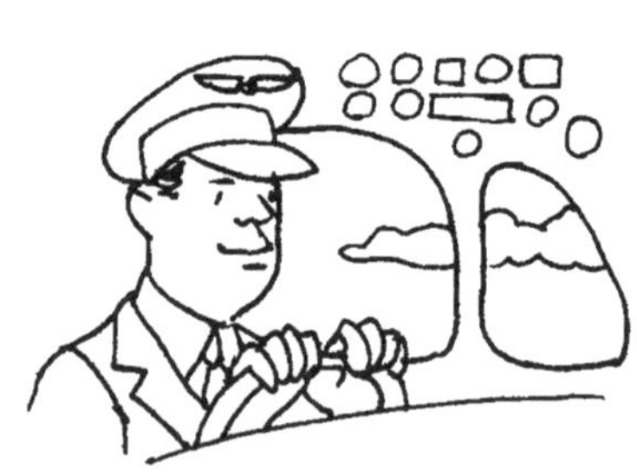

PILOT

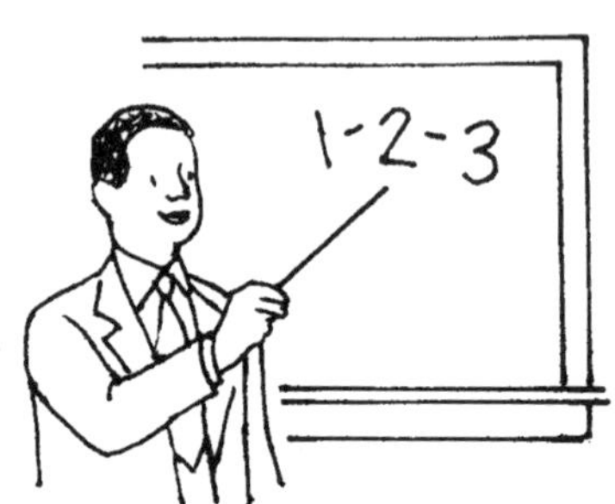

TEACHER

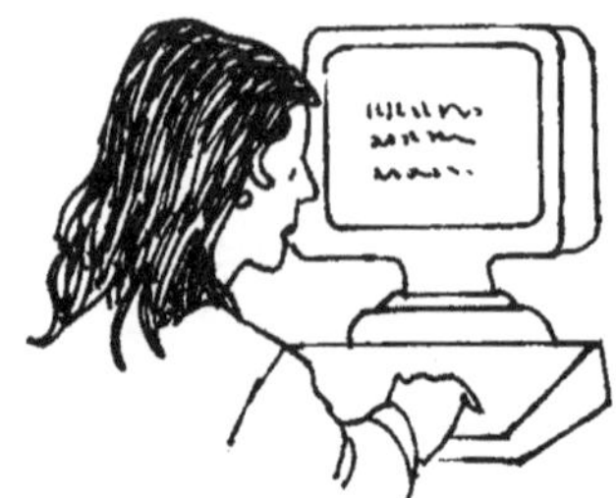

COMPUTER OPERATOR

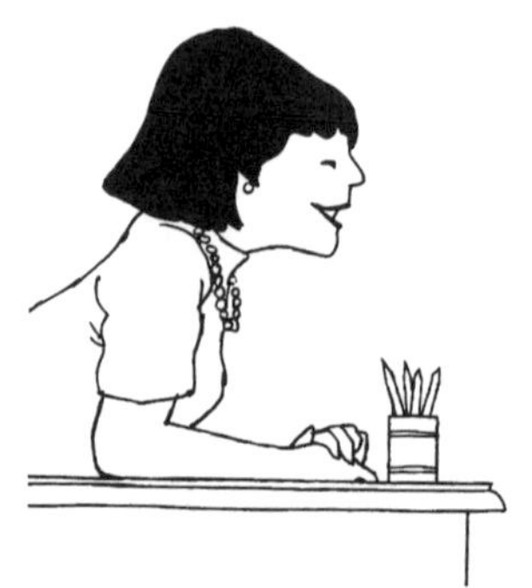

COUNSELOR

Name ______________________________

OCCUPATIONS AT SCHOOL

Directions: Circle the workers who might work at a school every work day. That means they are not called in just once in a while to do a job.

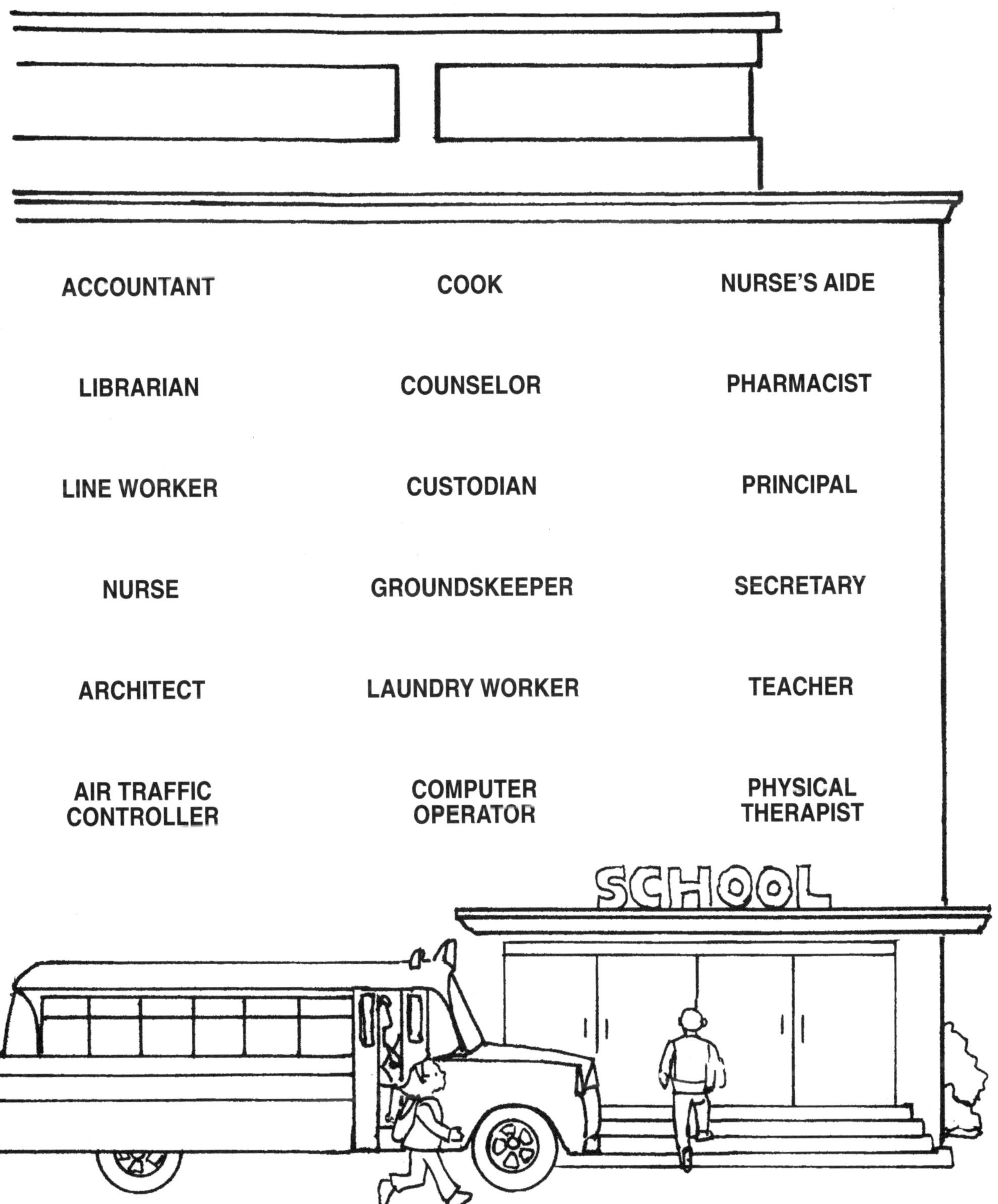

Name ______________________________

JOBS FOR BUILDING HOUSES

Directions: Circle the workers that would be needed to build or repair a house.

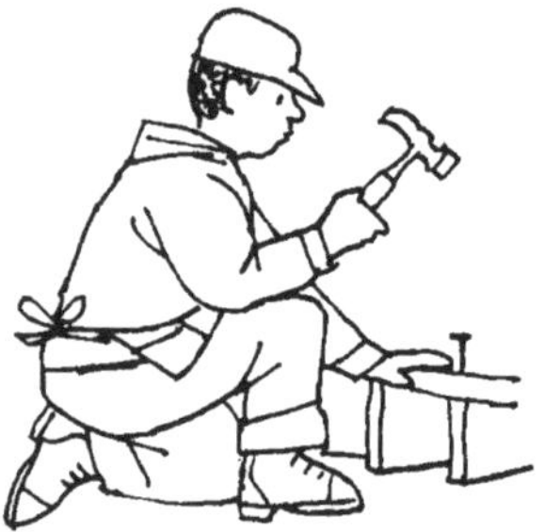

CARPENTER

COOK

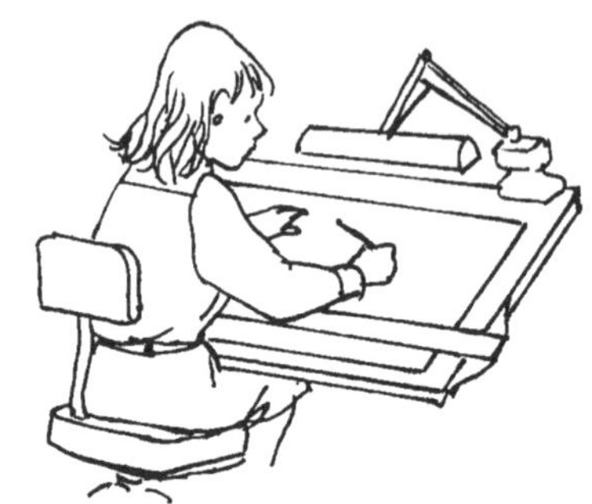

ARCHITECT

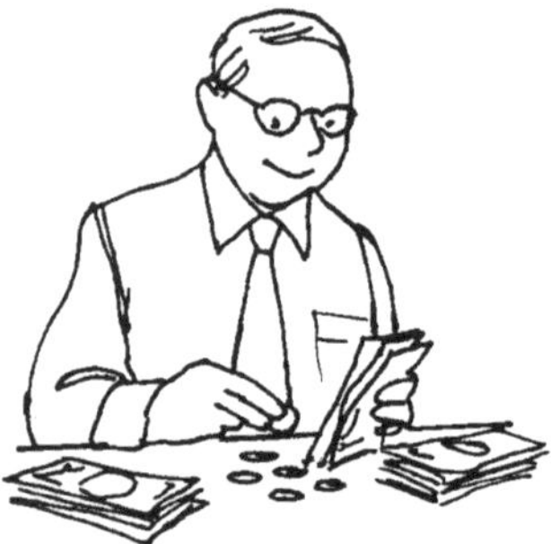

CASHIER

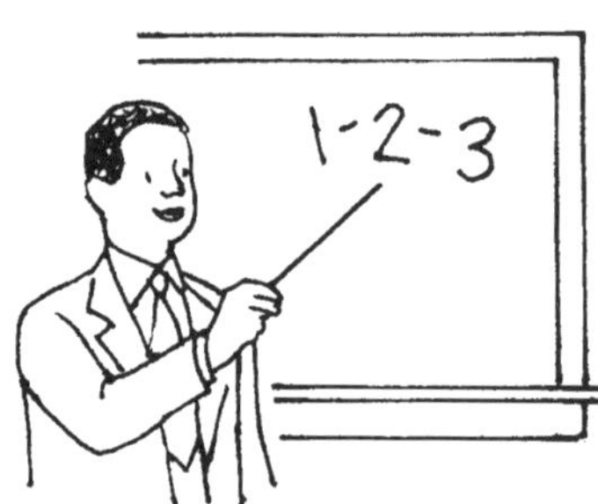

TEACHER

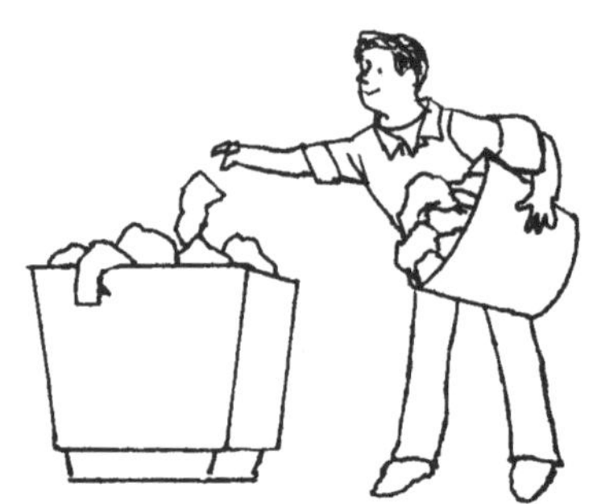

LAUNDRY WORKER

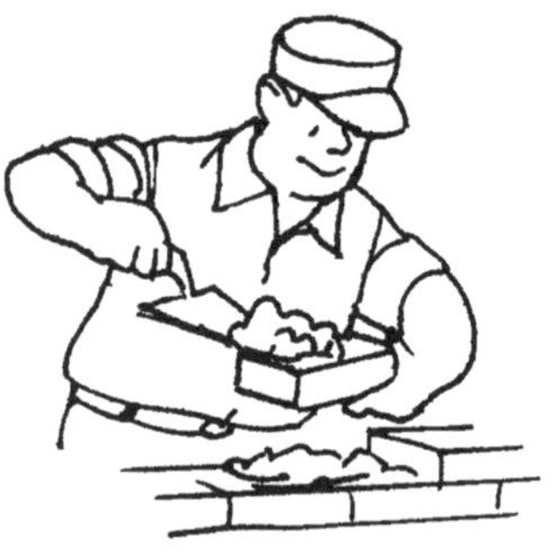

BRICKLAYER

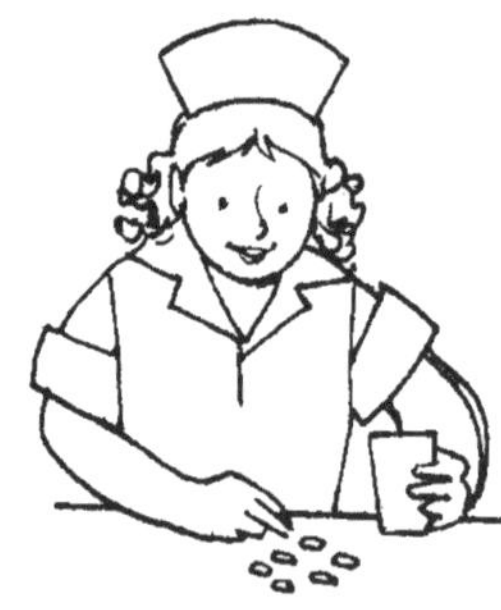

NURSE

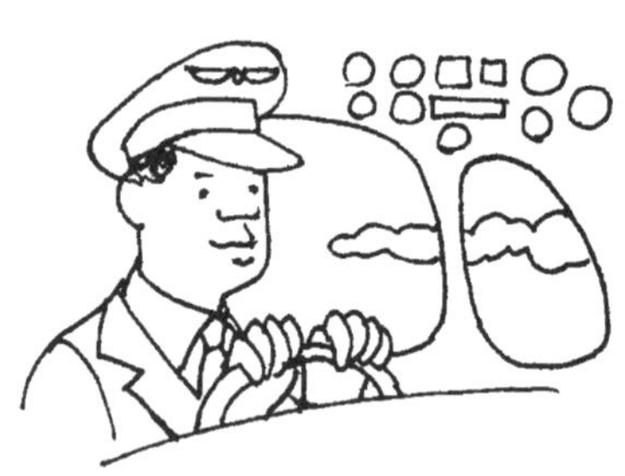

PILOT

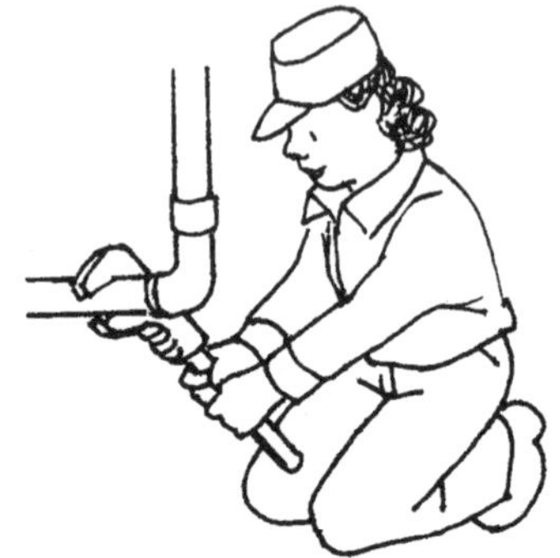

PLUMBER

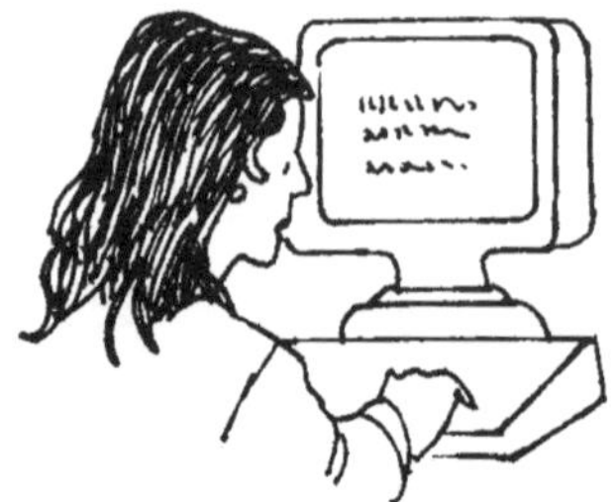

COMPUTER OPERATOR

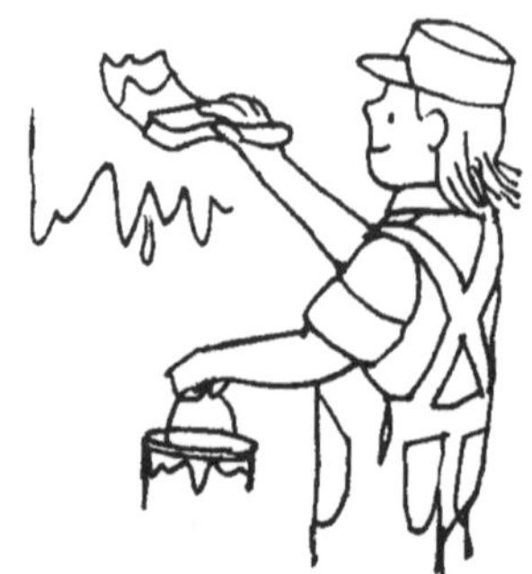

PAINTER

Name ______________________________

OCCUPATIONS FOR BUILDING HOUSES

Directions: Circle the workers who might work at building or repairing a house.

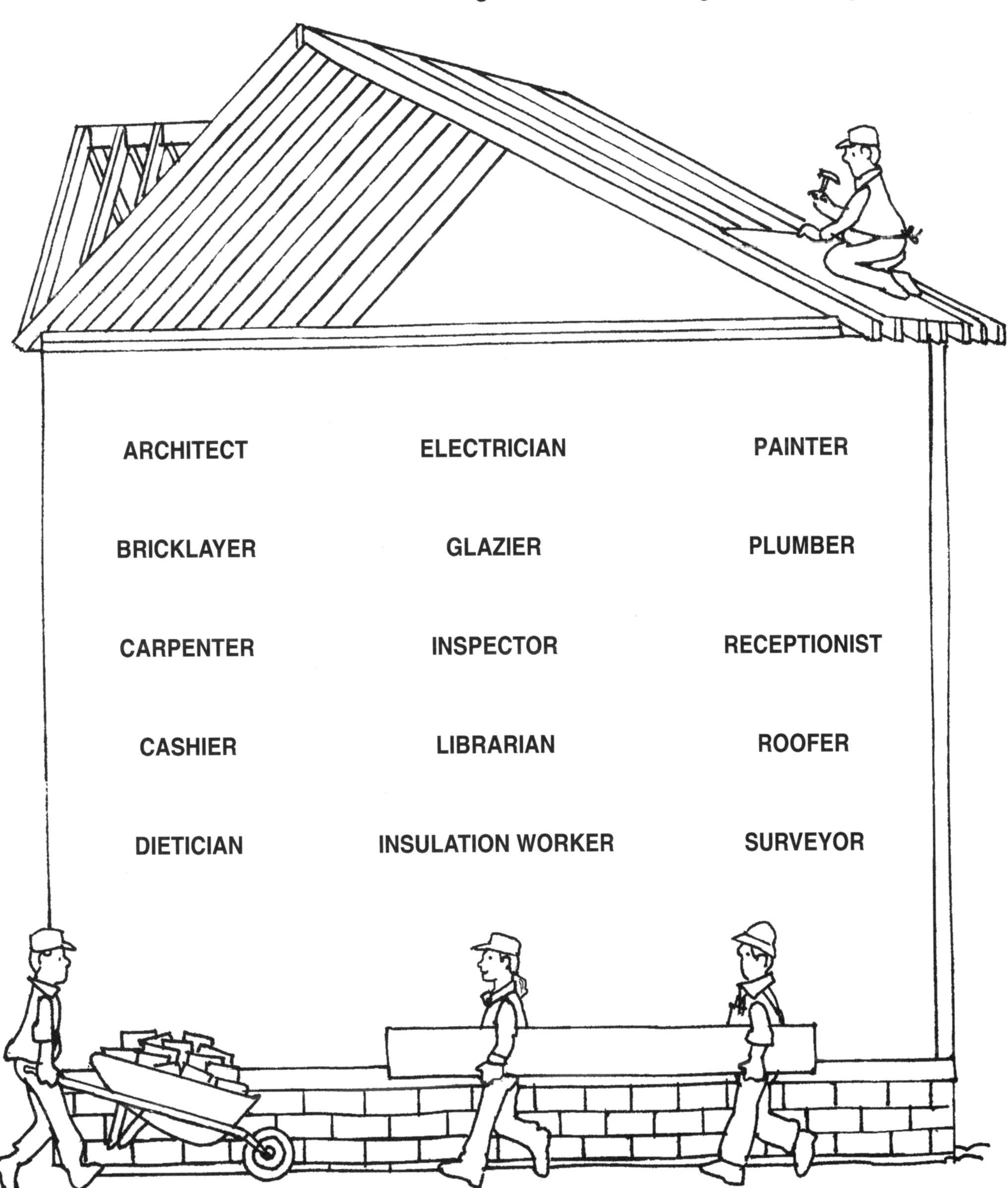

CHAPTER 6

INTEGRATING MATH AND LITERACY

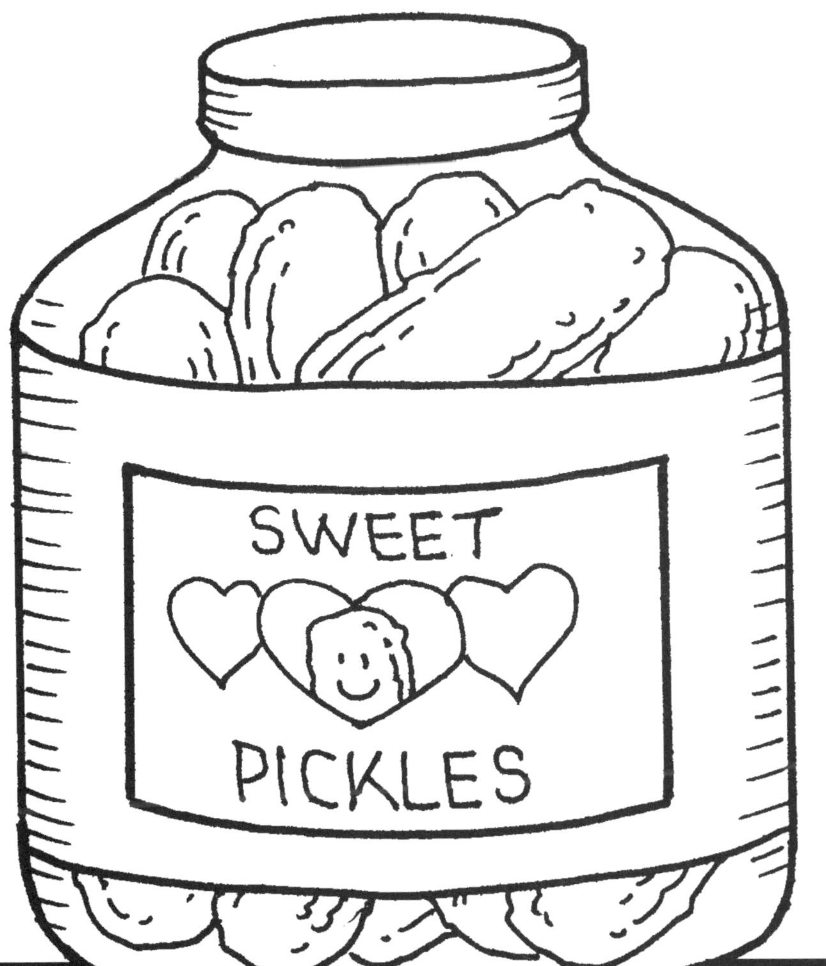

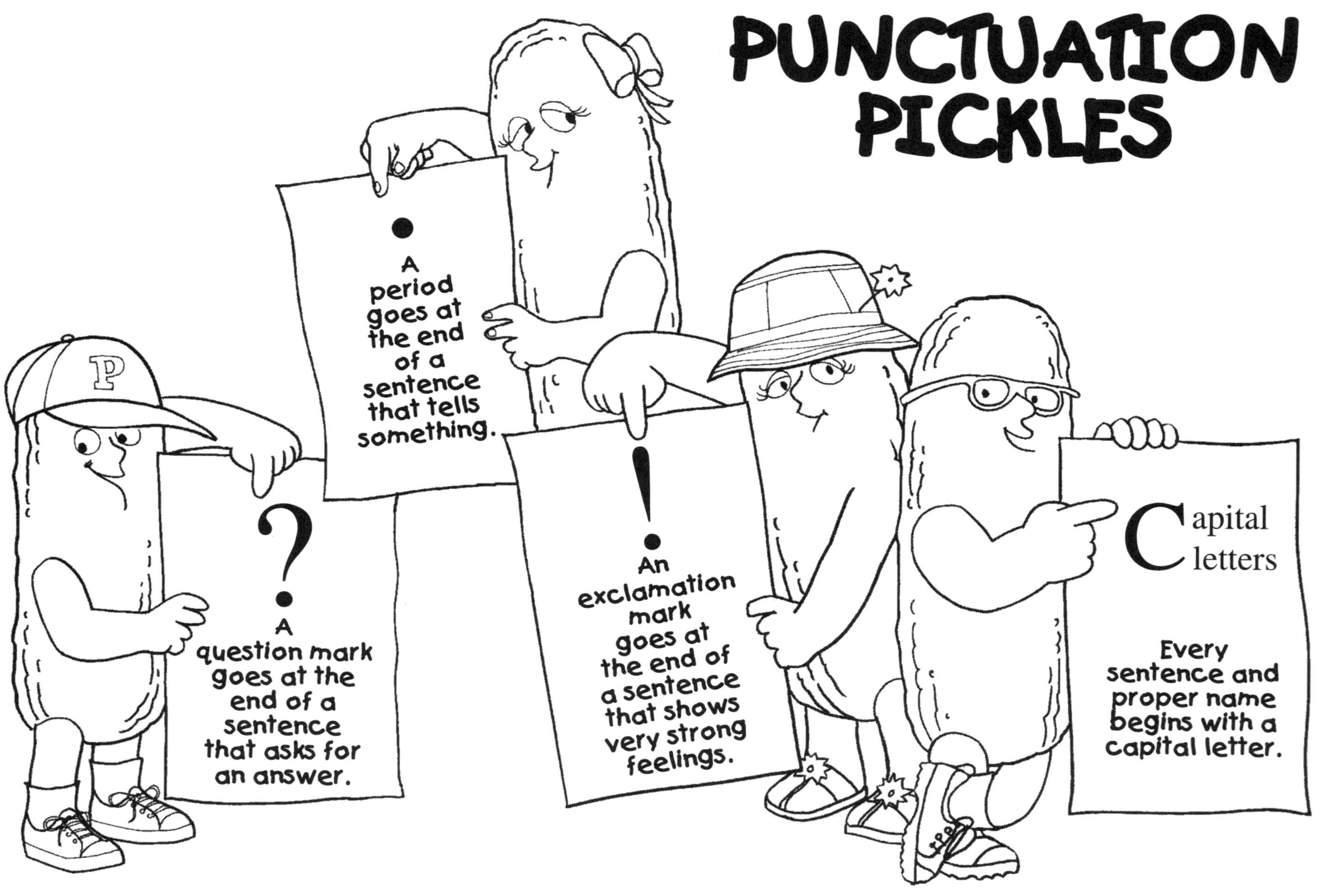
PUNCTUATION PICKLES
A period goes at the end of a sentence that tells something.
A question mark goes at the end of a sentence that asks for an answer.
An exclamation mark goes at the end of a sentence that shows very strong feelings.
Capital letters
Every sentence and proper name begins with a capital letter.

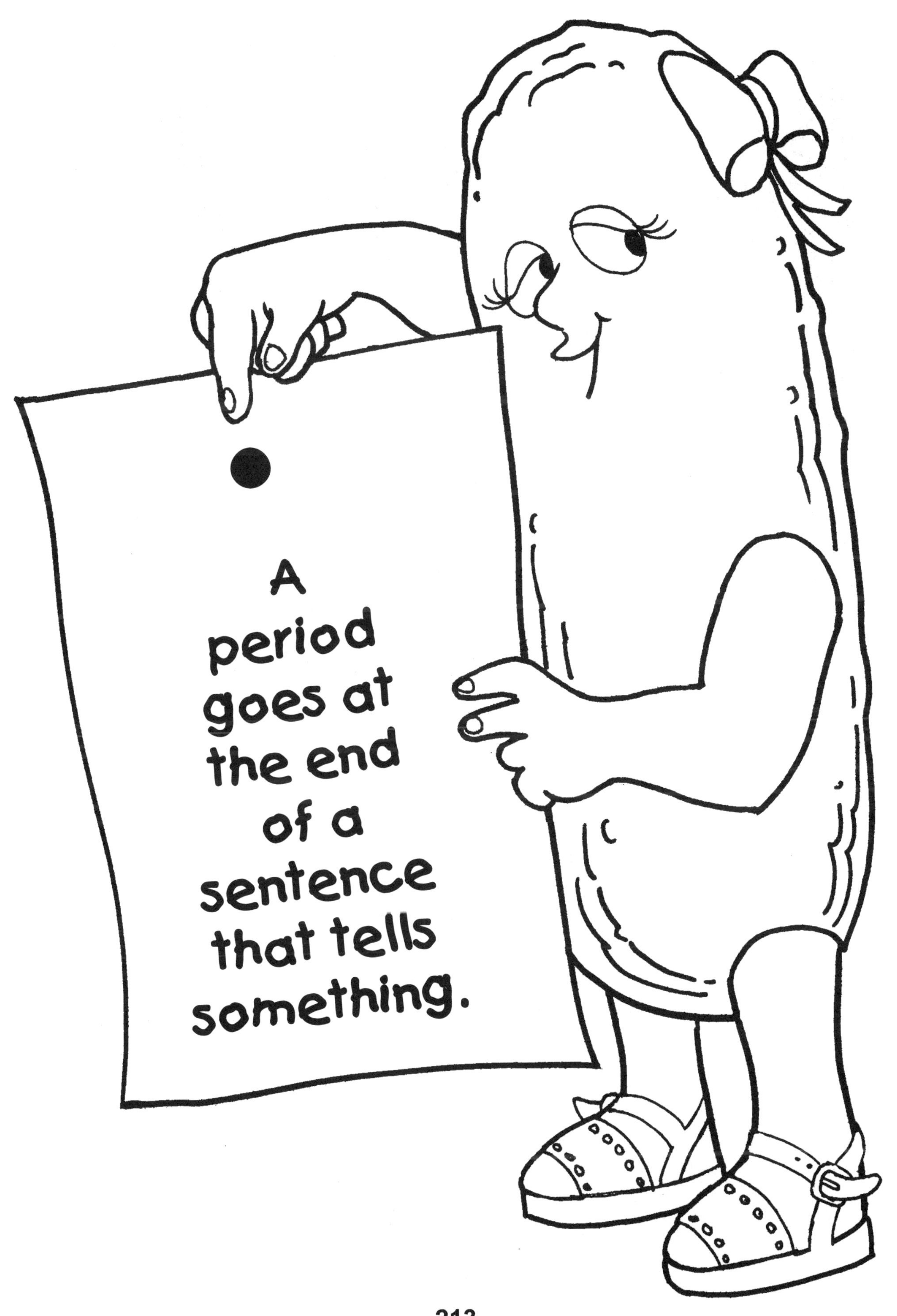
A
period
goes at
the end
of a
sentence
that tells
something.

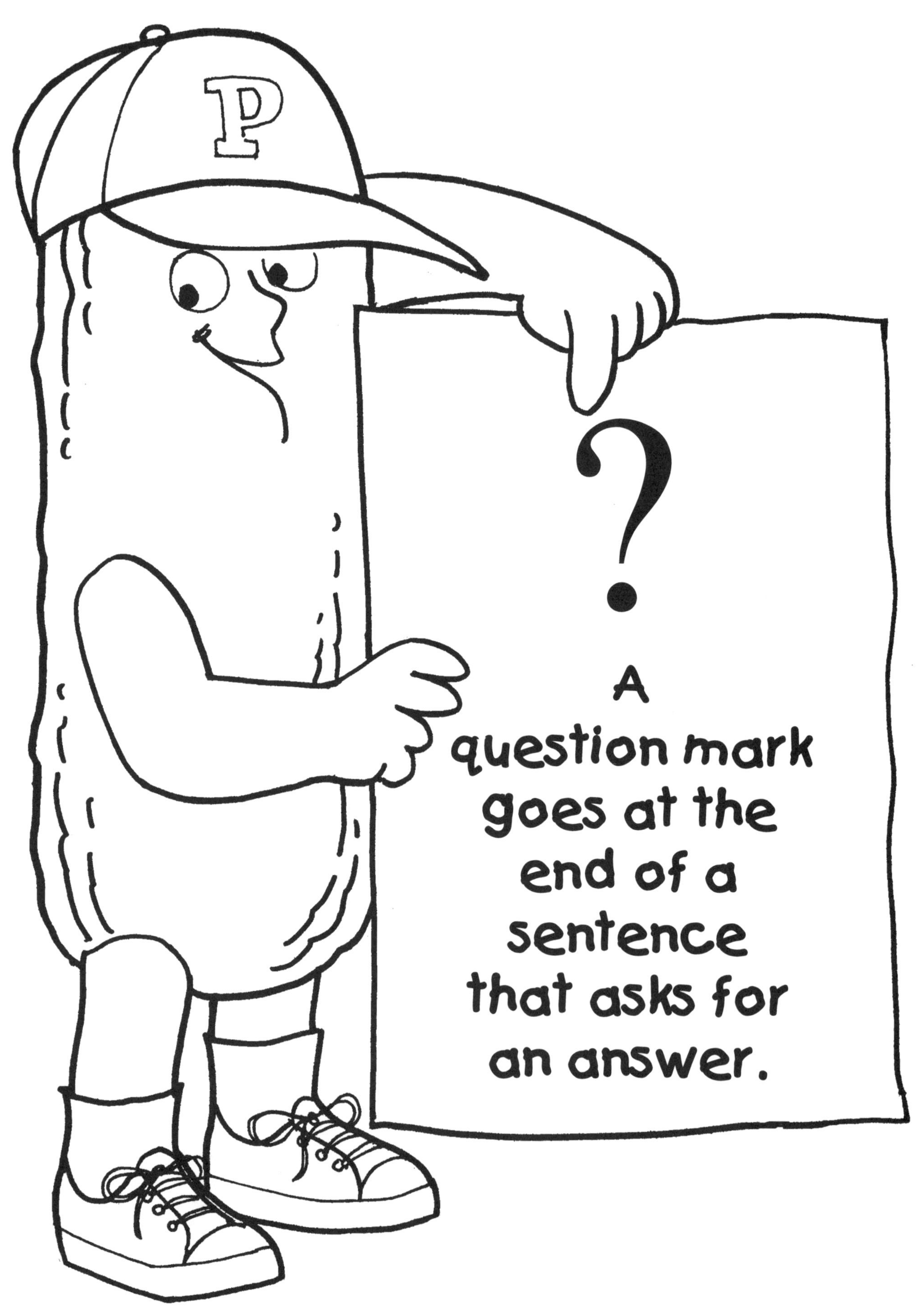
P
?
A
question mark
goes at the
end of a
sentence
that asks for
an answer.

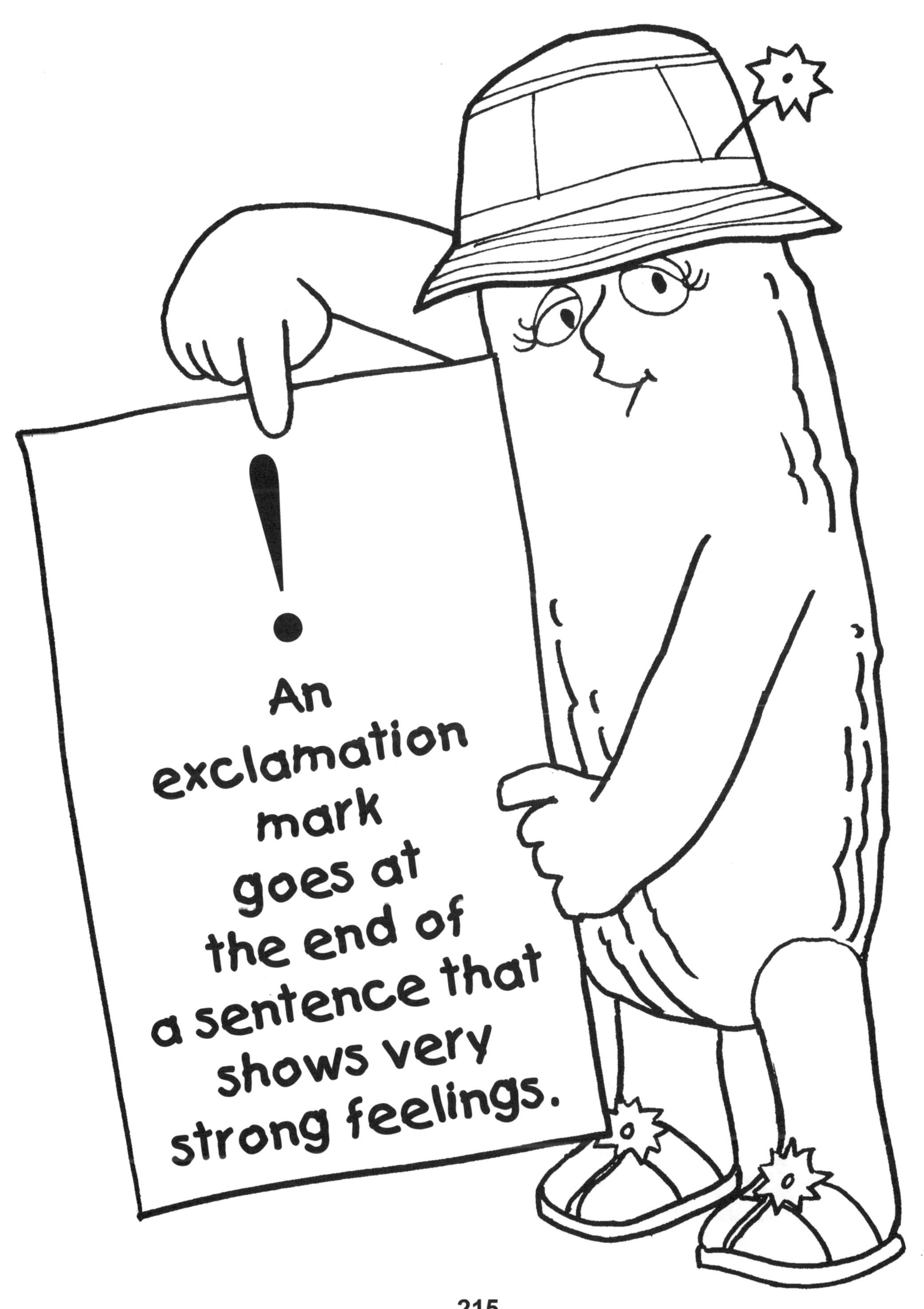
!
An exclamation mark goes at the end of a sentence that shows very strong feelings.

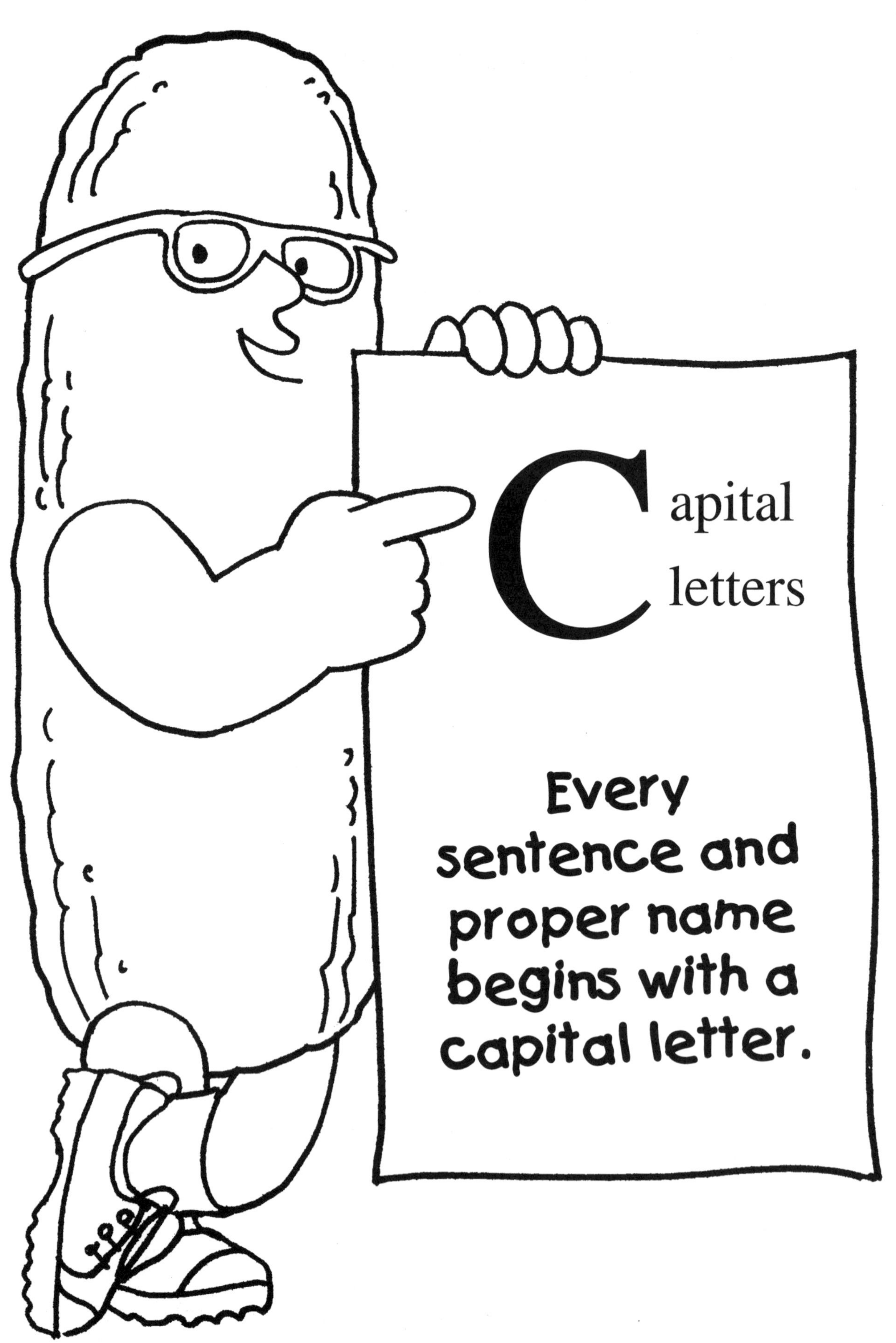
Capital
letters
Every
sentence and
proper name
begins with a
capital letter.

Name ______________________________

FINDING PUNCTUATION MARKS

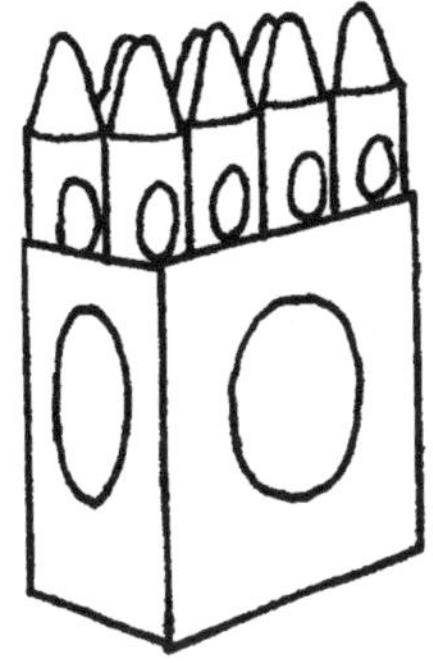

Directions:
Circle the periods with a green crayon or marker.
Circle the question marks with a blue crayon or marker.
Circle the exclamation marks with a red crayon or marker.
Circle the capital letter at the beginning of each sentence with a purple crayon or marker.

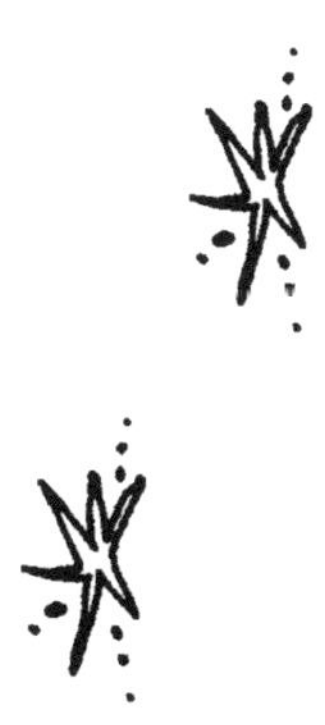

I like pickles, pickles, and more pickles!

Do you like sweet pickles?

Mom will go get pickles.

Thanks, Mom, for the pickles!

Sam, I broke the pickle jar!

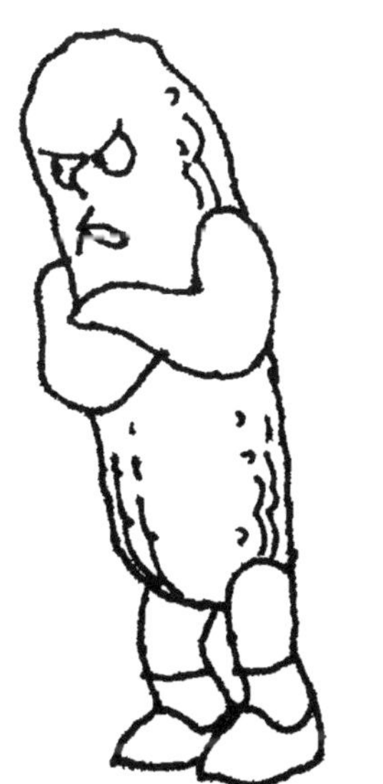

Sometimes I am happy.

Sometimes I am sad.

Are you sometimes sad?

Do you ever get mad?

It isn't right to hurt people, even when we are mad.

Name ______________________________

SENTENCES ABOUT PICKLES

Directions: Make these sentences correct. If you need help, use your Punctuation Pickles.

1. a pickle is green
2. do you like pickles
3. do you like sweet pickles
4. do you like sour pickles
5. mom, I broke the jar of pickles
6. grandmother makes pickles
7. there's a pickle in my soup
8. buy some pickles at the store
9. that cat is eating a pickle
10. is it a sweet pickle or a sour pickle

Name ______________________________

SENTENCES ABOUT ANGER

Directions: Make these sentences correct. If you need help, use your Punctuation Pickles.

1. everybody gets angry sometimes
2. is it all right to hurt people when you are angry
3. bad language gets you in big trouble with the principal
4. do you know whom to talk with when you are angry
5. do you like people who get angry all the time
6. when you are angry, take time to think about what you should do
7. do you stay angry for a long time
8. it is not okay to destroy things when you are angry
9. it is okay to let others know you are angry
10. show your anger in a way that does not hurt people or things

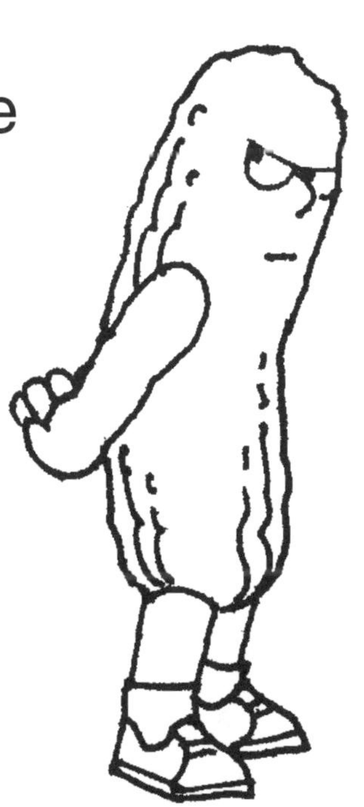

Name ______________________________

SENTENCES ON TATTLING/REPORTING

Directions: Make these sentences correct. If you need help, use your Punctuation Pickles.

1. yellow means thinking time is short
2. do you stop to think
3. red means stop
4. tattling is a flop
5. green means go
6. an adult needs to know
7. is this a tattle or a report
8. mary ran out into the street
9. that is a report
10. sam has 10 surprises on his desk
11. he touched one
12. is that a tattle or a report
13. that is a tattle

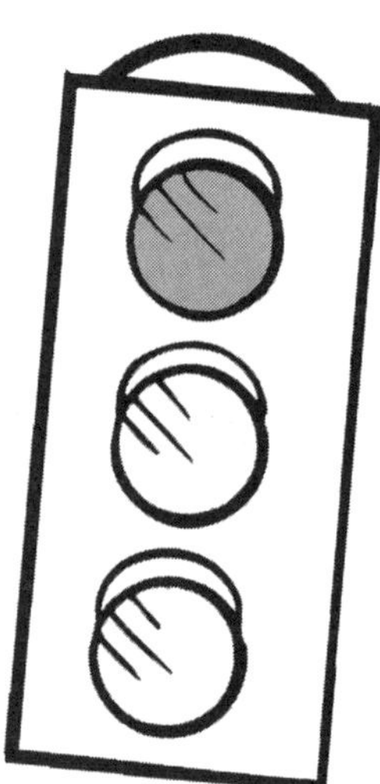

Name ______________________________

SENTENCES ON SAFETY

Directions: Make these sentences correct. If you need help, use your Punctuation Pickles.

1. can medicine from a store be bad for you

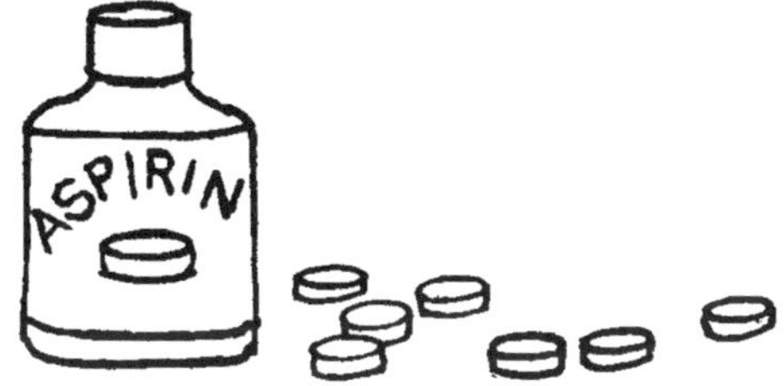

2. yes it can
3. never take medicine without a parent's help
4. what should you do if you find pills on the ground
5. tell an adult
6. what should you do if a friend passes out and there is no adult around
7. call 911
8. can you tell a friend you do not want to drink alcohol

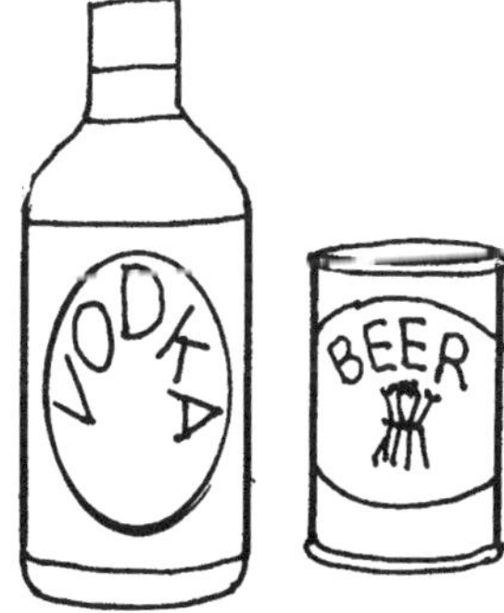

9. yes I can
10. is tobacco good for your body

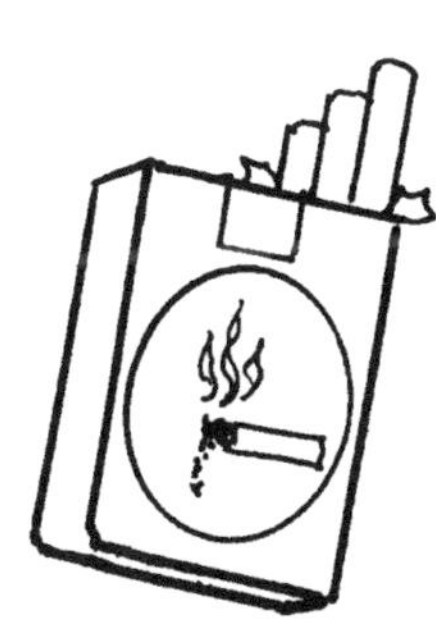

11. chewing tobacco or smoking tobacco hurts your body

TEN PICKLE JARS

Sung to the tune of
100 Bottles Of Soda (Pop) On The Wall

Ten pickle jars on the shelf.
Ten pickle jars.
Some are sweet and some are sour.
Ten pickle jars on the shelf.

Ten pickle jars on the shelf.
Ten pickle jars.
We took one down and ate it for lunch.
Nine pickle jars on the shelf.

Nine pickle jars ... (repeat 2nd verse)
Eight pickle jars ... (repeat 2nd verse)
Seven pickle jars ... (repeat 2nd verse)
Six pickle jars ... (repeat 2nd verse)
Five pickle jars ... (repeat 2nd verse)
Four pickle jars ... (repeat 2nd verse)
Three pickle jars ... (repeat 2nd verse)
Two pickle jars ... (repeat 2nd verse)
One pickle jar ... (repeat 2nd verse)

No pickle jars on the shelf.
No pickle jars.
Some were sweet and some were sour.
But now we ate them all!

Name ______________________________

PICKLE MATH

How many pickles are here?

There are ________ pickles.

If we eat one pickle, how many pickles will be left?

________ pickles will be left.

How many pickles are here?

There are _____ pickles.

Circle the pickle that is fifth in line.

How many pickles are here?

There are _____ pickles.

Circle the largest pickle.

How many pickles are here?

There are _____ pickles.

Circle the smallest pickle.

Name ______________________________

SWEET AND SOUR PICKLE PROBLEMS

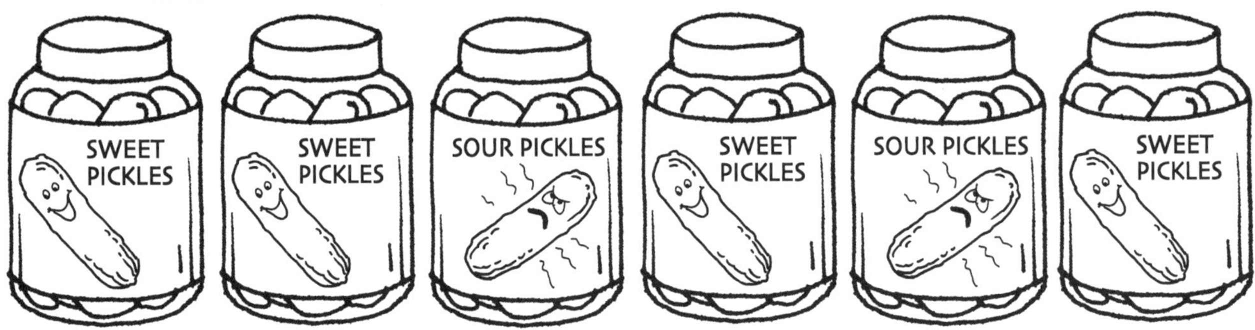

1. Count the jars of pickles. How many jars are there? _______

2. How many are jars of sweet pickles? _______

3. How many are jars of sour pickles? _______

4. If we bought two more jars of pickles, how many jars would we have?

   6 pickle jars
   \+ 2 pickle jars
   = _______ pickle jars

5. If we drop a jar and it breaks, how many jars will we have left?

   6 pickle jars
   – 1 pickle jar
   = _______ pickle jars

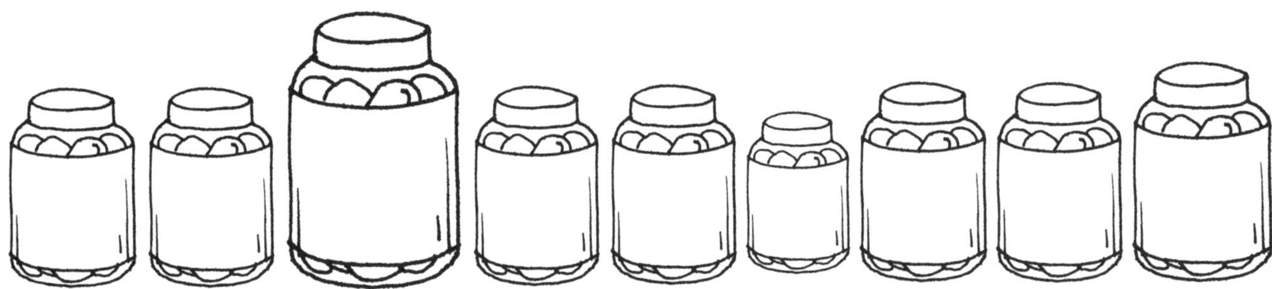

6. Count the pickle jars. How many jars are there? _______

7. Circle the largest pickle jar.

8. Underline the smallest pickle jar.

9. Put an ✘ on the jar that is second in line.

Name ____________________________

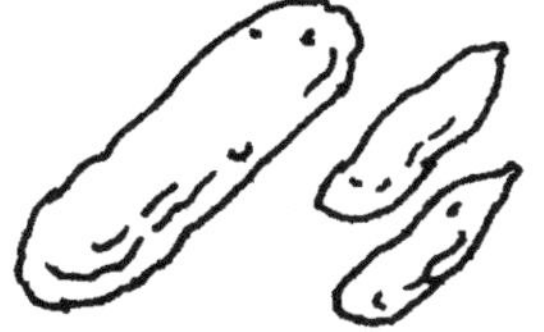

MRS. SMITH'S PICKLES

1. Mrs. Smith bought two jars of pickles for her class. In one jar, there were 15 pickles. The other jar had 14 pickles. How many pickles did Mrs. Smith have in all? ________

2. Mrs. Smith has 24 students in her class. If she gives each student a pickle, how many will she have left? ________

3. Mrs. Smith paid $1.04 for one jar of pickles and $1.53 for the other jar of pickles. How much did the two jars cost together? ________

4. Mrs. Smith bought some grapes for 30¢ and a jar of pickles for $1.40. How much did Mrs. Smith owe for the pickles and the grapes? ________

5. Mrs. Smith put eight pickles on a big plate. She put two small plates on Sam's desk. She asked Sam to put half of the pickles on each plate. How many pickles did Sam put on each plate? ________

6. After Mrs. Smith put the eight pickles on Sam's desk, she put the rest on the reading table. How many pickles did she put on the reading table? ________

A vote was taken to see which kind of pickles the students liked. Count the boxes to see how the students voted. Write your answer on the line that follows each row of boxes.

Dill Pickles □□□□□□□□□ ________

Sweet Pickles □□□□□□□□□□□ ________

No pickles □□□□ ________

7. Did all the students in Mrs. Smith's class vote? ________

8. How many students did not like pickles? ________

9. Which kind of pickles got the most votes? ________

Name ______________________________

PICKLES FOR LUNCH

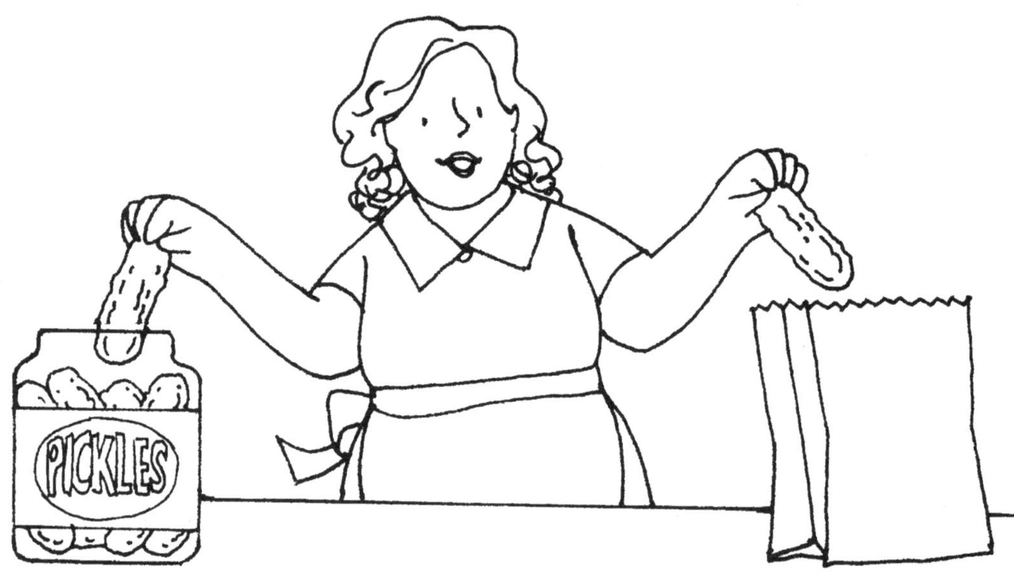

1. Bag lunches were being made for a kindergarten field trip. Each lunch was to get one pickle. There were 22 students in one kindergarten class and 23 in the other class. How many pickles would be needed? _______

2. The ladies making the lunches had 50 pickles in a gallon jar. How many pickles would be left after the kindergarten lunches were made? _______

3. The next day, each fifth-grade student in the lunchroom got two pickles. One class had 25 students. The other class had 24 students. How many pickles were needed for the fifth-grade students? _______

4. The ladies in the lunchroom had two jars of 50 pickles each. How many would be left after the fifth-grade lunch? _______

5. One day, the students had sliced pickles on their hamburgers. One table of eight students wanted to find out how many pickle slices were at that table. Three students had three pickle slices each. One student had five pickle slices. Four students had two slices each. How many pickle slices were at the table? _______

Name ______________________________

PICKLE COLLECTION

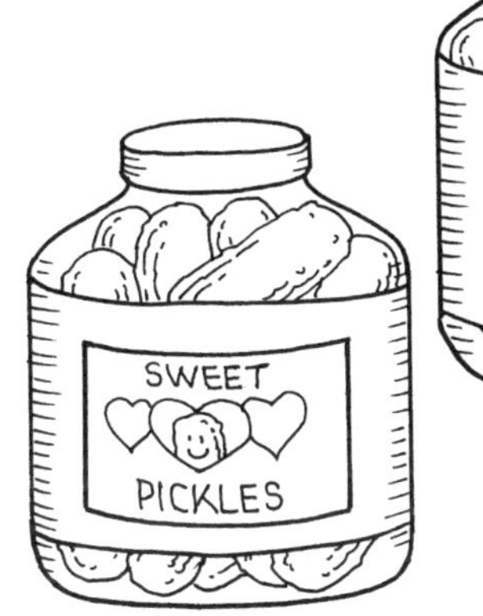

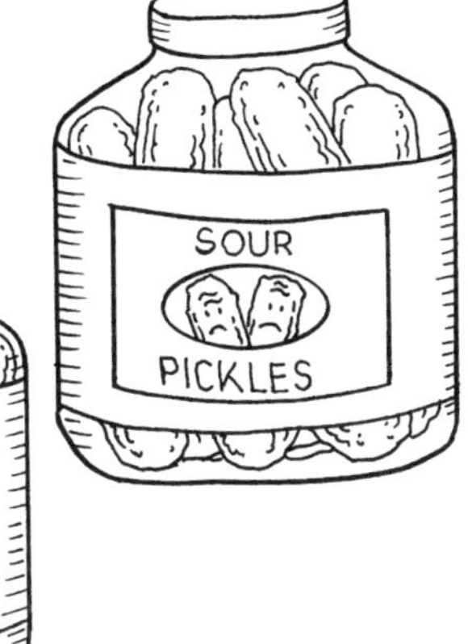

1. Students at Pickle Mountain School collected pickles to send to a food bank. They collected 25 jars of dill pickles, 14 jars of sweet pickles, and 12 jars of bread and butter pickles. How many jars of pickles did they collect? _______

2. Each jar of dill pickles had eight large pickles. How many dill pickles did they have? _______

3. There were nine teachers at Pickle Mountain School. Each teacher brought in three more jars of pickles. How many jars did the teachers add to the collection? _______

4. When the jars from the teachers were put with the student collection, how many jars were there in all? _______

5. When the students returned to school on Monday, they were surprised to find three cases of pickles on the porch. Each case contained 12 jars of pickles. How many jars of pickles were left on the porch? _______

6. When the truck came from the food bank, how many jars of pickles did the school have to donate? _______

7. The truck driver stopped at the senior center and left 26 jars of pickles for the Meals On Wheels program. How many did he have left to take to the food bank? _______

Name ____________________________

MR. BROWN'S PICKLE PROJECT

Mr. Brown's fourth-grade class did a project with pickles. Three students brought quart jars of homemade pickles bought at a local produce stand. For this lesson, they needed jars of pickles that did not have company labels.

First, they weighed the jars of pickles before they were opened. Then they weighed the juice, the jar, and the pickles separately.

Use the chart below to work the problems on this page. Show your work.

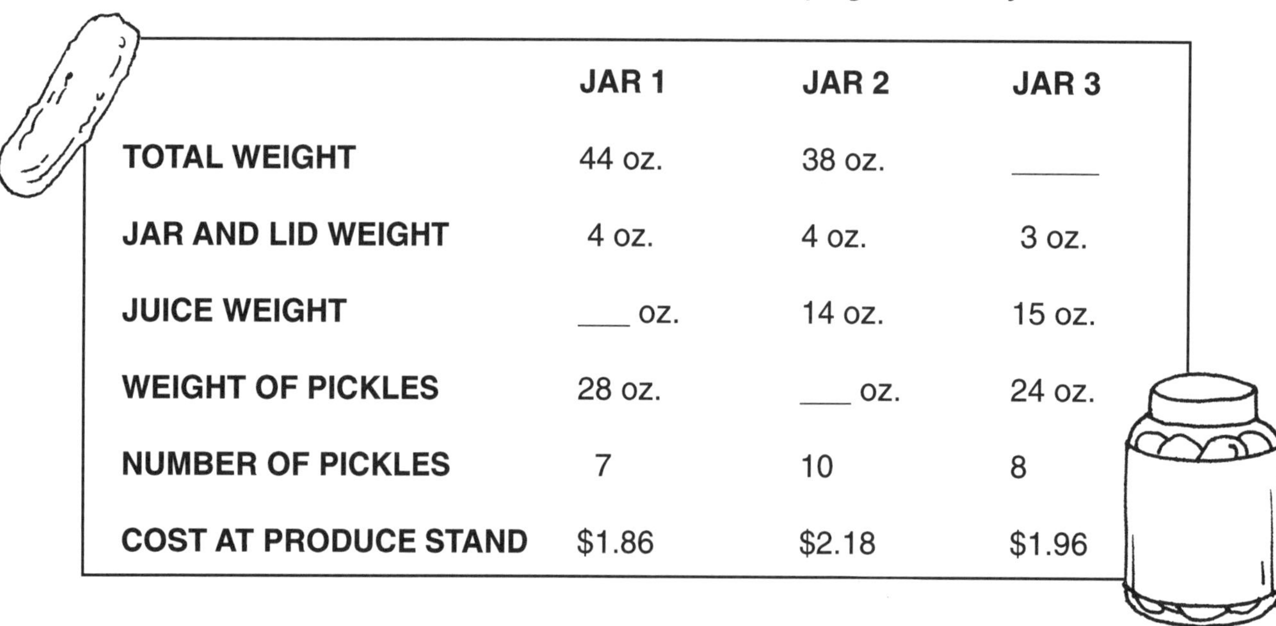

	JAR 1	JAR 2	JAR 3
TOTAL WEIGHT	44 oz.	38 oz.	____
JAR AND LID WEIGHT	4 oz.	4 oz.	3 oz.
JUICE WEIGHT	___ oz.	14 oz.	15 oz.
WEIGHT OF PICKLES	28 oz.	___ oz.	24 oz.
NUMBER OF PICKLES	7	10	8
COST AT PRODUCE STAND	$1.86	$2.18	$1.96

1. Use the information to fill in the blanks on the chart.
2. What is the average weight of an unopened quart jar of pickles? ______
3. What was the average weight of just the pickles? ______________
4. What was the weight of all of the juice? ____________________
5. Which jar had the smallest pickles? ________ How do you know? _____

   ____

   ____
6. What is the average number of pickles in a jar? ______________
7. What would the total cost of the three jars be? ______________

CHAPTER 7

VOCABULARY ACTIVITIES

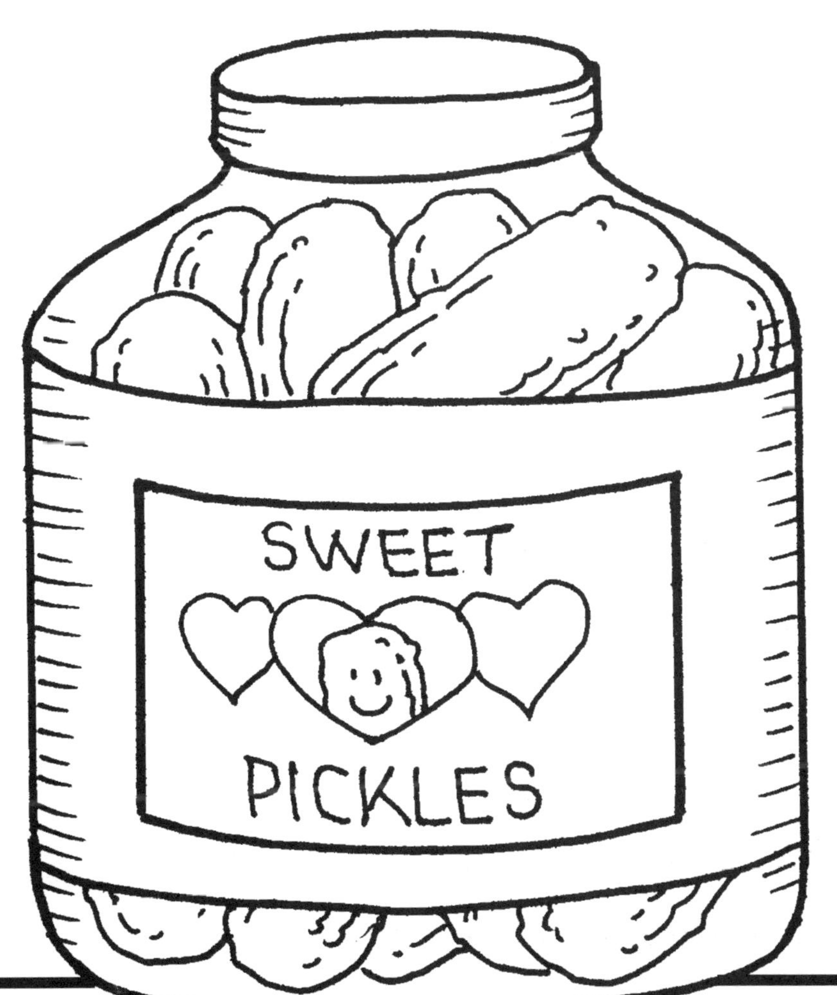

DISCOVERY LIST OF WORDS FOR
SWEET, SOUR, AND IN-BETWEEN FEELINGS

abandoned left all alone (I felt abandoned when everyone but me played soccer.)

accepted pleasantly received (He felt accepted when he was asked to help.)

adaptable able to change (When I didn't mind that our plans were changed, everyone said I was adaptable.)

admired to be looked at favorably (I felt admired when I won the contest.)

aggravated irritated (I was aggravated at the wind for blowing my papers around.)

alarmed suddenly cautious or scared (He was alarmed by a knock at the door in the middle of the night.)

amazed hardly able to believe a situation (I was amazed at the magician's tricks.)

angry mad (He was angry at her for spilling paint on his homework.)

annoyed bothered, only a little angry (I was annoyed when the fly kept buzzing around the table.)

anxious waiting for something to happen (I was anxious to see the circus.)

appreciated to be shown thanks (I felt appreciated when the teacher thanked me for helping.)

bashful shy (She felt bashful around adults.)

bewildered confused (He was bewildered by the stories he was hearing.)

bold not shy (I felt bold when I told the police officer what I had seen.)

bouncy happy and energetic (I felt bouncy when our team won the game.)

brave courageous (When I dove into the pool first, I felt brave.)

burdened carrying a heavy load (She felt burdened with all the bad news.)

capable able to do something (He felt capable of leading the games at the party.)

cautious careful (I was cautious when I crossed the street.)

charitable giving willingly (He was in a charitable mood when he donated to the Children's Fund.)

cheerful happy (She felt cheerful while playing with the children.)

confused unable to understand (I was confused by so many different kinds of directions.)

cooperative willing to work with others (We were all feeling cooperative as we worked on our school project.)

crabby not too pleasant (When I felt crabby, I didn't want anyone to bother me.)

creative imaginative (He was feeling very creative as he started to make the birdhouse.)

curious wanting to learn more (I was curious to see how my new videogame worked.)

dandy very fine (She was feeling just dandy when the test was over.)

defenseless unable to protect oneself (He felt defenseless when they were yelling at him.)

delighted thrilled (She was delighted when the flowers arrived.)

determined firm (I was determined to finish my homework before dinner.)

disappointed not as hoped for (I was disappointed when our game was called because of rain.)

discouraged losing hope (He was discouraged when he practiced and practiced and still couldn't make the team.)

disregarded not considered (She felt disregarded when no one would listen to her idea.)

downcast sad (I was downcast after I missed a word in the spelling contest.)

eager ready to do something (She was eager to start on the project.)

ecstatic very happy (He was ecstatic when he got an "A" on his test.)

elated highly joyful (I was elated when my parents said we were going to Hawaii.)

embarrassed feeling uneasy and hoping no one will notice (She was embarrassed when she dropped her lunch on the floor.)

energetic having plenty of physical ability to do a task (He felt energetic when he started moving the firewood.)

excited stirred up (I was excited about the new puppy.)

excluded left out (I was excluded from the group that took a trip.)

exhausted very tired (He felt exhausted after mowing the lawn.)

fantastic great (She felt fantastic when she made the team.)

fearful scared (I was left with a fearful feeling when the phone rang but no one would talk.)

forgiven having your apology accepted; set free from the burden of doing something wrong (After ruining his paper, she felt forgiven when he asked her to play.)

free not restricted by something (I felt free when I finished the paper.)

friendly ready to share kind things with another person (He was in a friendly mood when his classmate came over to play.)

frightened scared (She was frightened when the car in front of her had a accident.)

furious very mad (I was furious when a student made us miss the assembly.)

gallant brave and kind (He felt gallant when he saved the kitten caught in the tree.)

generous willingly giving more than required (Dad was in a generous mood and gave the waitress a large tip.)

gloomy cheerless; not looking good (I was feeling gloomy and didn't even notice the rabbit in my yard.)

glorious wonderfully magnificent (I felt glorious when our team won the championship.)

grateful thankful (She was grateful for the new box of crayons.)

grumpy in a bad mood (He woke up grumpy this morning.)

guilty deserving to be blamed (I was feeling guilty about taking the money without asking.)

happy full of joy (She was happy to see sunshine.)

helpful ready to give assistance (She felt helpful when she worked with the first-graders in reading.)

helpless unable to give assistance (We felt helpless as we watched the ball get hit by a car.)

hopeful expecting good to happen (They were hopeful that the garage sale would be a success.)

horrified unpleasantly shocked (They were horrified at the sight of the burning building.)

humiliated feeling no good (He was humiliated when the group of boys bullied him.

impatient unable to wait in a calm manner (Waiting in the line that didn't move made me feel impatient.)

important of great value (He felt important when he was asked to run for class president.)

industrious ready to get a lot done (I felt industrious as I started my science project.)

infuriated very angry (They were infuriated when they saw their project had been destroyed.)

inquisitive curious (He was inquisitive and kept asking questions.)

irritable easily upset (I had a headache and was irritable.)

jealous upset that someone else has what you want (He was jealous of the boy next door's new bike.)

jolly happy and laughing (We all felt jolly as we rode the rides at the amusement park.)

joyful happy (The kids were joyful when summer vacation began.)

jumpy nervous (I was jumpy when the lights went out.)

kind nice (He was kind to give some seed to the birds.)

kingly in a royal position (He felt kingly when he had the honor of ringing the bell to start the play.)

knowledgeable informed about a topic (She felt knowledgeable about snakes.)

let down disappointed (We felt let down when the promised box didn't arrive.)

lighthearted carefree; cheerful (The girls were lighthearted as they looked forward to a free day.)

lonely feeling alone, left out (Hearing the children playing outside, the sick boy felt lonely.)

lovable deeply cared about (After I told the truth, I felt lovable again.)

mad angry (We were mad at the people who threw trash into our yard.)

magnificent wonderful (We felt magnificent when we won the game.)

marvelous wonderful (We felt marvelous when we saw our project on television.)

merry happy (She felt merry as she danced around the room.)

mighty strong (He felt mighty as he lifted the bricks.)

miserable very unhappy (We all felt miserable when we had the flu.)

mournful sad about a great loss (Our whole family was mournful when our dog died.)

needed to be tied down to a duty; to be wanted by someone (I wanted to go outside, but I felt needed in the kitchen.)

neglected not taken care of (She felt neglected when she didn't get a turn.)

nervous uneasy about circumstances (I was nervous when I had to go to the principal's office.)

obligated having to do something (I felt obligated to pay back the money I borrowed.)

odd different from others; a feeling that is different from a person's normal feeling (I felt odd in my jeans when the other girls showed up in dresses.)

optimistic expecting a good outcome (I was optimistic as I sat down to take the test.)

overjoyed super happy (Sam was overjoyed when he found his lost puppy.)

overwhelmed having too much to do (The girl was overwhelmed by the amount of homework.)

patient understanding about inconveniences or delays (He was patient while he waited in the long line.)

patriotic feeling loyalty to one's country (We felt patriotic as we sang our national anthem.)

peaceful calm (I felt peaceful lying on the grass and watching the clouds.)

pessimistic expecting a bad outcome (Since it was getting late, he was pessimistic about getting a good seat at the movie.)

playful ready to have fun (Mom was in a playful mood when she put the plastic spider in my cereal.)

protected kept from harm (I felt protected when I saw the police officer coming down the street.)

proud having a good opinion of oneself, another person, or thing (I was proud of the job I did on my book report.)

puzzled unable to put the facts together (The man was puzzled when he saw three cars in his driveway.)

qualified able to do the task (She felt qualified to use the computer.)

quiet	keeping one's thoughts to oneself (I was quiet when the others talked so much.)
refreshed	rested and re-energized (We felt refreshed after a swim in the pool.)
rejected	not accepted (I felt rejected when I didn't get the part in the school play.)
relaxed	comfortable (I felt relaxed when I listened to the music.)
respectful	showing consideration (I felt respectful when I opened the door for my teacher.)
rushed	hurried (He felt rushed to get his work done before the bell rang.)
sad	unhappy (I was sad when I lost my kitten.)
safe	protected (We all felt safe when Mom and Dad got home.)
scared	afraid (I was scared when the lightning knocked out our power.)
secretive	keeping information from someone (We were secretive about Mary's surprise birthday party.)
stressed	having a lot on one's mind (Having two tests in one day made me feel stressed.)
surprised	responding to an unexpected event (The teacher was surprised when we got her a birthday cake.)
talkative	having a lot to say (She was very talkative after the excitement of the day.)
tearful	ready to cry (Leslie was feeling tearful when she broke her new toy.)
terrific	very, very good (We felt terrific when we won first prize.)
thankful	grateful (I felt thankful that no one was hurt in the car accident.)
timid	shy (She was timid when asked to speak in front of the class.)
tolerant	allowing for the differences of others (She was tolerant when she chose her friends because of the kind of persons they were, not by their race or ability.)
understand	to know what something means (I understand the homework assignment.)
ungrateful	not appreciative (He was ungrateful when he didn't get the present he wanted.)
unhappy	sad (I was unhappy when I couldn't go to the amusement park with my friends.)

upbeat	in a good, energetic mood (Everyone at the party was upbeat.)
useful	able to be of help (Doing my share of the work made me feel useful.)
valiant	brave (The boy was valiant when he took care of his little sister during a thunderstorm.)
valuable	worth a lot (I felt valuable when the teacher asked me to help another student in math.)
vicious	mean (The boy was vicious when he hurt the little girl's feelings.)
victorious	celebrating an accomplishment (We all felt victorious when the school won a blue ribbon.)
welcomed	accepted in a kind way (Jill felt welcomed when she went to her new school.)
whiny	complaining a lot (Margie was whiny when she didn't get her own way.)
wishful	hoping something will happen (He was wishful as he looked at all of the bikes in the store.)
wonderful	great (I felt wonderful going high in the swing.)
worried	being concerned that something bad will happen (Curt was worried about what the class would be like with the substitute teacher.)
X-rayed	looked at very closely (I felt X-rayed by the time my mom said I looked clean enough to go.)
youthful	feeling young and playful (The dog was 15 years old, but she still seemed youthful.)
yucky	lousy (He felt yucky after he ate five bags of popcorn.)
zany	clowning around (Craig was feeling zany when he pretended to be a Jack-in-the-Box and tried to scare everyone.)
zealous	eager to participate (I felt zealous about being in the walk-a-thon for juvenile diabetes.)
zippy	energetic (She felt so zippy that we couldn't keep up with her.)
zonked	senseless; feeling unconnected to what is happening (I felt zonked after reading the mystery book for three hours.)

DISCOVERY LIST OF WORDS FOR
SWEET AND SOUR FEELINGS

A

adaptable able to change (I was feeling adaptable and didn't mind the change of plans.)

angry mad (He was angry when a bully ripped up his homework.)

B

bashful shy (She felt bashful when she had to talk to adults.)

bold brave; daring (I felt bold when I told the police officer what I had seen.)

C

confused unable to understand (I was confused about which pages to read.)

curious wanting to learn more (I was feeling curious about how my new toy worked.)

D

delighted thrilled (She was delighted with her new outfit.)

disappointed not as hoped for (I was disappointed when I didn't get to go to the movie.)

E

embarrassed feeling uneasy and hoping no one has noticed (I was embarrassed when I dropped my tray in the lunchroom.)

excited stirred up (I was excited about my new puppy.)

F

friendly ready to share kind things with another person (He was in a friendly mood when his classmate came over to his house to play.)

frightened scared (She was frightened when the lightning struck close to her home.)

G

grateful thankful (She was grateful for the new box of crayons.)

grumpy in a bad mood (He woke up grumpy this morning.)

H

happy full of joy (She was happy to see the sunshine.)

helpful ready to give assistance (We were glad Tom was in a helpful mood when we came home with the groceries.)

I

important of great value (I felt important when I was asked to read to the class.)

irritable easily upset (Sherry was irritable today and I wanted to avoid her.)

J

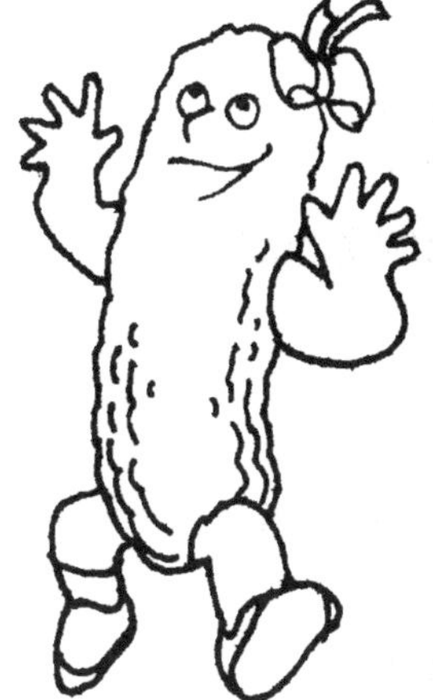

jolly happy and laughing (We all felt jolly on the merry-go-round.)

jumpy nervous (I was jumpy when the storm knocked out our lights.)

K

kind nice (Bob was feeling kind when he helped his neighbor work in the yard.)

L

lonely feeling all alone; left out (Hearing the children play outside made him feel lonely.)

M

mad angry (We were mad at the people who threw trash into our yard.)

mighty strong (Brad felt mighty as he lifted the heavy bricks.)

N

needed to be tied down to a duty or wanted by someone (I wanted to go outside, but I felt needed inside to help my mother.)

nervous uneasy; fearful (I was nervous when I had to speak in front of the class.)

O

overjoyed super happy (Sam was overjoyed with his new bike.)

overwhelmed having a lot to do at once (He was overwhelmed by the amount of homework he had.)

P

patient waiting without getting upset (Mike was patient in the lunchroom line.)

proud having a good opinion of oneself, another person, or thing (The boy was proud of the job he had done.)

Q

quiet keeping thoughts to oneself (I was quiet when the others talked so much.)

R

relaxed comfortable (Mary was relaxed when she lay on the grass, looking at the clouds.)

respectful showing consideration (The boy was respectful when he held the door for his teacher.)

S

safe protected (We felt safe when we reached home in the thunderstorm.)

scared afraid (Missy was scared of the barking dog.)

T

terrific very, very good (We felt terrific when we won the game.)

thankful grateful (I felt thankful for the presents I got for my birthday.)

U

understand	to know what something means (I understand my math assignment.)
unhappy	sad (I was unhappy when my friend moved away.)

V

valuable	worth a lot (I felt valuable when the teacher asked me to be a messenger.)
vicious	very mean (The bullies were vicious to the boy they didn't like.)

W

whiny	complaining a lot (Chris is whiny when she doesn't get her own way.)
wonderful	great (I felt wonderful when we rode the ferris wheel.)

X

X-rayed	looked at very closely (I felt X-rayed when Mom noticed all the good things about me.)

Y

youthful	feeling young and playful (Although she was 15, the dog still seemed youthful.)
yucky	lousy (Brad felt yucky when he had the flu.)

Z

zany	acting like a clown (She felt zany as she jumped on the trampoline.)
zippy	energetic (Mickey was so zippy that we couldn't keep up with him.)

Name ______________________________

YOUR NAME

Directions: Look at the word "pickles" below. Each letter has a feeling word after it. Write your first name, just like the word "pickles." Then write a feeling you sometimes have that begins with each letter of your name. Use your feeling vocabulary word list to help you when you can't think of a word. If you have time, do your last name, too.

P **Patriotic** ____ ______________________

I **Industrious** ____ ______________________

C **Cheerful** ____ ______________________

K **Kind** ____ ______________________

L **Lonely** ____ ______________________

E **Energetic** ____ ______________________

S **Safe** ____ ______________________

____ ______________________

____ ______________________

____ ______________________

____ ______________________

____ ______________________

____ ______________________

Name ______________________________

VOCABULARY SEARCH

Directions: Find the hidden words. The words are hidden across and down. Circle each word you find. When you are finished, use the lines below to write the definitions of two words in the word search list.

ADAPTABLE
ALARMED
ANNOYED
BOUNCY
CURIOUS
EAGER
ECSTATIC
FEARFUL
FURIOUS
GRATEFUL
GUILTY
MARVELOUS
OPTIMISTIC
OVERWHELMED
SAFE
SECRETIVE
SECURE
TOLERANT
UPBEAT
WORRIED
X-RAYED
ZANY
ZIPPY

____

____

____

____

Z A N Y B
C L L N M O L
U X L A S A U M
P R O R A R N S
Z B A Q M F V C E U
A E Y N E E E Y C L
T A E O D V L X R R
O T D A N N O Y E D
L V E A M F U K T F
E X C D F W S O I E
R D S A U S O V V A
A G T P R E P E E R
N R A T I C T R Z F
T A T A O U I W I U
A T I B U R M H P L
W E C L S E I E P D
J F N E C K S L Y E
G U I L T Y T M W H
V L W O R R I E D
E A G E R C D
C U R I O U S

Name ______________________________

SYNONYMS AND ANTONYMS

Directions: Find words that mean the same as the words listed below. Words that mean the same thing are called *synonyms*.

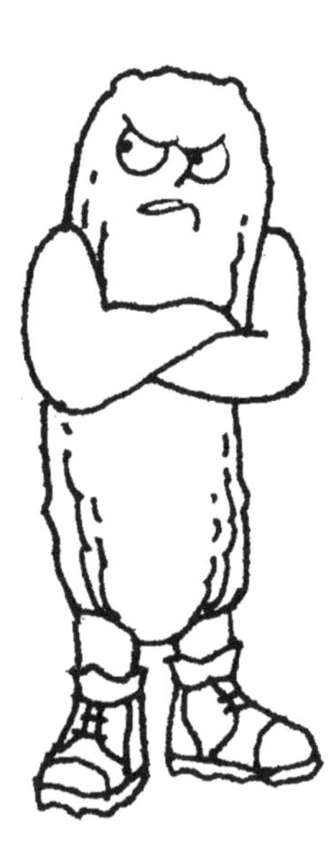

angry ______________________________

jumpy ______________________________

cheerful ______________________________

curious ______________________________

downcast ______________________________

frightened ______________________________

grateful ______________________________

magnificent ______________________________

welcomed ______________________________

Directions: Find words that mean the opposite of the words listed below. Words that have opposite meanings are called *antonyms*.

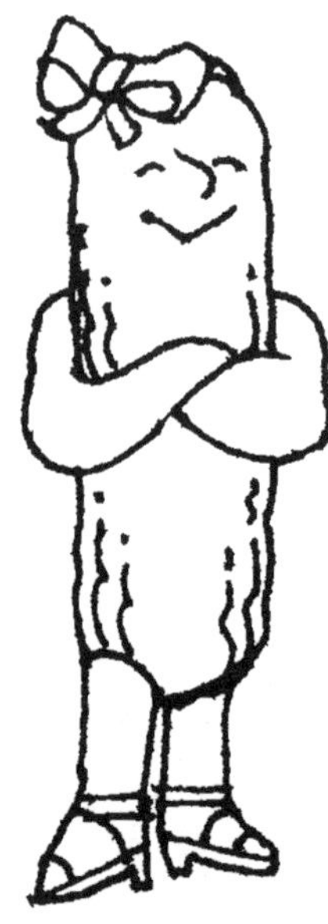

bashful ______________________________

cheerful ______________________________

humiliated ______________________________

optimistic ______________________________

safe ______________________________

vicious ______________________________

Name ________________________________

HOW MANY WORDS CAN YOU WRITE?

1. Write all the words you can that have something to do with being happy.

____

____

____

2. Write all the words you can that have something to do with being sad.

____

____

____

3. Write all the words you can that have something to do with being energetic.

____

____

____

4. Write all the words you can that have something to do with being angry.

____

____

____

5. Write all the words you can that have that have something to do with being afraid.

____

____

____

Name ______________________________

FIND THE WORD

Directions: Use your vocabulary word list to find the word that completes the sentence. The first letter of the word is there to help you.

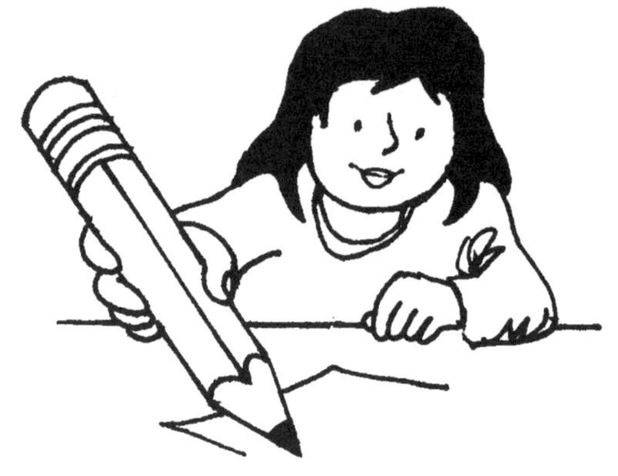

1. I did not want to talk when I felt **b** ____________________ .
2. I was **e**________________________ when I opened the present.
3. I was **g**________________________ for the sandwich.
4. I was **i**________________________ when my friend left.
5. I was **p**________________________ of the blue ribbon.
6. I felt **t**________________________ at the swimming pool.
7. I felt **y**________________________ when I ate too much.
8. After a good night's sleep, I felt **z**____________________ .
9. I was **f**________________________ when the thunder woke me.
10. I was **r**________________________ reading under the tree.

Name ______________________________

SWEET AND SOUR WORDS

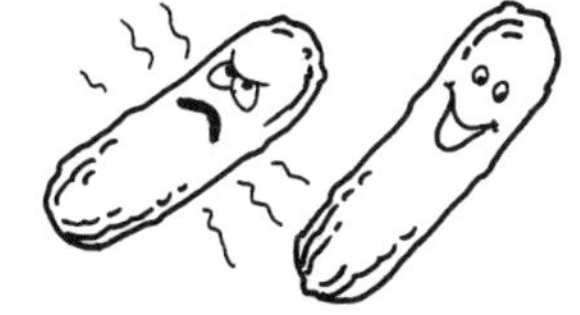

Directions: Use your vocabulary word list to help you complete this activity sheet.

Write five words that describe sweet pickle feelings.

1. ______________________
2. ______________________
3. ______________________
4. ______________________
5. ______________________

Write five words that describe sour pickle feelings.

1. ______________________
2. ______________________
3. ______________________
4. ______________________
5. ______________________

Pick one word from your list and write it on the line below.

____

Draw a picture of how you look when you feel like the word you wrote.

Name ______________________________

SWEET AND SOUR FEELINGS CROSSWORD

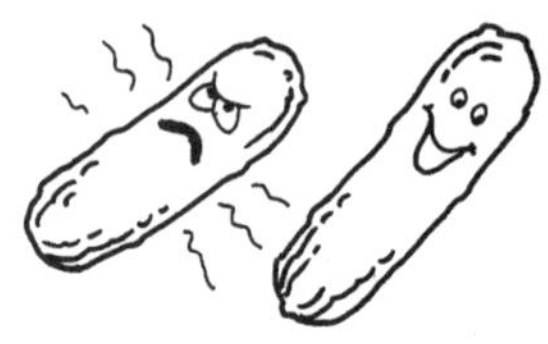

Directions: Complete the crossword puzzle below. Use your word list to help you.

ACROSS

3. grateful
6. feeling left out
7. protected

DOWN

1. in a bad mood
2. wanting to learn more
4. mad
5. nice

Name ______________________________

FEELINGS CROSSWORD

Directions: Complete the crossword puzzle below. Use your word list to help you.

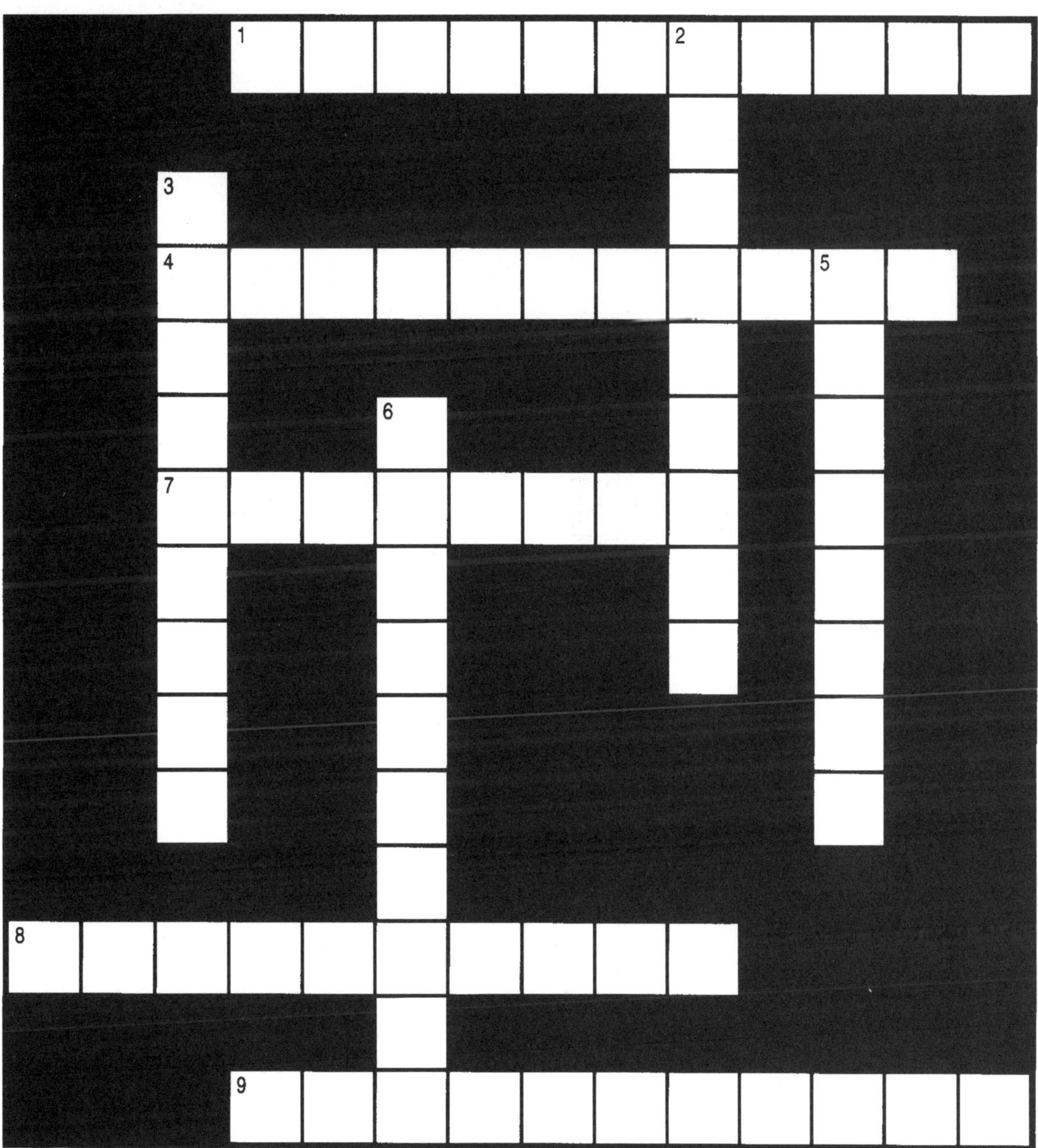

ACROSS

1. having a lot to do at once
4. losing hope
7. allowing for the differences of others
8. celebrating an accomplishment
9. ready to get a lot done

DOWN

2. very tired
3. able to change
5. very happy
6. confused

CHAPTER 8

PARENT INVOLVEMENT

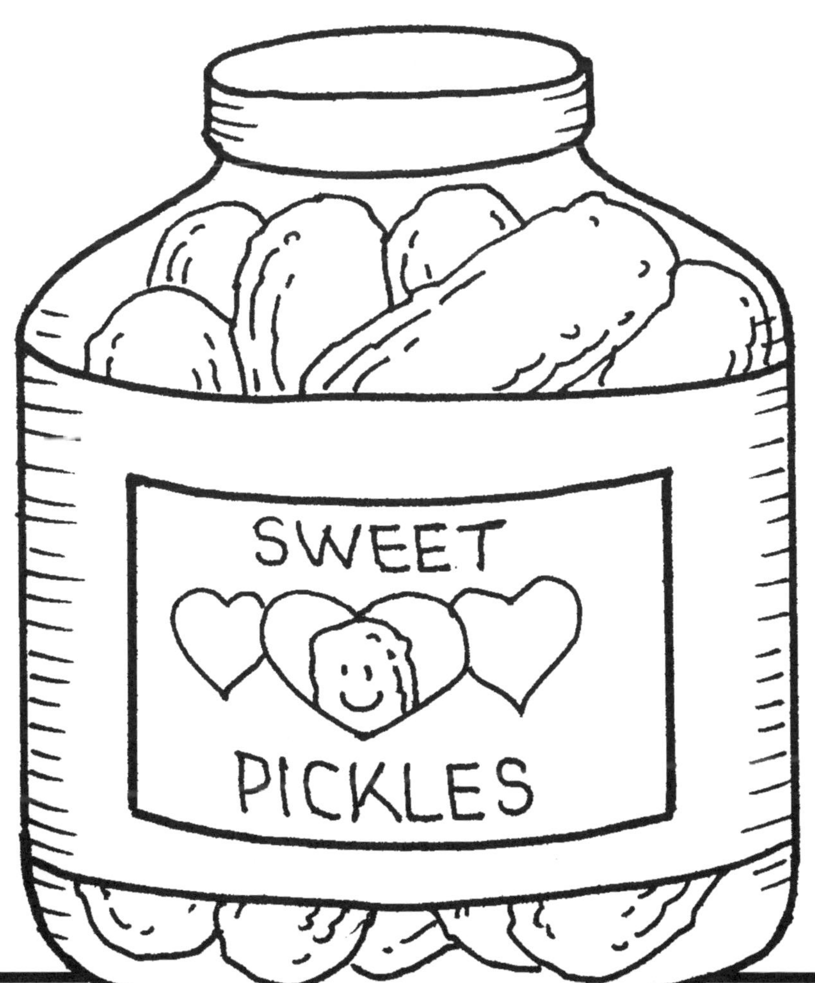

TAKE A TRIP THROUGH COOKBOOKS

Look through cookbooks you have or can borrow for the word *pickle*. Make a list of all the different kinds of pickles you can find.

______________________________ ______________________________

______________________________ ______________________________

______________________________ ______________________________

______________________________ ______________________________

______________________________ ______________________________

______________________________ ______________________________

Answer the following questions:

What is one liquid ingredient you found in all (or almost all) of the recipes?

____

Did you find *pickle* in recipes for things other than cucumbers?

____

What spice did you find most often?

____

Are pickles ready to eat as soon as they are put in a jar?

____

What pickles would have to stay in the jar longest before they were ready to eat?

____

Has anyone in your family ever made pickles?

____

TAKE A TRIP TO THE GROCERY STORE

Take this paper and a pencil to the pickle aisle at your grocery store and look at all the pickles.

List the different shapes you find (slices, etc.)

____

____

____

____

____

____

List the different varieties you find (zesty, dill, etc.)

____

____

____

____

____

____

Are there vegetables other than cucumbers in the pickle section? If so, what are they?

____

____

____

____

____

____

____

____

____

How many ounces is the smallest jar of pickles you can find?

____

How many ounces is the largest jar of pickles you can find?

____

How much is the most expensive jar of pickles you can find?

____

Find two kinds of pickles you might like to buy. What would they cost together?

____

P-I-C-K-L-E-S

How many smaller words can you make using only the letters in the word PICKLES? You may only use each letter once in each word. Write your words below.

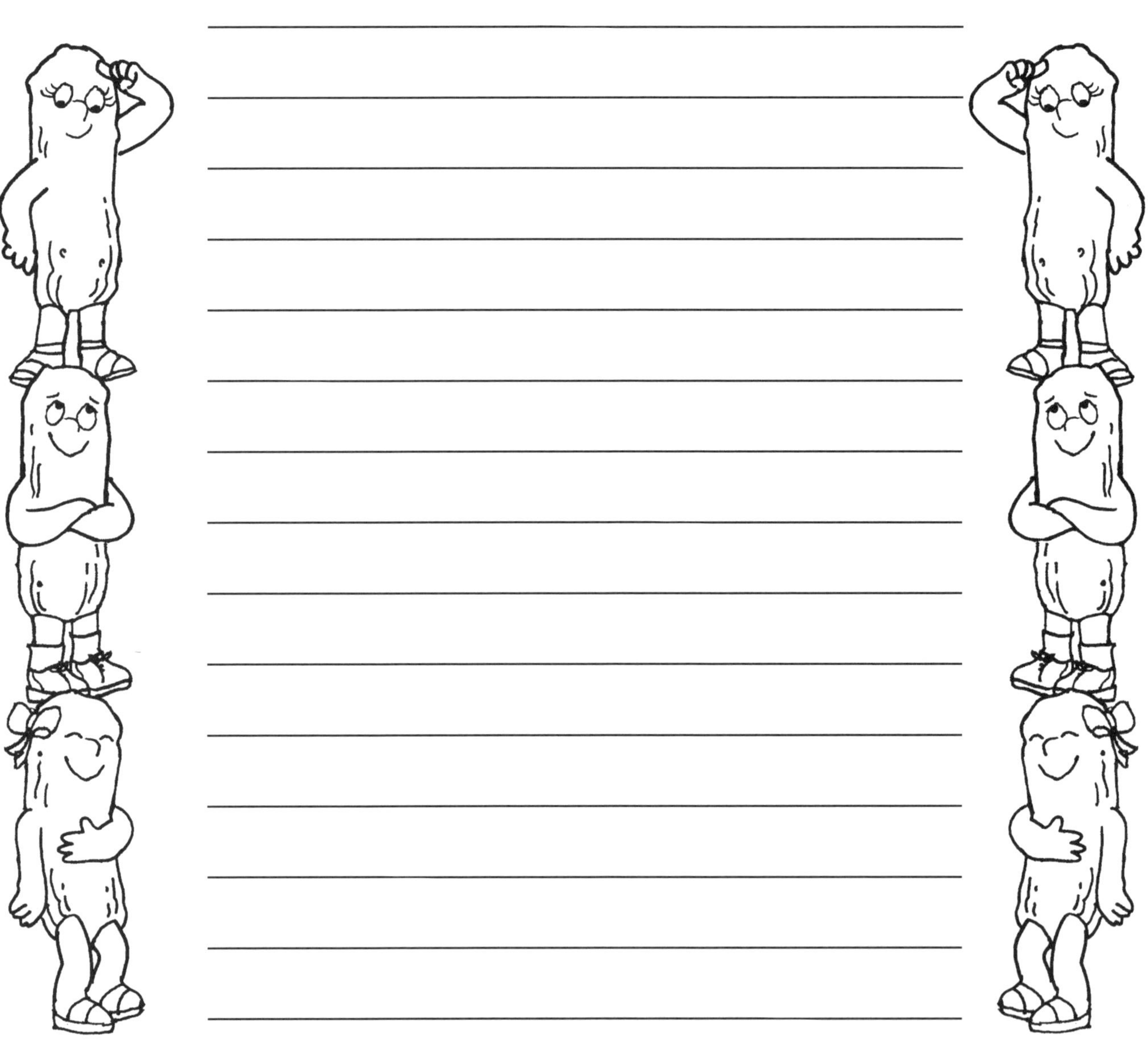

Note To Parents: To use this activity with other words, try Dill Pickles, Sour Pickles, or Sweet Pickles. If you have younger children, write the letters to the word PICKLES on separate pieces of paper or use refrigerator magnet letters. Then let your child move the letters around to make new words.

COOKING WITH PICKLES

Pickle Pudding

1 package (4-serving size) pistachio instant pudding
3/4 cup milk
1 tablespoon sweet pickle juice

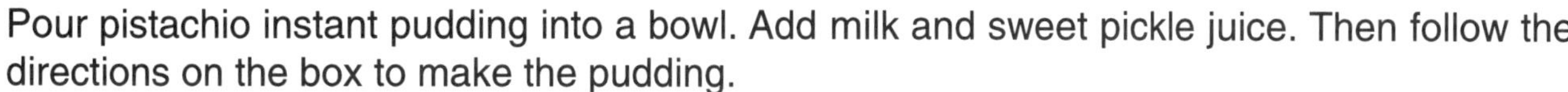

Pour pistachio instant pudding into a bowl. Add milk and sweet pickle juice. Then follow the directions on the box to make the pudding.

Pickle Chocolate Chip Cookies

1 package (4-serving size) pistachio instant pudding (or use vanilla pudding and add a little green food coloring)
1 cup quick biscuit mix
1/4 cup vegetable oil
1 egg, slightly beaten
3 tablespoons sweet pickle juice
1/2 cup mini-chocolate chips

Preheat the oven to 375°

Combine the pudding and biscuit mix in a bowl. Stir in the oil, egg, and pickle juice and blend well. Add the mini-chocolate chips. Drop from a teaspoon an inch apart onto an ungreased baking sheet. Bake about 12 minutes, until slightly browned. Remove from the baking sheet and cool on wire racks. Makes about 2 dozen cookies.

Peanut Butter And Pickle Cookies

1 cup creamy peanut butter
1 egg
2 cups quick biscuit mix
2 tablespoons sweet pickle juice
1 can *sweetened* condensed milk
3 tablespoons green decorating sugar crystals

Preheat the oven to 350°

Mix all the ingredients together until smooth. Drop by slightly rounded teaspoonsful onto an ungreased cookie sheet, about one inch apart. Bake 6 to 8 minutes. Makes about 5 dozen small cookies.

APPROPRIATE WAYS TO HANDLE ANGER

Everybody gets angry and sometimes there can be good reasons to be angry. Getting angry can give you the energy to take care of a problem. There are three things we cannot do when we are angry: hurt someone, destroy things, or use words that will get us in trouble with the principal, our teacher, or our parents. It's also important not to get mad over every little thing or to stay mad for a long time. Use this word search to find things that might help when you are angry. If you know what to do, it is easier for you to deal with the situation that made you angry.

Directions: Find the hidden words or phrases and circle them. Answers with more than one word are in stairstep style. Example:

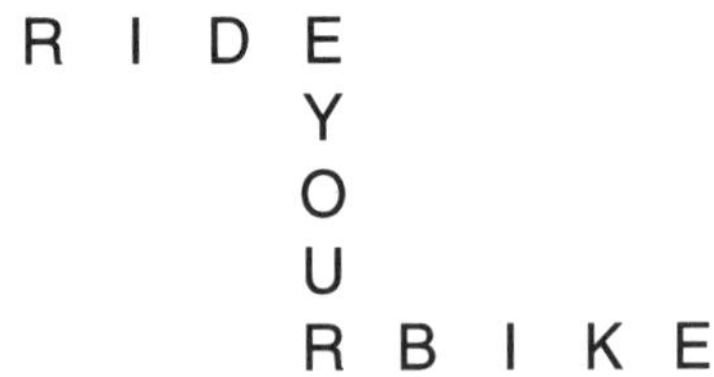

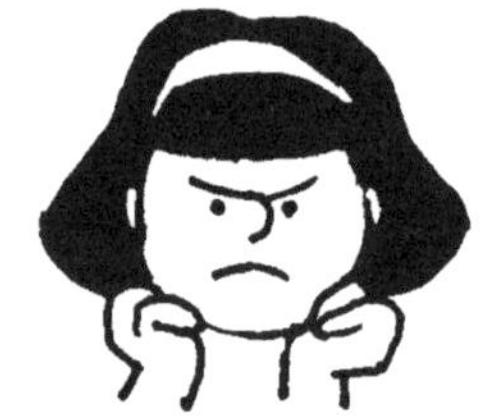

WALK
TAKE TIME TO CALM DOWN
CLEAN
DECIDE IT'S NOT A BIG DEAL
FIND SOMETHING FUNNY
TALK TO A FRIEND
EXERCISE
MAKE A SACK FOOTBALL
RIDE YOUR BIKE
WRITE SOMEONE (BUT DON'T MAIL THE LETTER)
LISTEN TO MUSIC
CRY
DRAW
RUN

```
T A L K X C G T A K E O M T Z L R S T U
B C D T E F G H I J T M A K E I M N O P
C Q R O A S T U V W I X Y U A S A C K E
Z F A H F I W H T J M K L P S T U F F S
D M W O R P Q R D S E T O V W E Y Z O B
I C D E I F G H E I J K C L M N T O O R
S T U V E X E R C I S E A W X Y Z M T C
K D C F N G H I T J K L L M N O P U B S
D V R I D E W X D F Y Z M D O W N S A X
E D Y E F Y G H E I T S J K L M N I L C
C T H E R O S T U N V N W X Y Z A C L L
I B C P W U E F G D S O M E T H I N G E
D K L R R R B I K E K E N T A P Q R F A
E I T S I Z Q R T U V W B X Y Z K V U N
L A Z N T Q A B C D E F I G H I J K N L
E L N O E S O M E O N E G D H A L Y N Z
A L C T A B I G J K L M N P Q R S T Y V
W A L K P H A D E A L D F G H J K R U N
```

SACK FOOTBALL

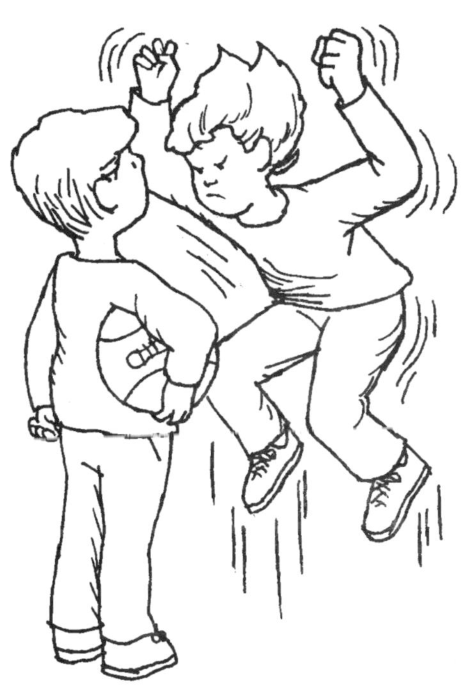

Energy from anger can be powerful. As adults, we can show children how to use that energy in a non-threatening way. Sometimes the problem causing the anger cannot be solved until some of the energy is used up. As adults, we can pull weeds, scrub the tub, clean the refrigerator, shop for groceries, exercise, or sit down and use our thought processes before we explode our anger onto another person in an unacceptable way.

We teach children that it is okay to get mad, but that they can't hurt someone, destroy things, or use words that will get them in trouble with the principal, their teacher, or their parents.

Sometimes a child needs time away from others in order to calm down. That time-out should not be a punishment, but an opportunity to get away from the cause of the anger.

Here's an idea that might be helpful for letting a child release some of the energy produced by anger. Your supervision is important, but give the child some distance from the cause of the anger.

Do you have an abundance of shopping bags? Stuff one bag with other bags and tape it closed. Or use a paper bag stuffed with wadded paper. Now your bag is ready for a hard workout and lighthearted fun. Toss it. Hit it. Kick it. Squeeze it. Stomp on it. Throw it away (or recycle).

RESPONSIBILITIES FOR ALL

It takes everyone's help to make sweet pickle days in a family. Use this chart to see who has responsibilities at your house. Complete this chart at home with an adult.

Write each family member's name in a block at the top of a column. Check the jobs each one does.

Going to work to earn money								
Cleaning the house								
Picking up toys								
Making beds								
Doing laundry								
Paying bills								
Cooking meals								
Doing dishes								
Buying food								
Doing yard work								
Caring for the car								
Repairing things								
Driving children to activities								
Taking care of trash and recycling								

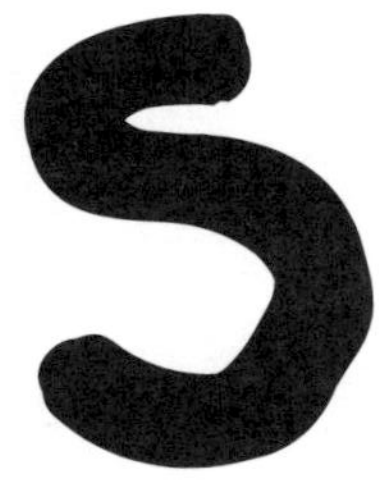

SPEND TIME WITH YOUR CHILDREN.

SPEND SPECIAL TIME WITH EACH CHILD.

You don't have to go anywhere to have special time alone with a child. It may be a reading time, an outside activity, or a cooking project.

Talk with your child, read to your child, and sing to your child before he or she learns to walk.

Make good use of the time you spend together. When you're at the store or in the kitchen or laundry area, involve your child. You child can learn to do things, increase his or her vocabulary, and have a good time with you.

Even though I am encouraging you to spend time with your child, I do not mean to make you think children always need adult attention. It is also important for children to have some independent time for creative play. And it goes without saying that moms and dads need some independent time, too.

Sit down and play games with your children. Start when they are toddlers. Playing games builds relationships and teaches many life skills.

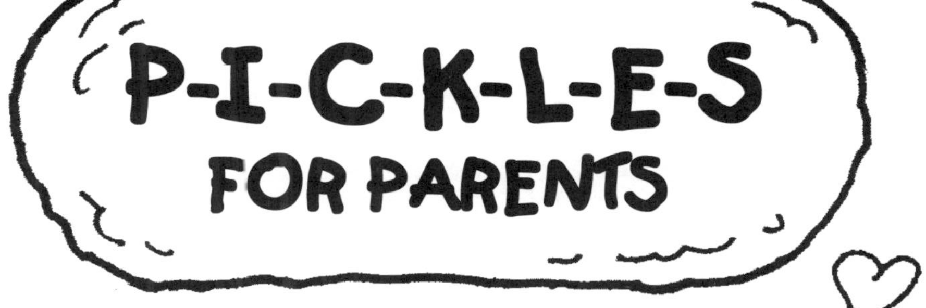

P Prepare yourself for the ups and downs.

I Individual differences should be respected.

C Cooperate to find solutions.

K Kindle trust and responsibility.

L Limit your battles and limit your responses.

E Encourage expression of feelings.

S Spend time with your children.

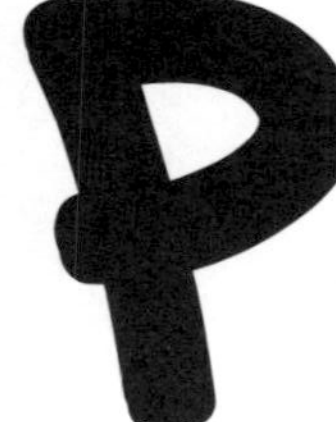

PREPARE YOURSELF FOR THE UPS AND DOWNS OF PARENTING.

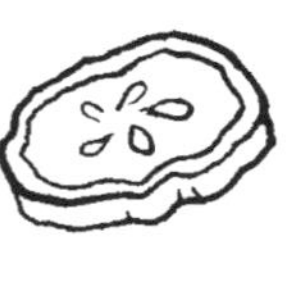

Do you remember the story of the ant and the grasshopper? The ant prepared for the winter, but the grasshopper did not consider the rough times ahead. As parents, we need to consider that there may be rough times ahead. Almost every parent I know has had ups and downs with their children.

Sometimes it helps just to know what behaviors are a normal part of growth and development. Being around other parents can give you added strength to make it through the rough times. You need to find other adults who are supportive, not critical. We are not alone in our love and concern for our children.

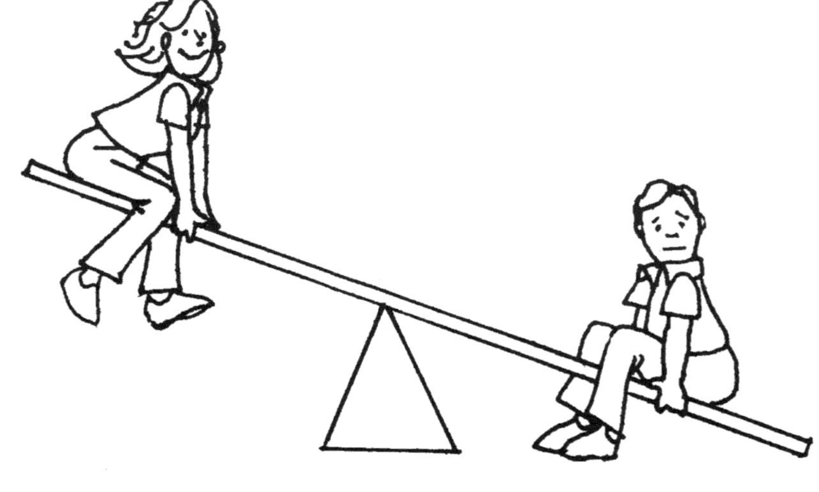

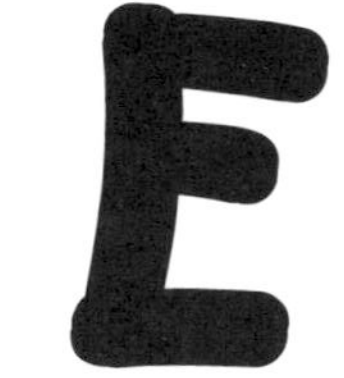

ENCOURAGE EXPRESSION OF FEELINGS.

Learning words for degrees of feelings can help us cope. Perhaps the most useful are words for levels of anger. You may simply be *annoyed* at someone, but when you use the word *angry,* you may raise the intensity of the feeling and *become* angry. A person may also be frustrated or scared, and voice those feelings as anger. That makes others respond to the anger rather than to the real feeling.

To help children express feelings, we must stop and listen. Sometimes it is hard for us to slow down long enough to do that. Listen and acknowledge the feeling without telling children they should not feel that way.

Before ending with the letter "E," I want to talk about times a child may not be able to express feelings. There are cases where our children are being treated as failures or discipline problems because of something that is beyond their control. Check with a medical doctor to rule out physical causes of these problems.

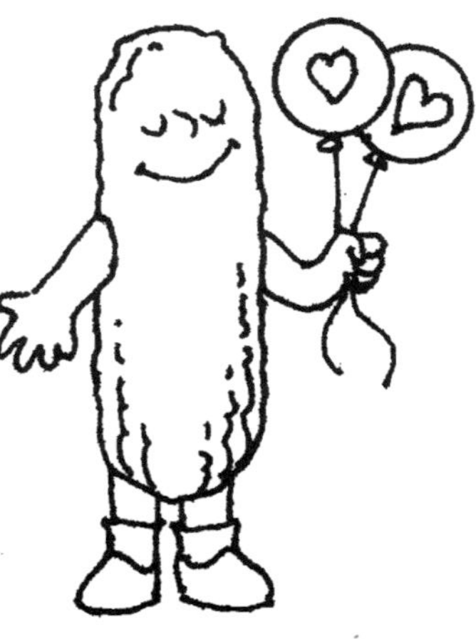

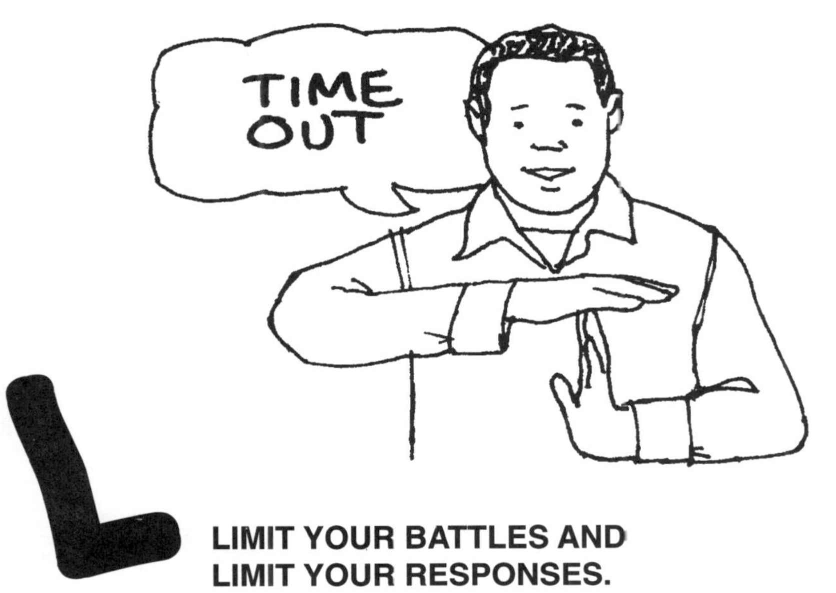

L LIMIT YOUR BATTLES AND LIMIT YOUR RESPONSES.

Limit the number of battles you have with your children and limit the ways you respond in battle situations. You, as the adult, can determine how and when to tackle the issue. You would not reach into a hot oven unprepared, but you may jump into a heated situation without thinking things through. In fact, you may even turn up the heat! Take a little time to think before you react.

First, limit the times of your responses. Wait until the timing is right to deal with your anger.

Second, limit the methods of your responses. Use the method that expresses your point of view without putting the child down.

Third, limit the length of your responses. Briefly say what needs to be said. Your child may hear *more* when you say *less*.

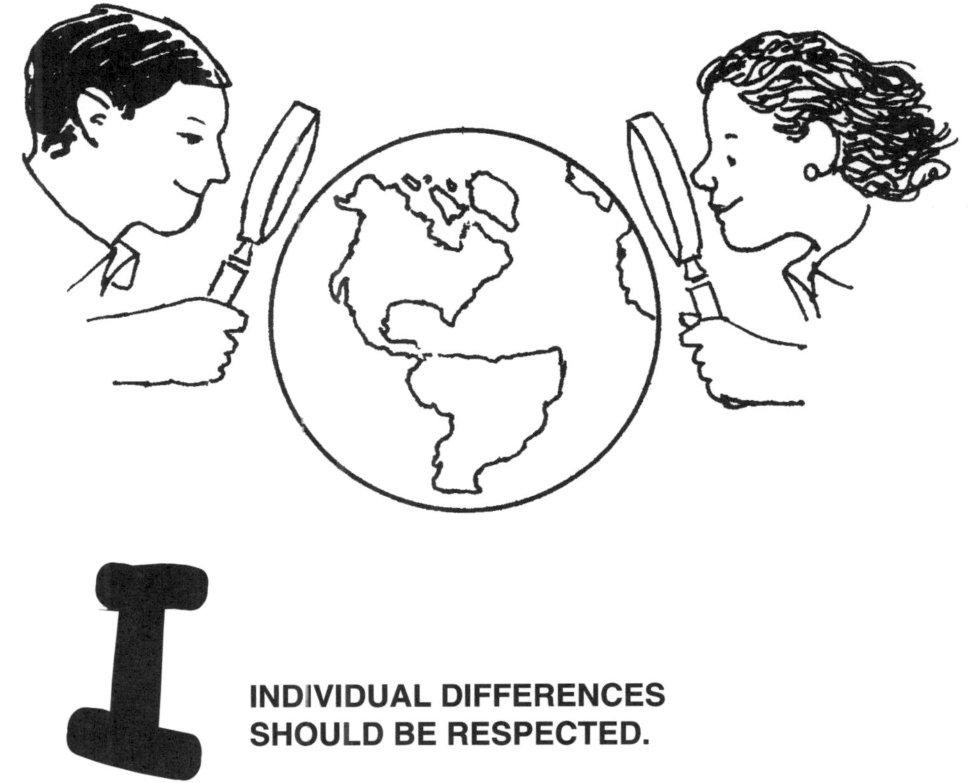

I INDIVIDUAL DIFFERENCES SHOULD BE RESPECTED.

At school, we teach our children they are special because they are unique.

It really is okay that we aren't all good at the same things and that we don't all like the same things.

Have you ever noticed how two people really do see the world from different points of view? They are not attempting to be disagreeable. Their individual differences put a different light on the same situation.

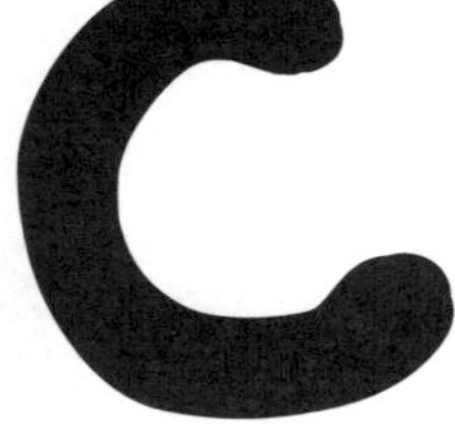

COOPERATE TO FIND SOLUTIONS.

Conflict-management is an important part of our school program. Students are taught that conflicts are a natural part of being around other people. Handling these conflicts can be constructive or destructive.

The negotiating point is the focus of C: Cooperate to find solutions. When you negotiate, you are cooperating to find a solution. Neither you nor the child may get exactly what you want, but look what you gain when you come up with a solution together! Your child is learning skills that will last for a lifetime.

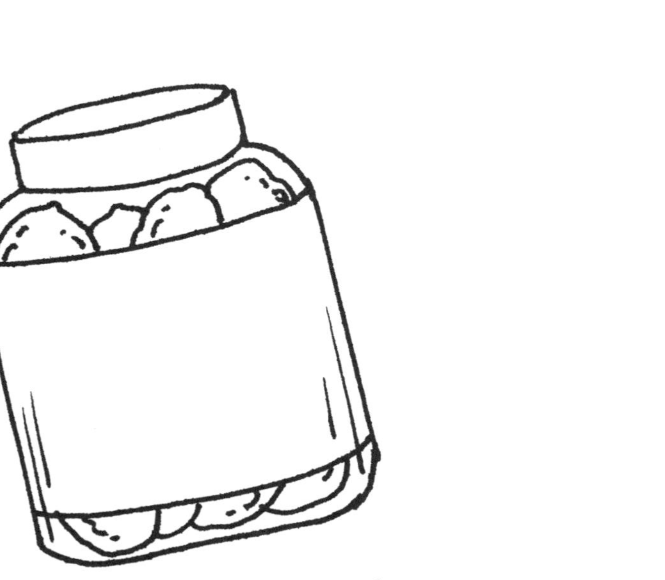

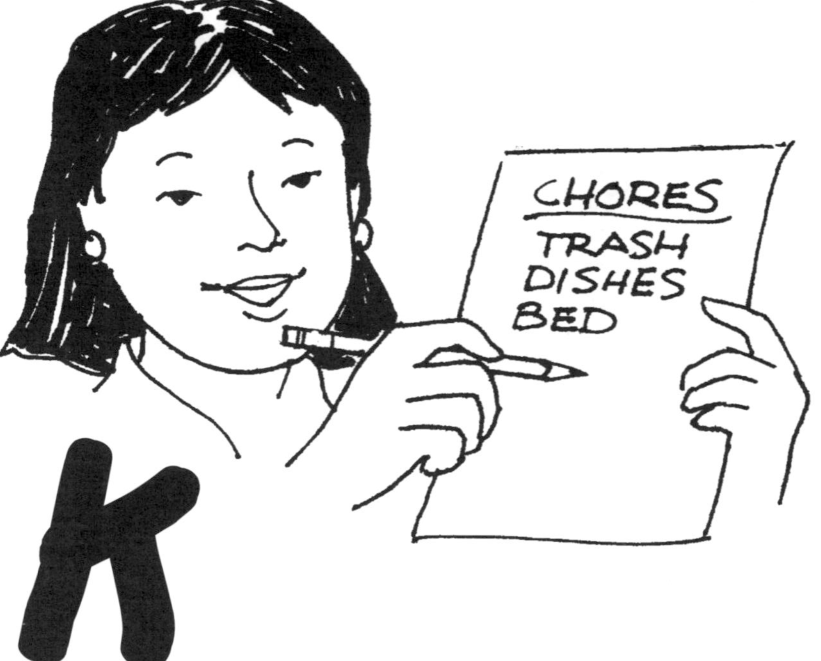

KINDLE TRUST AND RESPONSIBILITY.

Children need to feel useful and learn responsibility while they are young. Even preschoolers can be expected to accept responsibility. The key is to assign appropriate age-level responsibilities. A preschooler would not be given the responsibility of driving the sit-down lawn mower. But a preschooler could be given the responsibility of emptying wastebaskets.

Not only do our children need to have responsibilities, they need to learn to be responsible for their own behavior.

Children must learn to be responsible so we can trust them. But we must trust them so they have the chance to be responsible.

GUIDELINES FOR PLAYING GAMES

(These apply most, but not all, of the time.)

Unless you have lots of time, play games that can be completed in less than 10 minutes. You can always play again if everyone is having fun. Save lengthier games like *Monopoly* for snow days, vacations, or special weekends.

Avoid games that send someone all the way back to the beginning when almost at the end.

Avoid games with pieces that break or require batteries.

Puzzles can be fun. Start out with puzzles that don't have too many pieces and purchase more complicated ones as your family shows an interest.

Avoid games that make more noise than you can tolerate.

Benefits of Playing Games With Your Children

- ✔ Games encourage conversation.
- ✔ Games help teach vocabulary.
- ✔ Games teach patience.
- ✔ Games teach the importance of following rules.
- ✔ Games teach cooperation in setting up, playing, and cleaning up.
- ✔ Games give children a chance to see how parents react in a competitive situation. They see parents both win and lose.
- ✔ Games can build fond memories for children.
- ✔ Simple games like tic-tac-toe can be played anywhere, anytime. Keeping a deck of cards in the car or a tote bag is a good way of being prepared for waiting times.
- ✔ Games let children practice math, reading, thinking, and memory skills.
- ✔ Games teach children to enjoy activities they can share with their friends.

MATH SUGGESTIONS FOR PARENTS

Students seem to lose more math skills than reading skills during school vacations. Reading is everywhere, but you may need to provide math practice.

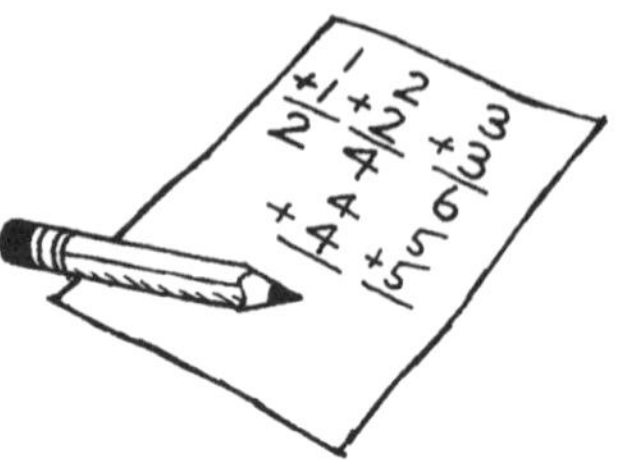

These suggestions were collected from educators as ways to help children develop math skills.

- ✔ Model aloud how you, as a parent, figure out math problems in everyday life. (There are 18 pieces of candy in this bag, and there are 26 children in your class. 18 and 18 is 36. If I buy two bags of candy, there will be enough for your class.)
- ✔ Play counting games with young children. Count flowers, red cars, pieces of candy, etc. Songs that count backwards help with the concept of subtraction.
- ✔ Make a grocery list from newspaper advertisements. Add up how much the items you've chosen will cost.
- ✔ Choose a simple recipe. Buy the items and add the cost before checking out. Go home and make the recipe!
- ✔ Cook with your child. Talk about measurements, temperature, and cooking time.
- ✔ Practice math facts in the car or while cooking.
- ✔ Use musical notes with an instrument to learn simple counting skills.
- ✔ Count how many stop signs or stoplights you see on the way to school, the store, etc. For a slightly older child, ask how many for a round trip or how many for five days of school. For even older children, add miles or figure gas mileage.
- ✔ Play Bingo. Play games. Most games use some math.
- ✔ Do math problems with small pieces of candy, raisins, cereal, etc. and eat them when finished. This will work for simple addition, subtraction, multiplication, and division.
- ✔ Preteens may use the checkbook method for keeping track of allowances or other monies earned and expenses.
- ✔ Play estimation games. How long do you think this string is? How much do you think those three items will cost? How many apples will fit in that box?
- ✔ Give young children their allowance in change. Teach them to put some in a place to save and allow them to spend the rest. With this money, they can practice counting, adding, and subtracting.

LIMIT THE WAY YOU RESPOND TO YOUR CHILDREN

When you are upset, try to remember to use "I" messages instead of "You" messages. When you find it possible to use this method, lines of communication may be a little clearer. An "I" message begins with "I" and describes your response to the situation. It shows your displeasure with your child's behavior, rather than your displeasure with your child. This may not seem like much of a difference to you, as an adult, but your child will definitely know the difference. Remember: Great kids sometimes do things that upset us. We wouldn't trade our children for anything, but we would trade a behavior once in a while. The following examples may be helpful:

"When I go to bed at night, there are no dirty dishes in the sink. I can't face dried-up food first thing in the morning. I don't care if you eat, just rinse the food off the dishes." Sentences like this work much better than, "You're such a slob. You eat whatever you want and leave the mess for me."

"I really thought those two bad grades would be gone from this report card. I believed you when you said you turned in all the assignments, but this shows there were 11 papers not turned in. Something different will have to be done. I have to be better informed about what's going on." This is a better way to handle this frequent, but touchy, subject than saying, "You are a liar. You don't even care about these grades."

"I'm disappointed that you didn't come home on time. It's frustrating when I need you home and have to just wait. The bank closed 10 minutes ago, and now I can't get this check cashed." This works better than, "You are so irresponsible. Can't you tell time?"

"I was really embarrassed when you screamed at me in the grocery store. I don't have enough money to get everything you want. Taking you to the store can be fun, but I need you to cooperate." This explains your feelings better than, "You were a baby in the store. How can you be so selfish as to cry over candy? You are so bad. I don't want to take you anywhere."

"I tripped over your toy trying to get to the phone. It really makes me angry when toys are left in the way." Say this instead of, "You don't care if I get hurt. You just leave things wherever you want."

CHAPTER 9

PICKLE RELISH

(Bits & Pieces)

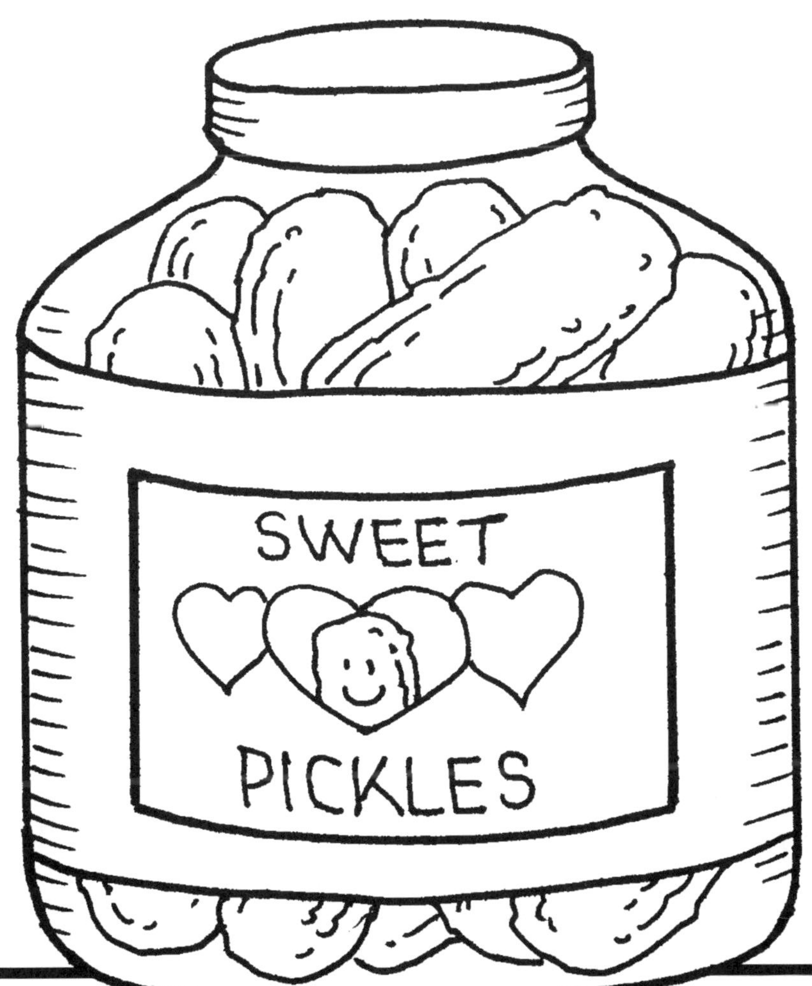

SAMPLE LESSONS FOR GRADES K-2

The following lesson plans are designed for 30-minute periods. As you know, the reactions and abilities of your students determine the number of things which can be accomplished in that amount of time. Therefore, these are guidelines to be adapted to your own personal situation. Throughout the lessons, you will see asterisks (*). These are sheets to be sent home for student review and parent education. For additional "pickle" materials available from the author, visit Pat Kienzle's website at: www.pickleladybooks.com.

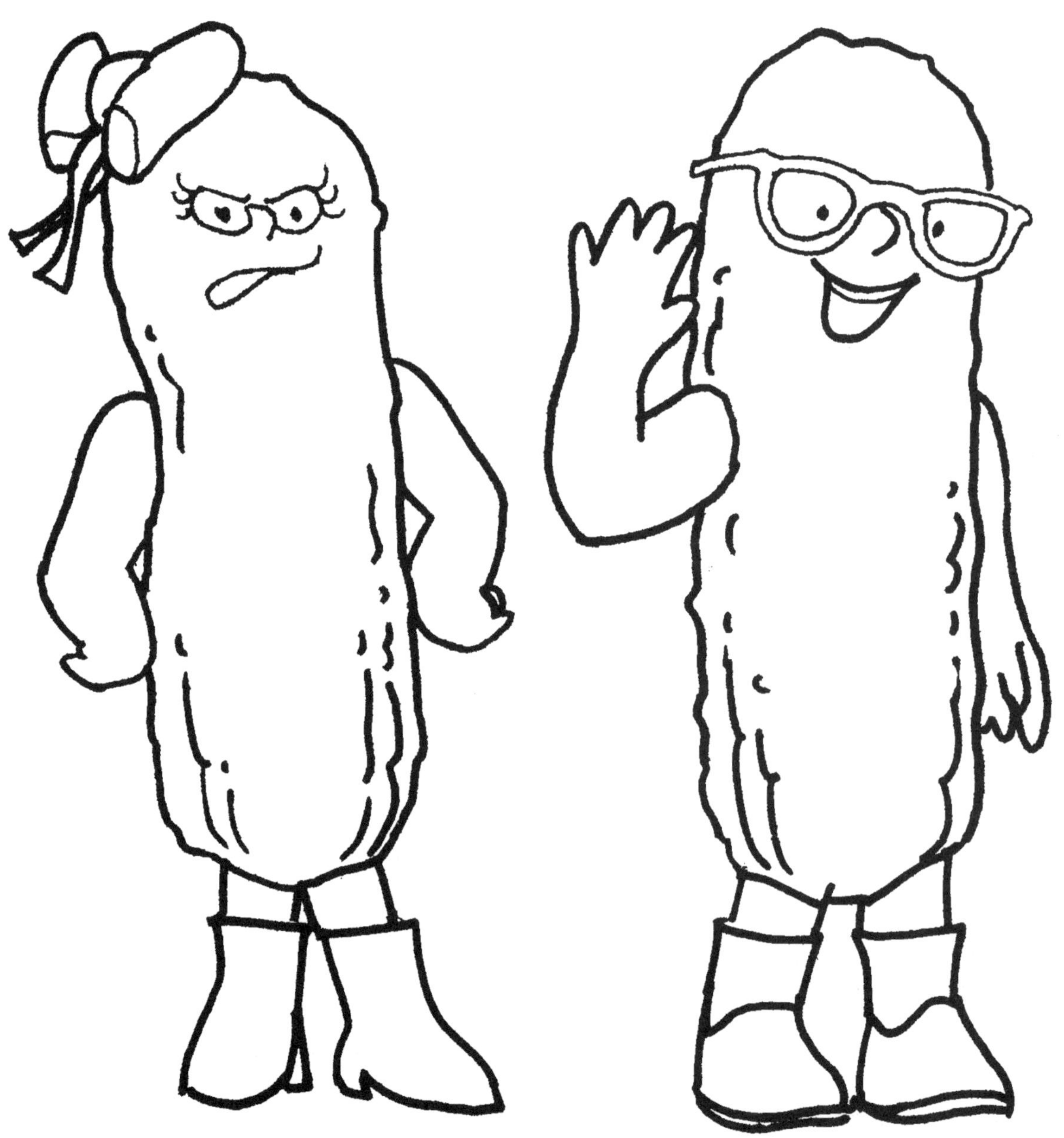

LESSON: INTRODUCING THE PICKLE THEME I

Materials Needed:

- ☐ Chalkboard and chalk or posterboard and marker
- ☐ Eight pieces of green construction paper, marker, scissors
- ☐ Jar of sweet pickles
- ☐ Jar of sour pickles
- ☐ Copy of *The Pickle Pledge* (page 39) for each student
- ☐ Optional: Jar of sweet gherkins
- ☐ Copy of *Pickle Things* by Marc Brown (ISBN 0-679-888469-6) or *Pickle Pop-Up* (page 63) for the leader
- ☐ Optional: Copy of *Secret Code #2* (page 61) for each second-grade student
- ☐ Completed copy of *Life Is Like A Pickle* (page 38) for each student

Pre-Lesson Preparation:

Reproduce copies of the activity sheets (see above list). Using the pickle illustrations found throughout the book or the blank pickle shapes on page 184, reproduce and cut out eight pickle shapes and label them: *happy, lonely, excited, proud, mad, scared, loved, sad.* On the chalkboard or posterboard, write: *Life is like a pickle. Sometimes it's sweet. Sometimes it's sour.*

Lesson:

1. Discuss the concept of sweet and sour pickles, explaining that all kinds of pickles are okay to eat even if you don't like the taste of them. Tell the students that sour pickles represent unpleasant feelings and sweet pickles represent pleasant feelings. Then read the posted theme from the chalkboard or posterboard and have students repeat it.

2. Show the students the cut-out pickles. Have them decide whether each one is sweet or sour, then place each one beside the appropriate jar of pickles. Have the students repeat the theme.

3. Give each student a copy of *The Pickle Pledge.* Teach the students the accompanying actions for *The Pickle Pledge* (page 40).

4. Kindergarten and first-grade students (optional activity): Teach the *sweet gherkin wave.* Show the students the jar of sweet gherkins. Relate their little fingers to the sweet gherkins in the jar. Ask them to wave their little "sweet gherkins" when they see you at school. This helps cut down on the students calling out, "Pickle Lady" or "Mr. Pickle."

5. Read the story *Pickle Things.* If the book is unavailable, play *Pickle Pop-Up.*

   Second-grade students (optional activity): Give each student a copy of *Secret Code #2.* Tell the students how much time they have to complete the activity sheet. Or allow the students to complete the activity sheet at home.

6. Recite the *Pickle Pledge* again. Collect the *Pickle Pledge* sheets for use in the next lesson.

7. *Distribute a completed copy of *Life Is Like A Pickle* to each student.

LESSON: INTRODUCING THE PICKLE THEME II

Materials Needed:

- ☐ Pickle jars and labeled pickles from *Lesson 1*
- ☐ Copy of *The Pickle Pledge* (from previous lesson–page 39) for each student
- ☐ Copy of *Actions For The Pickle Pledge* (page 40) for the leader
- ☐ Copy of *Pickle Routine* (pages 41-42) for the leader
- ☐ Copy of *Discussion Guide* (page 43) for the leader
- ☐ Copy of *Pickle Parade* (page 161) for each kindergarten or early first-grade student
- ☐ Copy of *Little Pickle Word Search* (page 49) for each older first-grade student or younger second-grade student
- ☐ Copy of *Sweet Pickle, Sour Pickle Word Searches* (page 50) for each advanced second-grade student
- ☐ Copy of *Pickle Things* by Marc Brown (ISBN 0-679-888469-6) or *Pickle Pop-Up* (page 63) for the leader or copy of *Ten Pickle Jars* (page 222) for each student and the leader
- ☐ Copy of *Parent Letter* (page 45) for each student

Pre-Lesson Preparation:

Reproduce copies of the activity sheets (see above list).

Lesson:

1. Using the jars of pickles and the cut-out pickles from the previous lesson, review the pickle theme: *Life is like a pickle. Sometimes it's sweet. Sometimes it's sour.*

2. Distribute a copy of *The Pickle Pledge* to each student. Recite *The Pickle Pledge,* using toys or actions to accompany the words. Refer to the *Pickle Routine* and *Discussion Guide* as guidelines for this part of the lesson presentation. (*Note:* The *Pickle Routine* and *Discussion Guide* may be incorporated into most K-1 lessons and used frequently in lessons presented to second-grade students.)

3. Discuss the *Parent Letter.*

4. Kindergarten/early first-grade students: Give each student a copy of *Pickle Parade.* Using the activity sheet, teach the students about properly walking in line. (Teachers may want copies of this activity to present on the first day of school.)

   Older first-grade/second-grade students: Give each student a copy of *Little Pickle Word Search* or *Sweet Pickle, Sour Pickle Word Searches.* Tell the students how much time they have to complete the activity sheets. Or allow the students to complete the word searches at home.

5. If there is enough time, end the lesson by re-reading *Pickle Things*, playing *Pickle Pop-Up*, or distributing copies of *Ten Pickle Jars* to each student and singing the song together.

6. *Distribute a copy of the *Parent Letter* to each student. Tell the students to take the letter home to their parents along with their copy of *The Pickle Pledge*.

LESSON: BULLYING

Materials Needed:

- ☐ Copy of *Pickle Routine* (pages 41-42) for the leader
- ☐ Copy of *Discussion Guide* (page 43) for the leader
- ☐ Copy of *Using "Pickle Cat"* (page 156) for the leader
- ☐ Copy of *Pickle Cat* (page 157) for each student and the leader
- ☐ Copy of *Pickle Gets Mad* (page 158) for each student and the leader
- ☐ Stuffed toy cat or full-bodied cat puppet
- ☐ Cat toy
- ☐ Stuffed toy dog or full-bodied dog puppet
- ☐ Drawing paper and crayons for each kindergarten or early first-grade student
- ☐ Copy of *Secret Code #3* (page 62) for each older first-grade student or second-grade student

Pre-Lesson Preparation:

Reproduce copies of the activity sheets (see above list).

Lesson:

1. Refer to the *Pickle Routine* and *Discussion Guide* as guidelines for this part of the lesson presentation.

2. Give each student a copy of *Pickle Cat* and *Pickle Gets Mad.* Present the *Using "Pickle Cat"* activity. After you have completed your presentation, discuss the dog's behavior. Explain that when the dog took the cat's toy, he was bullying Pickle Cat. Then say:

   "When the dog was a puppy, he liked to jump over things. Because of this behavior, his owners named him *Leapfrog.* But now, because he is such a bully, the other animals in his school have nicknamed him *Bullfrog.*"

3. Ask the students to name different ways a bully behaves. Then discuss some things they can do if they are being bullied by another person. Discuss when they should walk away or ignore the bully (if they are being teased or called a name) and when they should ask an adult for help (if they are being threatened or there is physical contact). Tell the students they may come to you (or another trusted adult) any time they feel scared or sad.

4. Kindergarten or early first-grade students: Give each student a piece of drawing paper and crayons. Tell the students to draw a picture of a cat and a dog getting along with each other.

   Older first-grade students or second-grade students: Give each student a copy of *Secret Code #3.* Tell the students how much time they have to complete the activity sheet. Or allow the students to complete it at home.

LESSON: CONFLICT RESOLUTION

Materials Needed:

- ☐ Copy of *Fight For A Frog* (pages 88-90) for the leader
- ☐ Copy of *Follow-Up Questions* (page 91) for the leader
- ☐ Copy of *Solving Conflicts At Pickle Mountain School* poster (page 92) for each student
- ☐ Chalkboard and chalk or posterboard and marker
- ☐ Copy of *Pickle Parade* (page 161) for each student

Pre-Lesson Preparation:

Reproduce copies of the activity sheets (see above list).

Lesson:

1. Discuss the meaning of *conflict*.

2. Read the story *Fight For A Frog* to the students. When you have finished reading the story, have the students answer the *Follow-Up Questions*.

3. Give each student a copy of the *Solving Conflicts At Pickle Mountain School* poster. Using the text on page 90 as a guide, review the *DINO* steps with the students. Make sure the students understand the meaning of the words *investigation* and *negotiation*.

4. Ask the students to tell you about how a person walking in a line could cause a conflict (fighting over a place in line, arguing over who will hold the door, pushing or hitting someone, etc.). Write their ideas on the chalkboard or posterboard. After completing the list, have the students use the *DINO* steps to think of ways to resolve or avoid the conflicts.

5. Give each student a copy of *Pickle Parade*. Discuss the activity sheet with the students, emphasizing how behaving appropriately and respecting others can help us all get along with one another.

LESSON: ANGER MANAGEMENT

Materials Needed:

- ☐ Copy of *Pickle Routine* (pages 41-42) for the leader
- ☐ Copy of *Discussion Guide* (page 43) for the leader
- ☐ Copy of *Using "Pickle Cat"* (page 156) for the leader
- ☐ Copy of *Pickle Cat* (page 157) for each student and the leader
- ☐ Copy of *Pickle Gets Mad* (page 158) for each student and the leader
- ☐ Stuffed toy cat or full-bodied cat puppet
- ☐ Cat toy
- ☐ Stuffed toy dog or full-bodied dog puppet
- ☐ Copy of *Sentences About Anger* (page 219) for each older first-grade student or second-grade student

Pre-Lesson Preparation:

Reproduce copies of the activity sheets (see above list).

Lesson:

1. Refer to the *Pickle Routine* and *Discussion Guide* as guidelines for this part of the lesson presentation.

2. After completing the *Pickle Routine*, say:

   "Today we are going to talk about anger."

   Give each student a copy of *Pickle Cat* and *Pickle Gets Mad*. Present the *Using "Pickle Cat"* activity. *(Note:* If you are presenting the activity to younger students, you may want to give the handouts to the teacher to distribute to the students to take home.)

3. Discuss with the students things that are okay to do when you are angry (talk, exercise, listen to music, relax).

4. Older first-grade/second-grade students: Give each student a copy of *Sentences About Anger*. Tell the students how much time they have to complete the activity sheet. Or allow the students to complete it at home.

LESSON: TATTLING/REPORTING

Materials Needed:

- ☐ Copy of *Thursday, The Third Day Of Third Grade* (pages 143-145) for the leader
- ☐ Copy of *Stoplight For Tattles And Reports* (page 181) for each student and the leader
- ☐ Red, yellow, and green crayon for each student
- ☐ Copy of *"When" Should You Tell? Pickles* (pages 177-178) for the leader
- ☐ Copy of *Playground Reporting* (page 179) for each kindergarten or early first-grade student
- ☐ Copy of *Secret Code (Tattling)* (page 182) for each older first-grade or second-grade student
- ☐ Copy of *Tattling/Reporting Guidelines* (page 180) for each student

Pre-Lesson Preparation:

Reproduce copies of the activity sheets (see above list). The leader should make a colored sample of *Stoplight For Tattles And Reports*.

Lesson:

1. Read the story *Thursday, the Third Day Of Third Grade* to the students.

2. Discuss the difference between tattling and reporting.

3. Give each student a copy of *Stoplight For Tattles And Reports* and a red, yellow, and green crayon. Show the students the colored sample activity sheet. Then have the students color their stoplight (top circle red, middle circle yellow, bottom circle green). Explain the meanings of the three colors. Have the students put their fingers on the appropriate color as you read the rhyme from the activity sheet. (If necessary, define a *flop* as *something that doesn't work out well,* like cake that didn't get the sugar added or a joke that no one thinks is funny.) Using the situations from the *"When" Should You Tell? Pickles*, have the children practice determining whether they should report a situation.

4. Kindergarten or early first-grade students: Give each student a copy of *Playground Reporting.* Tell the students how much time they have to complete the activity sheet. When the allotted time has elapsed, have the students share their answers with the class.

   Older first-grade/second-grade students: Give each student a copy of *Secret Code (Tattling).* Tell the students how much time they have to complete the activity sheet.

5. *Give each student a copy of the *Tattling/Reporting Guidelines* to take home. These guidelines can help parents understand what situations should be reported.

LESSON: DRUG/ALCOHOL EDUCATION

Materials Needed:

- ☐ Copy of *The Pickle Pledge* (page 39) for each student and the leader
- ☐ Copy of *Pickle Routine* (pages 41-42) for the leader
- ☐ Copy of *Discussion Guide* (page 43) for the leader
- ☐ Copy of *The Pickle Sweep* (pages 108-110) for the leader
- ☐ Copy of *Pickle Sweep Activity* (page 165) for the leader
- ☐ Paper strips labeled with actions
- ☐ Brooms and dustpans
- ☐ Copy of *The Pickle Sweep Song* (page 113) for each student
- ☐ Copy of *Sweep Out* (page 167) for each student

Pre-Lesson Preparation:

Reproduce copies of the activity sheets (see above list). Make the strips of paper as directed on page 165.

Lesson:

1. Recite *The Pickle Pledge* with the students.

2. Refer to the *Pickle Routine* and *Discussion Guide* as guidelines for this part of the lesson presentation.

3. Read *The Pickle Sweep* story to the students.

4. Present the *Pickle Sweep Activity.*

   After completing the activity, discuss the legal age for using tobacco products and drinking alcohol. Most students will know someone who smokes. Tell the students that smoking is unhealthy, but not against the law if you are of legal age. Tell them that most people who smoke wish they had never started. And tell them that smoking is unhealthy as well as expensive. Since second-hand smoke is also unhealthy, discuss ways to limit students' exposure to it. Consuming alcoholic drinks is not against the law for anyone of legal age, but consuming too much alcohol is dangerous. Driving with a blood alcohol content over the state limit is not only dangerous, it is illegal and can have severe consequences. They could hurt themselves or someone else.

   Remind the students that if they have any questions or concerns about drugs or alcohol, they can talk with you. They do not have to tell the whole class about their concerns or about someone they know who is using drugs or alcohol.

5. Give each student a copy of *The Pickle Sweep Song.* Teach the students *The Pickle Sweep Song* and sing it with them.

6. Give each student a copy of *Sweep Out.* Tell the students how much time they have to complete the activity sheet. Or allow the students to complete it at home. When everyone has completed the activity, have the students share their answers with the class. (*Alternative:* Copies may be given to the classroom teacher to distribute.)

LESSON: FEELINGS

Materials Needed:

- ☐ Copy of *Pickle Routine* (pages 41-42) for the leader
- ☐ Copy of *Discussion Guide* (page 43) for the leader
- ☐ Set of *Pickle Memory Game* cards (pages 70-71) for the leader
- ☐ Cardstock or heavyweight paper
- ☐ Optional: Laminator
- ☐ Chalkboard and chalk or posterboard and marker
- ☐ Copy of *Sonny's Birthday* (page 53) for each student and the leader
- ☐ Copy of *Kate's Cat* (page 54) for each student and the leader
- ☐ Copy of *Pickle Memory Game* (pages 70-71) for each student

Pre-Lesson Preparation:

Reproduce copies of the activity sheets (see above list). Reproduce on cardstock or heavyweight paper two copies of the *Pickle Memory Game*. Cut the cards apart and laminate them for durability. Read the directions for *Sonny's Birthday* (page 8) and *Kate's Cat* (page 9) and decide how you will present the stories to the students.

Lesson:

1. Refer to the *Pickle Routine* and *Discussion Guide* as guidelines for this part of the lesson presentation.

2. Discuss the meanings of the words printed on the *Pickle Memory Game* cards. Explain how different words can be used to express the same feeling. For example: happy/joyful, angry/mad, grateful/thankful, scared/afraid. List the pairs of words on the chalkboard or posterboard.

3. Give each student a copy of *Sonny's Birthday*. Read the story aloud, pausing to give the students an opportunity to name the pictures in the story. When you have finished reading the story, have the students name the different feelings described in it. Write the students' responses on the chalkboard or posterboard.

4. Give each student a copy of *Kate's Cat*. Read the story aloud, pausing to give the students an opportunity to name the pictures in the story. When you have finished reading the story, have the students name the different feelings described in it. Write the students' responses on the chalkboard or posterboard.

5. Using the completed deck of cards, have the students play the *Pickle Memory Game*. Give each student a copy of the *Pickle Memory Game* activity sheets. Tell the students they may use these sheets to make their own set of cards. (*Alternative:* Copies may be given to the classroom teacher to distribute.)

LESSON: MANNERS I

Materials Needed:

- ☐ Chalkboard and chalk or posterboard and marker
- ☐ Copy of *Grateful Gary's Gifts* (pages 98-100) for the leader
- ☐ Copy of *Follow-Up Questions* (page 101) for the leader
- ☐ Copy of *Sweet Pickle Tips For Opening Gifts* (page 164) for each student
- ☐ Wrapped gift box with tag
- ☐ Copy of song (page 162) for the leader
- ☐ Copy of *Secret Code (Manners)* (page 163) for each student

Pre-Lesson Preparation:

Reproduce copies of the activity sheets (see above list).

Lesson:

1. Discuss the meaning of the words *manners* and *politeness*.

2. Write the following rhyme on the chalkboard or posterboard:

   Politeness is to do and say
   The kindest thing in the kindest way.

   Recite the rhyme with the students.

3. Ask the students to tell you about manners they have been taught. Write their responses on the chalkboard or posterboard. Then tell the students you are going to read a story about using good manners.

4. Read the story *Grateful Gary's Gifts* to the students. When you have finished reading the story, have the students answer the *Follow-Up Questions*.

5. Give each student a copy of *Sweet Pickle Tips For Opening Gifts*. Show the students the wrapped box. Using the activity sheet, discuss the proper way to open a gift and show appreciation for it.

6. Discuss the proper way to act when going through a doorway. Say:

   "If I am going into the store and there are five people behind me, I will hold the door for the person behind me. Then that person holds the door for the next person. Sometimes we even pass along a smile. No one fights over who holds the door or who doesn't hold the door. Everyone takes a turn, and there are no sour pickles."

7. Teach the students the song on page 162.

8. Give each student a copy of the *Secret Code (Manners)*. Tell the students how much time they have to complete the activity sheet. Or allow the students to complete it at home. (*Alternative:* Copies may be given to the classroom teacher to distribute.) As the students are leaving, remind them to use good manners every day.

LESSON: MANNERS II

Materials Needed:

- ☐ Copy of *Penny Pauses* (page 132-134) for the leader
- ☐ Copy of the following questions for each student:

  Before you ask for something, ask yourself these questions:
  Does it cost a lot?
  Is there enough for lots of children?
  Does it look like it was meant to be given away?

- ☐ Selection of things it is appropriate or inappropriate to ask for: candy in a dish, stickers, used pencil, paper clip, fancy pen, stamp and stamp pad, ream of paper, coffee cup
- ☐ Copy of *"When" Should You Ask? Pickles* (page 173) for the leader
- ☐ Jar with label (page 172)
- ☐ Copy of *"When" Should You Ask? Pictures* (page 174) for each student

Pre-Lesson Preparation:

Reproduce copies of the activity sheets (see above list). Reproduce and cut apart the *"When" Should You Ask? Pickles* and place them in the jar with the label.

Lesson:

1. Review the manners discussed in the previous lesson.

2. Recite this rhyme with the students:

   Politeness is to do and say
   The kindest thing in the kindest way.

3. Tell the students that many children have not been taught about when it is okay to ask for something. Then name something visible in the room that a student could have inappropriately asked for.

4. Read the story *Penny Pauses* to the students. Then give each student a copy of the *before you ask for something* questions listed above. Tell the students to keep this sheet as a reminder of when it is okay to ask for something.

5. Using the collected items, guide the students in deciding whether it would be appropriate or inappropriate to ask for each item.

6. Display the *"When" Should You Ask? Pickles* jar. Have a student pick a pickle from the jar. Then have the student (or the leader) read the statement and answer the question printed on the pickle.

7. Give each student a copy of the *"When" Should You Ask? Pictures*. Tell the students how much time they have to complete the activity sheet. Or allow the students to complete it at home. (*Alternative:* Copies may be given to the classroom teacher to distribute.)

LESSON: CHARACTER EDUCATION I

Materials Needed:

- ☐ Copy of *How Pickle Mountain Got Its Name* (pages 80-82) for the leader
- ☐ Chalkboard and chalk or posterboard and marker
- ☐ Copy of *Character Education At Pickle Mountain School* (pages 93-95) for the leader
- ☐ Copy of *Three Care Rules* (page 97) for each student
- ☐ Crayons or markers for each student

Pre-Lesson Preparation:

Reproduce copies of the activity sheets (see above list).

Lesson:

1. Read the story *How Pickle Mountain Got Its Name* to the students. When you have finished reading the story, point out how the children did not just watch the farmer and feel sorry for him. When the children saw what was happening to the farmer's cucumbers, they started picking them up. Moms and dads and grandpas and grandmas also helped pick up the cucumbers. The whole community showed good character by being helpful and caring.

2. Have the students name the different character traits found in the story. List the students' responses on the chalkboard or posterboard.

3. Then tell the students that the children at Pickle Mountain School are still learning about good character. Read the story *Character Education At Pickle Mountain School* to the students.

4. Teach the students the song in the story (page 94).

5. Give each student a copy of *Three Care Rules* and crayons or markers. Tell the students to color and decorate the poster. (*Alternative:* Copies may be given to the classroom teacher to distribute.) When everyone has finished coloring and decorating the poster, tell the students they may take their posters home.

LESSON: CHARACTER EDUCATION II

Materials Needed:

- ☐ Copy of *How Pickle Mountain Got Its Name* (pages 80-82) for the leader
- ☐ Copy of *Character Education At Pickle Mountain School* (pages 93-95) for the leader
- ☐ Copy of *We Care About Each Other Pictures* (page 189) for each student
- ☐ Copy of *We Care About Ourselves Pictures* (page 191) for each student
- ☐ Copy of *We Care About The Earth Pictures* (page 193) for each student

Pre-Lesson Preparation:

Reproduce copies of the activity sheets (see above list).

Lesson:

1. Review the main ideas presented in *How Pickle Mountain Got Its Name* and *Character Education At Pickle Mountain School.*

2. Sing the song from the story (page 94) with the students.

3. Tell the students that today they are going to think of ways they care about others, themselves, and the earth.

4. Give each student a copy of the *We Care About Each Other Pictures.* Discuss the pictures illustrated on the activity sheet. Then instruct the students to circle the pictures that show that we care about each other.

5. Give each student a copy of the *We Care About Ourselves Pictures.* Discuss the pictures illustrated on the activity sheet. Then instruct the students to circle the pictures that show that we care about ourselves.

6. Give each student a copy of the *We Care About The Earth Pictures.* Discuss the pictures illustrated on the activity sheet. Then instruct the students to circle the pictures that show that we care about the earth.

7. Sing the song from the story again.

LESSON: CAREER EDUCATION

Materials Needed:

- ☐ Copy of *Pickle Routine* (pages 41-42) for the leader
- ☐ Copy of *Discussion Guide* (page 43) for the leader
- ☐ Copy of *Snow Days Secrets* (pages 139-140) for the leader
- ☐ Copy of *Follow-Up Questions* (page 141) for the leader
- ☐ Copy of *Jobs At School* (page 206) for each student
- ☐ Copy of *Jobs At A Pickle Factory* (page 200) for each student
- ☐ Copy of *Snow Days Secrets* picture (bottom of page 140) for each student
- ☐ Crayons or markers for each student

Pre-Lesson Preparation:

Reproduce copies of the activity sheets (see above list).

Lesson:

1. Refer to the *Pickle Routine* and *Discussion Guide* as guidelines for this part of the lesson presentation.

2. Tell the students you are going to read a story about secrets. Ask them to listen carefully to hear in the story of two places where people can go to work.

3. Read the story *Snow Days Secrets* to the students. Then discuss the *Follow-Up Questions*. (*Optional:* Review when to tell a secret with the *"When" Should You Tell A Secret?* activity [pages 172, 183-184].)

4. Ask the students to name the two places that people can go to work that were mentioned in the story (a school and a factory).

5. Give each student a copy of *Jobs At School*. Review the activity sheet, describing each job. Tell the students to circle the picture of each worker who might work at a school every work day.

6. Give each student a copy of *Jobs At A Pickle Factory*. Review the activity sheet, describing each job. Tell the students to circle the picture of each worker who might work at a large pickle factory every work day.

7. Give each student a copy of the *Snow Days Secrets* picture and crayons or markers. Have the students color the picture. (*Alternative:* Copies may be given to the classroom teacher to distribute.)

SAMPLE LESSONS FOR GRADES 3-4

The following lesson plans are designed for 30-minute periods. As you know, the reactions and abilities of your students determine the number of things which can be accomplished in that amount of time. Therefore, these are guidelines to be adapted to your own personal situation. Throughout the lessons, you will see asterisks (*). These are sheets to be sent home for student review and parent education. For additional "pickle" materials available from the author, visit Pat Kienzle's website at: www.pickleladybooks.com.

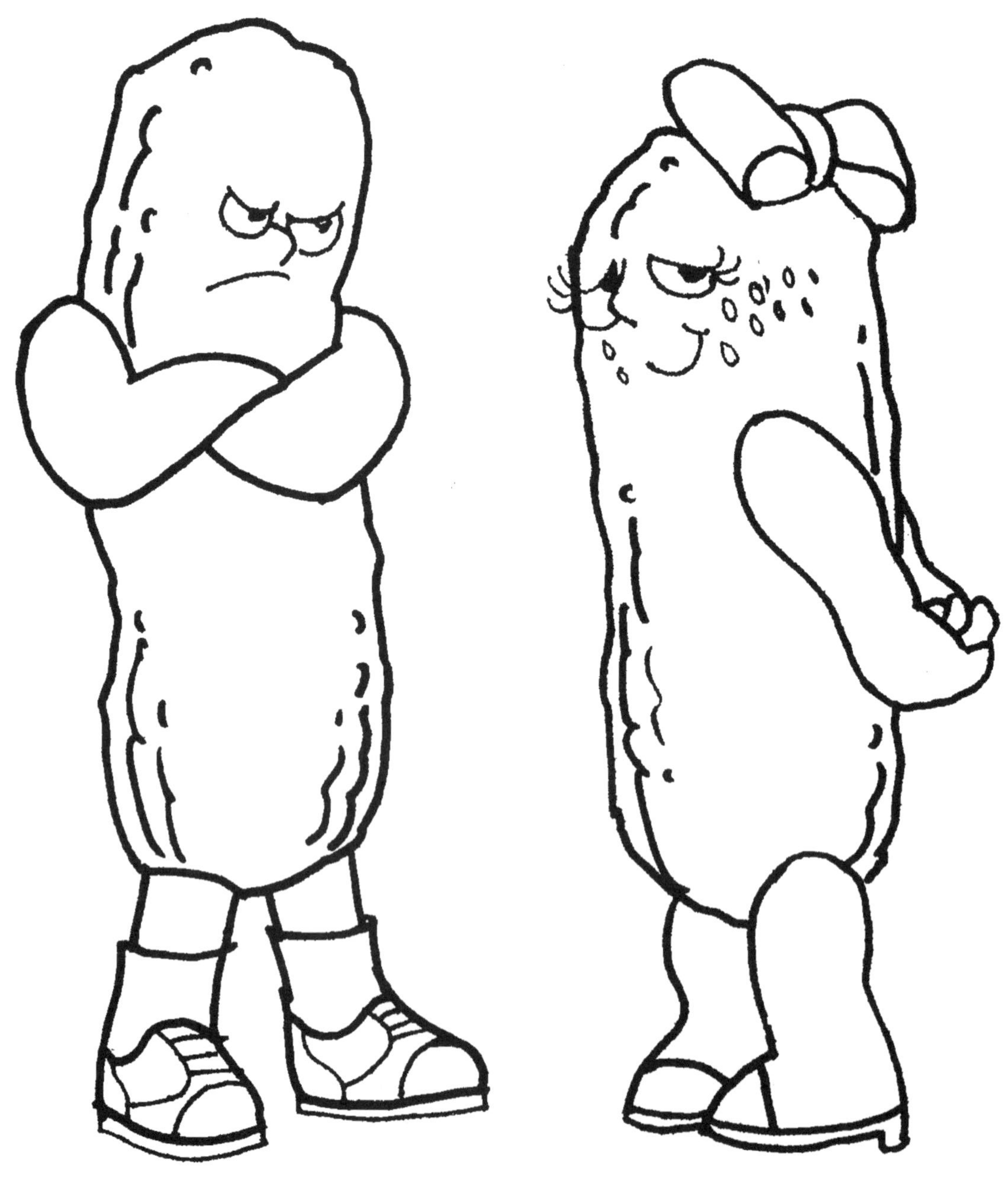

LESSON: ANGER MANAGEMENT

Materials Needed:

- ☐ Optional Activity: Copy of *Using "Pickle Cat"* (page 156) for the leader
- ☐ Optional Activity: Copy of *Pickle Cat* (page 157) for each student and the leader
- ☐ Optional Activity: Copy of *Pickle Gets Mad* (page 158) for each student and the leader
- ☐ Optional Activity: Stuffed toy cat or full-bodied cat puppet
- ☐ Optional Activity: Cat toy
- ☐ Optional Activity: Stuffed toy dog or full-bodied dog puppet
- ☐ Thesaurus
- ☐ Chalkboard and chalk or posterboard and marker
- ☐ Copy of *Appropriate Ways To Handle Anger* (page 256) for each student

Pre-Lesson Preparation:

Reproduce copies of the activity sheets (see above list).

Lesson:

1. Optional Activity: Give each student a copy of *Pickle Cat* and *Pickle Gets Mad.* Present the *Using "Pickle Cat"* activity.
2. Tell the students that when they were younger, they probably used only the words *mad* and *angry* to express how they felt when they were upset. Now they are ready to expand their vocabulary and learn words that can be used to describe different degrees of anger.
3. Ask one student to use the thesaurus to look up the word *angry.* Have him/her read aloud the words associated with *angry.* Then ask the students to name any other words they can think of that express anger. List the words on the chalkboard or posterboard. The list should include: *annoyed, irritated, fuming, mad, livid, irate, furious, enraged, outraged, infuriated.*
4. Write the following sentence on the chalkboard or posterboard: *The child was _________ when I walked into the room.* Have several students complete the sentence by using a word that means a slightly angry, then moderately angry, and finally extremely angry.
5. Tell the students it is important to be able to express feelings clearly. People can better understand how we are feeling when we use the appropriate words.
6. Give each student a copy of *Appropriate Ways To Handle Anger.* Then say:

   "Everybody gets angry sometimes. But it is important not to get mad over every little thing or to stay mad for a long time. A person who is too angry can do several things to calm down. By completing this word search, you will learn some techniques to help yourself calm down when you are angry."

   Tell the students how much time they have to complete the activity sheet. When the allotted time has elapsed, have the students name different situations in which they could use these calming techniques.
7. Remind the students that there are three things they cannot do when they are angry: hurt someone, destroy things, or use words that will get them in trouble with the principal, their teacher, or parents.

LESSON: BULLYING

Materials Needed:

- ☐ Optional Activity: Copy of *Using "Pickle Cat"* (page 156) for the leader
- ☐ Optional Activity: Copy of *Pickle Cat* (page 157) for each student and the leader
- ☐ Optional Activity: Copy of *Pickle Gets Mad* (page 158) for each student and the leader
- ☐ Optional Activity: Stuffed toy cat or full-bodied cat puppet
- ☐ Optional Activity: Cat toy
- ☐ Optional Activity: Stuffed toy dog or full-bodied dog puppet
- ☐ Chalkboard and chalk or posterboard and marker
- ☐ Copy of *Secret Code #3* (page 62) for each student

Pre-Lesson Preparation:

Reproduce copies of the activity sheets (see above list).

Lesson:

1. Optional Activity: Present the *Using "Pickle Cat"* activity. After you have completed your presentation, ask the students what name they might call the dog for taking the cat's toy (bully). Then say:

   "When the dog was a puppy, he liked to jump over things. Because of this behavior, his owners named him *Leapfrog*. But now, because he is such a bully, the other animals in his school have nicknamed him *Bullfrog*."

2. Then say:

   "To help yourselves understand bullies, think of a car windshield and the weather. When it is sprinkling, the wipers easily wipe the rain from the windshield. But in heavy rain, the driver may have to pull off the road because he or she can't see and it isn't safe to continue driving. Driving in a hailstorm is dangerous, and the driver may have to look for shelter. Sometimes bullying is like a light rain. At other times, bullying can be dangerous, like a hailstorm."

3. Write the following on the chalkboard or posterboard:

   Sprinkling rain: Teasing that can be ignored (easily wiped away)
   Heavy rain: Teasing that you can walk away from (pull off the road)
   Hailstorm: Threats or physical contact (dangerous)

4 Have the students name different bullying situations and the category under which each one would fit. List the students' ideas under the appropriate categories. Then say:

   "Because we are caring, responsible citizens, we should help when we see another student in the 'Hail Zone' or frequently in heavy rain. There are times when helping someone could put you in a difficult or dangerous situation. At such times, the best way to help is to notify a trusted adult."

5. Discuss what retaliation is and how it leads to more bullying.

6. Tell the students they may come to you (or another trusted adult) any time they feel scared or sad.

7. Give each student a copy of *Secret Code #3*. Tell the students how much time they have to complete the activity sheet. Or allow the students to complete it at home.

LESSON: CONFLICT RESOLUTION

Materials Needed:

- ☐ 4 Dictionaries
- ☐ Copy of *Fight For A Frog* (pages 88-90) for the leader
- ☐ Copy of *Follow-Up Questions* (page 91) for the leader
- ☐ Copy of *Solving Conflicts At Pickle Mountain School* poster (page 92) for each student
- ☐ Paper and pencil for each student

Pre-Lesson Preparation:

Reproduce copies of the activity sheets (see above list).

Lesson:

1. Have four students use the dictionaries to find the meaning of the words *conflict*, *investigation*, *negotiation*, and *mediation* and read the definitions aloud.

2. Read the story *Fight For A Frog* to the students. When you have finished reading the story, have the students answer the *Follow-Up Questions*.

3. Give each student a copy of the *Solving Conflicts At Pickle Mountain School* poster. Using the text on page 90 as a guide, review the *DINO* steps with the students. Tell the students that *O-Offering* refers to *mediation*.

4. Using the following examples, ask the students to determine whether each conflict was successfully resolved and if so, to name which *DINO* steps were used.

   Renaldo and Felicia each wanted to use the computer. They asked their teacher to help them decide who could use it first. Their teacher looked at her records to see who had most recently used the computer. *(Resolved: Steps D and O)*

   Juan and Carlos each wanted to use the computer. Their argument became so loud, their father told them to turn the computer off. *(Unresolved)*

   Kimberly and Lexa each wanted to use the computer. After listening to each other, they decided Lexa should finish her school assignment first. *(Resolved: Steps D, I, and N)*

   Gary and Gwen each wanted to use the computer. They worked out a schedule so they could each have time to finish their assignments. *(Resolved: Steps D and N)*

5. Distribute paper and a pencil to each student. Then ask the students to brainstorm or write a paragraph about ways of resolving the following problem. The paragraph may also be completed at home.

   The class could go on only one field trip. The possibilities were a trip to the state capitol with a stop at the toy museum or a trip to a butterfly farm with a stop at a candy factory.

LESSON: TOLERANCE

Materials Needed:

- ☐ Copy of *The "Unempty" House* (pages 127-129) for the leader
- ☐ Chalkboard and chalk or posterboard and marker
- ☐ Dictionary
- ☐ Art paper, pencils, and crayons or markers for each student group

Pre-Lesson Preparation:

Reproduce copies of the activity sheets (see above list).

Lesson:

1. Read the story *The "Unempty" House* to the students.

2. Ask the students to name some types of disabilities. Then have the students describe other ways in which people are different from one another (their appearance, the language they speak, their opinions, etc.). Write their ideas on the chalkboard or posterboard.

3. Have one student look up the meaning of the word *tolerance* in the dictionary and read the definition out loud. Referring to the list written on the chalkboard or posterboard, discuss the meaning of tolerance. Then have the students give examples of ways they show tolerance in relation to each word on the list.

4. Divide the students into small groups. Distribute art paper, pencils, and crayons or markers to each group. Then tell the students to select one way they can show tolerance at school and illustrate it on their paper. (*Note:* If there is not enough time for the students to finish their drawings, tell them they may finish them outside of class and bring them to the next lesson.) When everyone has finished drawing, have each group share its picture with the class. Display all the pictures in a prominent place in the classroom.

LESSON: ATTITUDE

Materials Needed:

- ☐ Copy of *What Are Bread And Butter Pickles?* (page 57) for each student
- ☐ Copy of *Bread And Butter Choices* (page 58) for each student
- ☐ Optional: Jar of Bread and Butter pickles
- ☐ Copy of *Secret Code #1* (page 60) for each student

Pre-Lesson Preparation:

Reproduce copies of the activity sheets (see above list). If possible, have some bread and butter pickles for students to sample. Mrs. Fanning's pickles (mentioned on page 57) are a product of GFA Brands, Inc. of Cresskill, N.J. They are distributed in the northeast, the west coast, and in some other parts of the country. Other brands of bread and butter pickles are readily available in stores.

Lesson:

1. Discuss the meaning of *attitude*. The *Thorndike-Barnhart Children's Dictionary* defines *attitude* as *a way of thinking, acting or feeling.* (*Note:* This is a good lesson if your character-education program uses the traits of *optimism* or *adaptability*.)

2. Tell the students that today they have the opportunity to learn how they can gain control over their own happiness.

3. Give each student a copy of *What Are Bread And Butter Pickles?* Read and discuss the first four paragraphs with the students, emphasizing the concept that sometimes things in life are not very sweet and not very sour. They are just sort of in-between. Have the students complete the activity sheet, then review their answers.

4. Give each student a copy of *Bread And Butter Choices*. Read the directions with the students, then have them complete the activity sheet. When everyone has completed the activity sheet, review the students' answers, emphasizing that having a good attitude toward any situation can make them feel better and have a better day. Explain that having a good attitude is one way they may gain control over their own happiness.

5. Have the students tell about times they were able to make a situation better by having a good attitude.

6. If bread and butter pickles are available, let the students taste them if they wish.

7. Give each student a copy of *Secret Code #1.* Instruct the students to complete the activity sheet at home. (*Alternative:* Copies may be given to the classroom teacher to distribute.)

LESSON: CHARACTER EDUCATION

Materials Needed:

- ☐ Chalkboard and chalk or posterboard and marker
- ☐ Dictionary
- ☐ Copy of *Character Education At Pickle Mountain School* (pages 93-95) for the leader
- ☐ Copy of *We Care About Each Other Phrases* (page 188) for each student
- ☐ Copy of *We Care About Ourselves Phrases* (page 190) for each student
- ☐ Copy of *We Care About The Earth Phrases* (page 192) for each student

Pre-Lesson Preparation:

Reproduce copies of the activity sheets (see above list).

Lesson:

1. Have the students name words that describe good character traits (*responsibility, compassion, perseverance, optimism, cooperation, respect,* etc.). Write the words on the chalkboard or posterboard.

2. Have one student look up the meaning of the word *character* in the dictionary and read the definition out loud. Ask the students to tell how the definition relates to each of the words listed on the chalkboard or posterboard.

4. Tell the students you are going to read a story, and that while you are reading, they should listen for another definition of character. Read the story *Character Education At Pickle Mountain School* to the students.

5. When you have finished reading the story, ask if anyone can name the meaning of character defined in the story *(acting with care)*. Have the students use the words written on the chalkboard or posterboard to describe ways they can demonstrate caring behavior toward other people.

6. Give each student a copy of *We Care About Each Other Phrases, We Care About Ourselves Phrases,* and *We Care About The Earth Phrases*. Have the students complete the activity sheets, then review their answers with the class. If there is not enough time to complete the activity sheets in class, have the students finish them at home.

LESSON: VOCABULARY EXPANSION FOR EXPRESSING FEELINGS I

Materials Needed:

- ☐ Copy of *Pickle Routine* (pages 41-42) for the leader
- ☐ Copy of *Discussion Guide* (page 43) for the leader
- ☐ Copy of *Discovery List Of Words For Sweet, Sour, And In-Between Feelings* (pages 230-236) for each student
- ☐ Copy of *Your Name* (page 242) for each student
- ☐ Copy of *Synonyms And Antonyms* (page 244) for each student
- ☐ Copy of *Vocabulary Search* (page 243) for each student

Pre-Lesson Preparation:

Reproduce copies of the activity sheets (see above list). If you have enough supplies, make a copy of the *Discovery List Of Words For Sweet, Sour, And In-Between Feelings* for each student to keep and refer to during writing activities. If you must take your sets from class to class, make extras and leave at least three sets with the classroom teacher.

Lesson:

1. Review the pickle theme: *Life is like a pickle. Sometimes it's sweet. Sometimes it's sour.*
2. Refer to the *Pickle Routine* and *Discussion Guide* as guidelines for this part of the lesson presentation. (*Note:* Although the *Pickle Routine* is not presented in every lesson, older students can review it several times during the school year.)
3. Tell the students:

   > "When you were younger, you used simple words to describe feelings. Now you are ready to expand your vocabulary."

4. Give each student a copy of the *Discovery List Of Words For Sweet, Sour, And In-Between Feelings.* To become familiar with the list, instruct the students to find the following words in the list. Then ask for a volunteer to read each word and definition out loud.

   Bewildered (page 230) Ecstatic (page 231) Glorious (page 232)
   Inquisitive (page 233) Optimistic (page 234) Tolerant (page 235)
   Zealous (page 236)

5. Give each student a copy of *Your Name.* This exercise will help students become more familiar with the word list. When everyone has completed the activity sheet, ask for volunteers to share their answers with the class. (*Alternative:* The activity sheets may be displayed on a bulletin board or made into a class book.)
6. Give each student a copy of *Synonyms And Antonyms.* Tell the students to use the word list to find words that mean the same as or the opposite of the words listed on the activity sheet. This activity works well when students work in pairs or small groups.
7. If you do not have a word list for each child to keep, collect them for use in the next lesson.
8. Give each student a copy of *Vocabulary Search.* Instruct the students to complete the activity sheet at home. (*Alternative:* Copies may be given to the classroom teacher to distribute.)

LESSON: VOCABULARY EXPANSION FOR EXPRESSING FEELINGS II

Materials Needed:

- ☐ Copy of *Discovery List Of Words For Sweet, Sour, And In-Between Feelings* (pages 230-236) for each student
- ☐ Copy of *Feelings Crossword* (page 249) for each student
- ☐ Optional: Completed copy of *Feelings Crossword* (page 249) for the leader
- ☐ Optional: Overhead projector, transparency, and marker
- ☐ Copy of *How Many Words Can You Write?* (page 245) for each student
- ☐ Paper and pencil for each student

Pre-Lesson Preparation:

Reproduce copies of the activity sheets (see above list). Optional: Make a transparency of a completed copy of the *Feelings Crossword.*

(*Note:* Since there is not enough time to complete the writing activity [see #5] in a 30-minute lesson, decide whether it will be an out-of-class assignment or performed during the next guidance lesson.)

Lesson:

1. If students do not have a copy from the previous lesson, give each student the *Discovery List Of Words For Sweet, Sour, And In-Between Feelings.*
2. Tell the students they are going to expand their vocabulary.
3. Give each student a copy of the *Feelings Crossword.* If possible, allow the students to work in pairs, small groups, or as a class. Tell the students how much time they have to complete the crossword puzzle. When the allotted time has elapsed, review the answers with the students and have them correct any mistakes. (If an overhead projector is available, show the students a transparency of the completed puzzle.)
4. Give each student a copy of *How Many Words Can You Write?* Have the students work in groups, assigning each group one question. If an overhead projector is available, use a transparency to compile each group's word list. Tell the students to complete their papers, using the lists from the transparency. As you review the lists with the students, discuss how some words—such as irritated, annoyed, and furious—relate to stronger feelings and describe different levels of anger.
5. Tell the students they are going to make up a crazy dream. It cannot be a nightmare, but it can have *some* scary moments. In the dream, their feelings can range from happy to sad to scared to happy to mad to sad to excited to any of the other feelings discussed in the lesson. But they cannot use the words *happy, scared, mad, sad.* The writing prompt could be: "You won't believe this crazy dream I had." Tell the students you will be anxious to see their stories and find out how many words from their vocabulary list they used. Distribute paper and a pencil to each student and tell them whether they will write the stories out of class or during the next guidance lesson. The completed stories would make a great bulletin-board display, especially if the students illustrate them.
6. If necessary, collect the word lists.

LESSON: CAREER EDUCATION I

Materials Needed:

- ☐ Copy of *All Jobs Are Important* (page 196) for each student
- ☐ Copy of *Packed Pickle Goes To The Hospital* (pages 103-105) for the leader
- ☐ Optional: Sample *Packed Pickle* (page 107) for the leader
- ☐ Copy of *Follow-Up Questions* (page 106) for the leader
- ☐ Copy of *Occupations List* (pages 197-198) for each student
- ☐ Copy of *Occupations At A Hospital* (page 203) for each student
- ☐ Optional: *Packed Pickles* (page 107)

Pre-Lesson Preparation:

Reproduce copies of the activity sheets (see above list). Make a *Packed Pickle* to display as you read the story. If you want the students to participate in the *Packed Pickle* activity (see #6), you wlll need additional *Packed Pickles.* (*Note:* You could ask a volunteer or parent to make several to share during the lessons or make one for each student.)

Lesson:

1. Discuss the interdependence of tasks and how we all rely on workers to perform those tasks. For example: I need gas to drive my car. In order for me to be able to purchase gas, what jobs must already have been performed? Where are the people who perform these tasks employed? Which employees come to work at that place every work day? Which employees would come occasionally to make deliveries or repairs?

2. Give each student a copy of *All Jobs Are Important.* Have the students complete the activity sheet alone or working with a partner. Tell the students how much time they have to complete the activity sheet. When the allotted time has elapsed, discuss the students' answers.

3. Read the story *Packed Pickle Goes To The Hospital* to the students. Show the students the sample *Packed Pickle* at the appropriate time in the story. When you have finished reading the story, have the students answer the *Follow-Up Questions.*

4. Give each student a copy of the *Occupations List* and a copy of *Occupations At A Hospital.* Tell the students they may refer to the *Occupations List* when completing the activity sheet. Instruct the students to circle the names of workers who might work at a very large hospital. (*Note:* Some answers may require your input or the student's justification. For example: The commercial driver could drive an ambulance rather than a big truck. The two people who obviously don't work in a hospital are an air traffic controller and a principal.) Tell the students how much time they have to complete the activity sheet.

5. When the allotted time has elapsed, collect the *Occupations Lists.* Save them for use in future lessons.

6. You may extend this lesson by distributing *Packed Pickles* to several students or to every student. Instruct the students to take them home for a weekend/week and get autographs and job titles of workers. (*Alternative:* The student may give the *Packed Pickle* to his/her parent to take to work to get autographs and job titles of workers.)

LESSON: CAREER EDUCATION II

Materials Needed:

- ☐ Students' *Packed Pickles* from previous lesson
- ☐ Copy of *Big and Bigger Field Trips* (pages 114-115) for the leader
- ☐ Copy of *Follow-up Questions* (page 116) for the leader
- ☐ Copy of *Occupations List* (from previous lesson—pages 197-198) for each student
- ☐ Copy of *Occupations At An Airport* (page 205) for each student
- ☐ Optional: Completed copy of *Occupations At A Hospital* (page 203) for the leader
- ☐ Optional: Completed copy of *Occupations At An Airport* (page 205) for the leader
- ☐ Optional: Overhead projector, transparencies, and marker
- ☐ Copy of *Occupations At School* (page 207) for each student

Pre-Lesson Preparation:

Reproduce copies of the activity sheets (see above list). Optional: Make a transparency of the completed *Occupations At A Hospital* and *Occupations At An Airport* activity sheets.

Lesson:

1. If the students were instructed to take *Packed Pickles* home, have them share with the class the signatures and job titles of the workers whose autographs they obtained. (*Note:* The *Packed Pickles,* along with notes of the places the students visited, make a great bulletin-board display.)

2. Read the story *Big And Bigger Field Trips* to the students. When you have finished reading the story, have the students answer the *Follow-up Questions*.

3. Give each student a copy of the *Occupations List* and a copy of *Occupations At An Airport*. Tell the students they may refer to the *Occupations List* when completing the activity sheet. Instruct the students to circle the names of workers who might work at an airport. (*Note:* Some answers may require your input or the student's justification. For example: A nurse *could* be employed at a large airport. The four people who obviously don't work at an airport are a counselor, a principal, a judge, and a librarian.) Tell the students how much time they have to complete the activity sheet.

4. Discuss how some occupations can be performed in different settings. Using the overhead projector and transparencies (if available), compare *Occupations At A Hospital* to *Occupations At An Airport* to determine which jobs could be performed in either place.

5. Give each student a copy of *Occupations At School*. Tell the students they may refer to the *Occupations List* when completing the activity sheet. Instruct the students to circle the names of workers who might work at a school. Tell the students how much time they have to complete the activity sheet.

6. Have the students tell what jobs they might like to have at a hospital, airport, or school.

7. Collect the *Occupations Lists* for use in future lessons.

8. If the students are sharing the *Packed Pickles,* allow other students to take one home for a weekend/week and to collect autographs and job titles of workers.

LESSON: CAREER EDUCATION III

Materials Needed:

- ☐ Students' *Packed Pickles* from previous lesson
- ☐ Copy of *Occupations List* (from previous lesson—pages 197-198) for each student
- ☐ Copy of *Occupations At A Pickle Factory* (page 201) for each student
- ☐ Copy of *Occupations For Building Houses* (page 209) for each student

Pre-Lesson Preparation:

Reproduce copies of the activity sheets (see above list).

Lesson:

1. If the students were instructed to take *Packed Pickles* home, have them share with the class the signatures and job titles of the workers whose autographs they obtained.

2. Give each student a copy of the *Occupations List*, *Occupations At A Pickle Factory*, and *Occupations For Building Houses*. Tell the students they may refer to the *Occupations List* when completing the activity sheets. Tell the students how much time they have to complete the activity sheets.

3. When the allotted time has elapsed, review the students' answers. Collect the *Occupations Lists* for use in future lessons.

4. Divide the class into teams and play the *Occupations List Game #2* (see instructions on page 25).

5. If the students are sharing the *Packed Pickles,* allow other students to take one home for a weekend/week and collect workers' autographs and job titles.

ASSISTANCE WITH LESSON PLANNING

This list will help you locate parts of *Pickle Packet II* that you can use with topics you are teaching.